STATISTICS: Textbooks and Monographs

A Series Edited by

D. B. Owen, Founding Editor, 1972–1991

W. R. Schucany, Coordinating Editor
Department of Statistics
Southern Methodist University
Dallas, Texas

D1158092

DRUG SA
ASSESSM
CLINICAL

R. G. Cor
for Biosta
University

A. M. Ksh
for Multiv
Experimen
University

Additional Volumes in Preparation

DRUG SAFETY ASSESSMENT IN CLINICAL TRIALS

edited by

GENE SOGLIERO-GILBERT

Pfizer Inc.
Groton, Connecticut

Marcel Dekker, Inc.   New York • Basel • Hong Kong

Library of Congress Cataloging-in-Publication Data

Drug safety assessment in clinical trials / edited by Gene Sogliero
-Gilbert.
    p.   cm. -- (Statistics, textbooks and monographs ; v. 138)
    Includes bibliographical references and index.
    ISBN 0-8247-8893-1
    1. Drugs--Testing. 2. Drugs--Testing--Statistical methods.
3. Drugs--Toxicology. I. Sogliero-Gilbert, Gene.
II. Series.
    [DNLM: 1. Drug Evaluation--methods. 2. Clinical Trials--methods.
QV 771 D7948 1993]
RM301.27.D79 1993
615'.1901--dc20
DNLM/DLC
for Library of Congress   93-8117
                                                   CIP

[Handwritten: RM301.27 .D79 1993]

The publisher offers discounts on this book when ordered in bulk quantities. For more information, write to Special Sales/Professional Marketing at the address below.

This book is printed on acid-free paper.

Marcel Dekker, Inc.
270 Madison Avenue, New York, New York 10016

Current printing (last digit):
10 9 8 7 6 5 4 3 2 1

PRINTED IN THE UNITED STATES OF AMERICA

To the memory of my father and mother,
Frank T. and Sarah (Taggart) Cianfarani

Preface

Although numerous journal articles have been written about drug safety, they are often difficult to obtain and highly specific—even the professional can find it hard to keep up with recent work in the field. In addition, there is a large population of intelligent, curious, and concerned adults who are not directly involved in clinical trials and who have limited time or resources, but would like to be better informed about drug safety assessment.

The purpose of this book is to bring together in one volume (1) aspects of medical understanding and interpretation of safety data; (2) computational techniques for processing, displaying, and summarizing large quantities of safety data; and (3) statistical issues that make safety data a challenge to analyze.

According to the dictionary, safety is defined as "freedom from danger, risk, or injury." To understand drug safety, one must, paradoxically, look carefully at all negative events that occur during the course of a clinical trial in which an experimental drug is administered. These negative events are compared to what might be expected when the patients are not receiving the treatment therapy.

The primary negative events that constitute the essence of the "safety profile for a drug" consist of "adverse reactions" (which include ordinary events such as headache or sleeplessness and more serious and unusual events such as rash or fainting) and "laboratory abnormalities." Adverse reactions, or side effects, are recorded at each visit after an investigator queries the patient about problems experienced since the last visit. Sometimes they are spontaneously reported by the patient. Because most of these events occur at random in the general population, disentangling the random events from the "drug-related" events is a challenge.

While laboratory abnormalities are, in a strict sense, adverse events, they are discussed in this book as a separate aspect of safety analysis. Laboratory test results represent objective scientific tests that are performed on body fluid samples, obtained at prespecified timepoints, from all patients in a study. As such, they constitute a reliable record of a drug's effect on the body.

Laboratory abnormalities that occur during the course of clinical trials are reviewed as to whether the abnormality is characteristic of the underlying disease syndrome or is caused by the medicine used as part of the assigned therapy. Performing, recording, displaying, analyzing, interpreting, and summarizing these tests constitute a major component of the cost and time that are invested in clinical trials.

Woven into the texture of this book are two different, but complementary, purposes of safety data collection. The first and most important is the medical interpretation of individual negative events with respect to the diagnosis and prognosis of each patient. For this purpose, every abnormal laboratory or adverse event conveys vital information about a patient's condition. Prior to the development of large-scale clinical trials as we know them, laboratory tests were done to aid the doctor in confirming a diagnosis or for monitoring the patient's progress in fighting a disease. They will always be used for this purpose, especially for patient care in hospitals or clinics.

The second purpose of collecting safety data came about with the careful planning of large-scale clinical trials, the development of reliable data bases, and the steady improvement and increased use of computers. With information from large groups of patients receiving the same drug under controlled conditions, subtle changes occurring in many patients might be overlooked. When looking at the study as a whole, however, within the context of comparative studies and by careful data processing and statistical analysis, these subtle changes might be identified as statistically significant, with one drug displaying a safety advantage over another drug.

In addition to the coverage of these two types of nontherapeutic events recorded from clinical trials, the manifestation of toxicity as learned from preclinical toxicology is discussed. Such required preclinical studies in animals are the precursor to clinical trials in humans.

I wish to express my sincere thanks to all the contributors. Without their collective vast experience and technical knowledge, this book would not have been possible. My deep gratitude to Marjorie Dougan for helping me coordinate the many tasks inherent in bringing this book together.

Finally, I wish to thank the Central Research Division of Pfizer Inc. for providing the physical and intellectual environment that made this book possible.

Gene Sogliero-Gilbert

Contents

Contributors

Janet M. Begun Department of Biostatistics and Data Management, Pharmaceutical Product Development, Inc., Morrisville, North Carolina

J. F. Bion Department of Anaesthesia & Intensive Care, Queen Elizabeth Hospital, The University of Birmingham, Edgbaston, Birmingham, England

M. I. Bowden Department of Anaesthesia & Intensive Care, Queen Elizabeth Hospital, The University of Birmingham, Edgbaston, Birmingham, England

Christy Chuang-Stein Clinical Biostatistics Unit I, The Upjohn Company, Kalamazoo, Michigan

Yechiel A. Hekster Department of Clinical Pharmacy, University Hospital, Nijmegen, The Netherlands

Piet M. Hooymans Department of Clinical Pharmacy and Toxicology, Maasland Hospital, Sittard, The Netherlands

Robert Janknegt Department of Clinical Pharmacy and Toxicology, Maasland Hospital, Sittard, The Netherlands

Ellen D. Kelso Medical Regulatory Affairs, Lilly Research Laboratories, Eli Lilly and Company, Indianapolis, Indiana

Deborah S. Kirby Department of Clinical Research, Central Research Division, Pfizer Inc., Groton, Connecticut

Gary G. Koch Department of Biostatistics, School of Public Health, University of North Carolina, Chapel Hill, North Carolina

William C. Maier Department of Biostatistics and Data Management, Pharmaceutical Product Development, Inc., Morrisville, North Carolina

James T. Mayne Department of Drug Safety Evaluation, Central Research Division, Pfizer Inc., Groton, Connecticut

Noel R. Mohberg Clinical Biostatistics Unit I, The Upjohn Company, Kalamazoo, Michigan

Lawrence K. Oliver Clinical Research Laboratories, The Upjohn Company, Kalamazoo, Michigan

Karl E. Peace Biopharmaceutical Research Consultants, Inc., Ann Arbor, Michigan

Norman E. Pitts* Department of Clinical Research, Central Research Division, Pfizer Inc., Groton, Connecticut

David S. Salsburg Department of Clinical Research, Central Research Division, Pfizer Inc., Groton, Connecticut

Judith E. Schmid Department of Biostatistics and Data Management, Pharmaceutical Product Development, Inc., Morrisville, North Carolina

Gene Sogliero-Gilbert Department of Clinical Research, Central Research Division, Pfizer Inc., Groton, Connecticut

Max W. Talbott Medical Regulatory Affairs, Lilly Research Laboratories, Eli Lilly and Company, Indianapolis, Indiana

Naitee Ting Department of Clinical Research, Central Research Division, Pfizer Inc., Groton, Connecticut

Lonni Zubkoff-Schulz Department of Clinical Research, Central Research Division, Pfizer Inc., Groton, Connecticut

---

*Retired.

1

Preclinical Drug Safety Evaluation

James T. Mayne

Pfizer Inc.
Groton, Connecticut

I. BACKGROUND

The quest for improved medicines has resulted in a tremendous international effort dedicated to the discovery and development of new drug entities. In most Western countries, by far the largest portion of this effort is located in the pharmaceutical industry. By 1989, according to the Pharmaceutical Manufacturers Association (PMA), the annual research and development expenditures of member pharmaceutical companies had exceeded the total annual funding provided by the National Institutes of Health. The yearly research and development expenditures of the U.S. pharmaceutical industry alone were estimated at 6.5 billion $U.S. in 1990, while the estimated mean development cost per approved drug in the U.S. was approximately $231 million in 1987 dollars [1,2]. Of this cost per compound, approximately 8%, or $18.5 million, was spent on toxicology and preclinical safety testing [3]. Dollars alone may not be the most appropriate unit of scale to provide a suitable perspective on the magnitude of this endeavor.

The drug development process strives to achieve a balance between the advancement of novel effective therapies and the need to assure that these drugs are free of unacceptable toxicity in the intended patient population. The costs of nonhuman safety studies typically run into the millions of dollars for a single compound; more for drugs with unique characteristics and patient populations.

1

These safety studies are conducted such that relevant information on safety is collected from several model systems according to defined exposure conditions prior to the first comparable exposure in human subjects. For example, reproductive toxicology studies are conducted in animals before women of childbearing potential are entered into clinical trials. In this sense, all toxicology studies may be considered preclinical toxicology studies. For the purposes of this chapter, however, the term *preclinical toxicology* will be used to describe those key safety studies conducted prior to the administration of the first dose to human subjects.

II. PRECLINICAL STUDIES AND GOVERNMENT REGULATORY AGENCIES

It is the responsibility of any group interested in testing a new drug in humans to first investigate any potential toxicity in nonhuman models. An adequate toxicology database is essential not only as a basis for an accurate prediction of the response of human subjects but also as a source of information for the proper design of safe, informative phase I trials. All relevant data must be compiled and analyzed as an integrated safety database before the nature of potential toxicities and their relevance to human safety can be understood. This process is generically described as risk assessment and is intended to minimize the risk of drug-induced toxicity incurred by clinical subjects enrolled in phase I studies.

In the United States, the authority for regulating these efforts is entrusted to the Food and Drug Administration (FDA). The regulatory document submitted to the FDA by the sponsor of a new drug is the Investigational New Drug Application (IND), which serves as the primary information source for regulatory evaluation of preclinical safety. As part of this document, an integrated summary of the safety database is presented along with the individual safety study reports. The primary objective of the FDA in reviewing an IND is "to assure the safety and rights of [human] subjects" [4]. Regarding toxicology studies in particular, the general guidelines set forth in the *Federal Register* state that "an integrated summary of the toxicological effects of the drug in animals and in vitro" is to be submitted [4].

These few words have played a major role in shaping the way preclinical toxicology studies are done. It would be impossible to present an exact generic formula for the collection of preclinical safety data. Each investigational drug is unique; therefore, an acceptable safety package must be designed and conducted on a case-by-case basis. In addition, slightly different approaches to preclinical safety testing have evolved at different research institutions over time. The FDA has consistently and intentionally encouraged a case-specific approach to safety evaluation by not issuing specific study requirements. Rather, it is incumbent on the applicant to design an appropriate safety evaluation program for each experimental drug.

III. DESIGN OF PRECLINICAL TOXICOLOGY STUDIES

As stated above, each investigational drug is unique. Therefore a thorough understanding of the chemical, pharmacological, and pharmacokinetic properties of an experimental drug is necessary for successful study design.

A. Chemical Background Data

A wide variety of basic chemical information should be available before critical toxicology studies are initiated. This information is reviewed by the toxicologist and may provide guidance toward proper toxicology study design and conduct. For example, the chemical structure and molecular weight are useful for predicting potential metabolism and elimination routes. In addition, solubility and partition coefficient data may provide insight into the absorption and distribution of the drug. The pK_a and salt form, if any, also can be used to predict the extent of drug absorption expected after oral exposure. Stereochemistry is also a consideration, since different enantiomers of racemic drugs may have widely different bioactivities. Information about potential pharmaceutical formulations for use in human clinical subjects is also very useful, since the formulation may contain vehicles or excipients that could modify absorption, activity, and toxicity [5,6]. Data on the purity of the test compound are critical since relatively minor impurities may induce their own toxicity or modify the toxicity of the test drug. In addition, the chemical stability of the test drug, under the environmental conditions to be used for dose preparation and storage, should be evaluated to verify that the doses used in safety studies are delivered as intended.

B. Pharmacology Background Data

Perhaps the most useful information for the proper design of toxicology studies is data describing the basic pharmacological properties of the test drug. The tremendous advances of recent years in the fields of pharmacology, medicinal chemistry, and molecular biology have combined to produce exciting new investigational drugs with unprecedented potency and selectivity. While these advances have revolutionized the drug discovery process, they represent an evolving challenge to the toxicologist. Microgram doses producing efficacy at nanomolar plasma drug concentrations are now commonplace. It is therefore essential that toxicologists review and understand all available pharmacology data because toxicity is increasingly a function of pharmacological properties. A simple understanding of the therapeutic indication is not sufficient.

Pharmacology data are routinely collected from in vitro and whole-animal studies. Information useful to the toxicologist includes pharmacological activity data, often obtained from in vitro test systems. These data may take the form of median inhibitory concentration (IC50) values for an enzyme inhibitor, or receptor binding affinity (K_m) constants for a receptor antagonist, or simple activity units for a compound designed to mimic endogenous substances. Of equal or greater utility are whole-animal efficacy data, which often are reported as dose–response curves and a median effective dose (ED50, Fig. 1). These data are particularly helpful since they represent the effects of the test drug in living biological systems over a range of doses, in a manner analogous to toxicology studies. Extrapolation of relevant data for toxicological evaluation is simplified when efficacy data are available in the same animal species and by the same route of exposure as will be used in toxicology studies.

C. Pharmacokinetic/Pharmacodynamic Background Data

Many advances of value to the toxicologist have occurred in the area of pharmacokinetics/pharmacodynamics. Promising new techniques, such as the advent of physiology-based pharmacokinetics, give investigators access to simple but powerful mathematical models of the major components of pharmacokinetics; i.e., absorption, distribution, metabolism, and elimination [7]. These newer methods may contribute additional insight into understanding interspecies differences, with the potential for allowing more rational animal model selection and data interpretation [8,9].

A conference, cosponsored by the FDA, entitled "The Integration of Pharmacokinetic, Pharmacodynamic and Toxicokinetic Principles in Rational Drug Development," was held in April 1991 [10]. A portion of this conference was devoted to a review of strategies for the effective incorporation of phar-

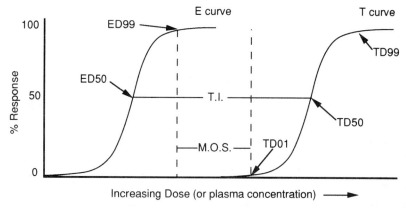

Figure 1   Dose–response curves. E curve = efficacy dose–response; T curve = toxicity dose–response; ED99/TD99 = pharmacological/toxic dose that produces a 99% response; ED50/TD50 = pharmacological/toxic dose that produces a 50% response; TD01 = toxic dose that produces a 1% response; T.I. = therapeutic index; and M.O.S. = margin of safety.

macokinetic/pharmacodynamic data into preclinical safety studies. The proceedings of this conference focused on the usefulness of pharmacodynamic data (absorption extent and route, tissue distribution and protein binding, metabolism, and elimination pathways) for the interpretation of toxicology study results. The use of pharmacokinetic data to substantiate the extent and duration of systemic exposure of toxicology study animals to test compound was also highlighted.

Of primary interest to the toxicologist are the pharmacokinetic data generated in species used in toxicology studies. These data may then be compared to similar data from in vivo efficacy studies to aid in toxicology dose selection. Doses selected for toxicological investigation on the basis of relative plasma concentration data between species are often more directly applicable to the risk assessment process. These data also may detect nonlinear or saturation kinetic behavior of the drug. Nonlinear kinetics indicate that systemic exposure does not change in proportion to dose, such as when there is a superproportional relationship between plasma levels and dose. This type of drug kinetics can complicate the establishment of dose–response relationships. For example, under superproportional kinetics, plasma drug levels increase greatly after relatively minor increases in dose, leading to very steep dose–response curves, decreasing the separation between toxic and nontoxic doses. On the other hand, supraproportional kinetics occur when plasma drug levels increase very little following relatively large increases in dose, impairing identification of threshold doses for different responses [11]. It is important that pharmacokinetic data used for interpretation of toxicology results be collected at toxicologically relevant doses, since kinetic characteristics can change as a function of dose, as described above.

A useful set of pharmacokinetic parameters (assuming oral administration) in relevant species would include bioavailability or fraction of total dose absorbed (F, requires comparison to intravenous data), maximum plasma concentration achieved after a single dose (C_{max}), the time after dosing when C_{max} occurs (T_{max}), the absorption rate constant (K_a), the elimination rate constant (K_{el}, usually estimated from intravenous data), the plasma half-life ($t_{1/2}$), the volume of distribution (V_d), and the clearance rate (Cl). In addition, multidose kinetic data such as time to steady state may be obtained from toxicology studies. Several excellent texts have been devoted to the derivation and use of these data [12,13]. When properly applied, these data provide guidance for critical toxicology study design elements such as dose selection and timing of key functional assessments (electrocardiogram, blood pressure, etc.) relative to dosing [7,9,13].

D. General Design Considerations

Some of the elements that go into the design of preclinical safety studies are common to a variety of study protocols. Dose and species selection are perhaps the most critical steps, although additional decisions are made regarding the numbers of animals and some groups used, the route and duration of administration, and the number and type of control groups. Many of these decisions are dependent on the anticipated design of early human studies.

General toxicology study design guidelines, commonly referred to as the "Red Book," were last published by the FDA in the early 1980s [14]. Although these guidelines were originally released by the Bureau of Foods and were intended as "principles for the safety assessment of food additives and color additives," the scientific basis for these guidelines has been applied to the design of safety studies with other types of compounds. Similar guidelines have been drafted by regulatory bodies in Europe and Japan [20,21].

Because of the importance of preclinical safety studies, great care is taken to ensure proper design, conduct, and interpretation. Studies to be submitted for regulatory agency review are conducted according to strict guidelines known collectively as "Good Laboratory Practices" (GLP) as set forth by the FDA [15]. These guidelines strive to assure that data collected during safety studies are accurately obtained and thoroughly documented, and that the results and conclusions drawn from these data are substantiated by the raw data record. By certifying safety studies as "conducted in compliance with Good Laboratory Practices," the drug sponsor assures the regulatory agency that data were properly reported and that these raw data are archived and available for review. Although compliance with GLP guidelines places a burden on the drug sponsor, adherence to these guidelines means that regulatory agencies are presented with a more consistent data file, which speeds regulatory review of drug applications.

1. Dose Selection

The doses selected for use in toxicology studies generally are intended to define a dose–response curve, where toxicity is the response of interest (Fig. 1). Dose is usually defined in units of mg/kg, or the amount of test drug in mg administered per kg body weight for each study animal. When other animal toxicology data are unavailable, the toxicologist refers to pharmacology data, pharmacokinetic data, projected clinical doses and intended clinical plasma levels, and other data as described above. A central concept in toxicology is that the "safety" of a test compound cannot be adequately understood until its toxicity is understood. Therefore, at least one dose level is usually selected that is intended to produce some degree of toxicity. Additional dose levels are selected to further define a dose–response relationship. These doses are sometimes spaced at log-based intervals to fit the log function associated with most dose–response curves as shown in Fig. 1. For drug safety testing, it is desirable to establish a "margin of safety" (Fig. 1), which is the dose range between the maximum dose required to produce a desired pharmacological effect and the lowest dose that produces evidence of toxicity. For this reason, lower doses are usually included in the study design that are expected to cause no adverse effects. Ideally, the biological properties of the experimental drug allow a great deal of separation between pharmacologically active doses and toxic doses; however, this is not always the case in practice.

Vehicle selection for whole-animal toxicology studies is intended to approximate projected clinical dose formulations. For orally delivered drugs, this often means simply dissolving the test drug in water or suspending it in a liquid slurry using methylcellulose or some other suspending agent. Clinical formulations are sometimes used if they are available at the time of toxicology testing and if they substantially improve the similarity between test animal exposure conditions and human exposure conditions. Generally, elaborate formulations with multiple excipients are avoided in early toxicity studies to avoid confounding toxicology data interpretation.

2. Animal Model Selection

Another critical stage in the design of preclinical toxicology studies is animal model selection [16]. For preclinical toxicology studies, this usually means defining the species and strain to be used in animal studies. These are referred to as animal models because the primary goal of this selection is to choose test animals that will "model" or predict human responses as closely as possible. Although great strides have been made in our ability to predict whole-animal responses based on data from studies using alternative test systems such as tissue culture, it is currently not possible to artificially reproduce the vast and complex intricacies of intact biological systems. Until adequate alternative systems are available, animal testing will be a necessary component of preclinical drug safety evaluation.

Criteria considered in the selection of animal models in toxicology studies include previous experience with the species and its responses, any physical/physiological/biochemical characteristics unique to the model, the species used in pharmacological profiling of the test compound, interspecies differences in the pharmacokinetics or metabolism of the test compound, and environmental or nutritional influences on toxicity [17,18]. Generally, a described by FDA in the Goldenthal guidelines (Table 1), multiple-dose subchronic preclinical toxicity studies are conducted in a minimum of two different species, at least one of which is a nonrodent. An equal number of each sex are used per dose group. In general, young and still growing animals are used in these studies. An exciting new facet of animal model selection has been the introduction of transgenic animal strains designed to express useful genetic traits. An example of this technology would be mice into which the human DNA sequence coding for drug-metabolizing enzymes had been inserted, creating a mouse model that would metabolize test drugs more similar to humans. Several such transgenic strains are already available commercially, and hold the promise of dramatically increasing the predictive value of animal testing. A more thorough discussion of animal

Table 1 FDA Guidelines for Preclinical Animal Toxicity Studies to Support Oral or Parenteral Clinical Studies

Desired duration of human admin.	Development phase	Preclinical study design	
		Species	Duration
Several days	I, II,	2 (1 rodent, 1 nonrodent)	2 weeks
	III, NDA		2x human < 3 months
Up to 2 weeks	I	2 (1 rodent, 1 nonrodent)	2 weeks
	II		2-4 weeks
	III, NDA		Up to 3 months
Up to 6 weeks	I, II	2 (1 rodent, 1 nonrodent)	6 weeks
	III		3 months
	NDA		3-6 months
7 weeks or longer	I, II	2 (1 rodent, 1 nonrodent)	1x human duration
	III		6 months[a]
	NDA[b]		6 months[a]

[a] Assumes USFDA adoption of 6-month studies as recommended by ICH conference (currently under review).
[b] Does not include reproductive, carcinogenicity, or genetic toxicity studies.
Source: Adapted from Ref. 60.

selection is beyond the scope of this chapter; however, much has been written elsewhere on this subject [16,19].

3. Numbers of Dose Groups and Animals

Selection of the number of animals per dose group to be included in preclinical toxicity studies attempts to achieve a balance between minimizing animal use and providing a sufficient sample population size for meaningful interpretation. A power calculation may be employed to estimate optimal dose group size if response incidence and severity can be estimated. Most guidelines suggest a minimum of 10 animals per sex per dose group for rodent studies, and a minimum of 3–4 animals per sex per dose group for nonrodent studies [20,21]. At least three drug-treated groups are usually included in subchronic studies. Additional groups may be added depending upon the range of doses desired and how extensively the dose–response relationship is to be defined. Study animals are always randomly assigned into dose groups, preferably using a body weight–based blocked randomization.

4. Route, Frequency, and Duration of Administration

The route of test drug administration in preclinical toxicity studies should closely reflect phase I clinical exposure conditions. For orally delivered drugs, this usually means intragastric gavage of study animals with solutions or suspensions of test drug. Drugs with intravenous indications would be delivered intravenously to animals, and other delivery routes such as oral capsules, intraperitoneal or subcutaneous injections, or intravenous infusions may also be used to more closely model early clinical conditions. The concentration of test drug in samples collected from actual formulated dosing material is measured several times over the course of a study to verify the dose delivered. Test drugs are also commonly administered as an admix in the feed, although this approach has several disadvantages and is usually reserved for animal studies of longer duration. Accurate estimation of the actual dose consumed in an "in-feed" study is more difficult than with other routes of administration, since it is obviously dependent on the feeding behavior of the test animals, which may be affected by the test drug. The concentration of drug in the feed is adjusted daily or weekly to compensate for variation in food consumption. In addition, validation of the concentration of test drug in feed is often more involved than when simple liquid vehicles are used.

Test drug is commonly administered 7 days a week in multidose preclinical studies, to maximize exposure during the study period. The frequency of oral dosing is most often once daily in preclinical studies, although other regimens such as twice per day (bid) or three times per day (tid) may be used to produce higher plasma drug levels or to more closely approximate projected clinical regimens. Intravenous administration may be as a single bolus, multiple daily bolus deliveries, or as a constant rate infusion, depending again on the pharmacokinetic characteristics of the test drug and the dosing regimens intended for use in human subjects.

Selection of the proper duration of administration is also largely dependent on clinical study designs. Conceptually, the goal is to ensure the safety of phase I clinical subjects by exposing animals to test drug for a period of time in excess of the maximum duration of exposure planned for early clinical studies. The FDA has published recommendations on toxicology study length relative to planned duration of exposure in humans. These are also contained in the Goldenthal guidelines presented in Table 1. Generally, studies conducted to document safety for an IND submission are of 3 months or less in duration.

5. Number and Type of Control Groups

Control groups are included in all preclinical toxicity study designs to help the toxicologist distinguish normal background variation from test drug–induced responses. Untreated controls also serve as study monitors to identify changes induced by diet, stress, or other environmental factors and to prevent such changes from being mistakenly attributed to the test drug. Control animals are matched as closely as possible to drug-treated animals prior to dosing to maximize the probability that any differences found between controls and treated animals were in fact produced by the test drug. The number of animals used in control groups is also a function of the statistical power necessary to detect differences between controls and treated animals, which is in turn dependent on the amount of variation in the response.

"Positive" controls are control groups treated with an agent other than the test drug that produces a known and consistent response. Test drugs may be compared to existing compounds with similar toxicological, pharmacological, or chemical characteristics by using positive controls.

IV. PRECLINICAL SAFETY STUDY TYPES

The various toxicology studies conducted in preparation for phase I clinical trials may be categorized for the sake of description, although there may be considerable crossover between categories. These categories would typically include pharmacology profiling studies, acute toxicity studies, multidose toxicity studies, mechanistic toxicity studies (for lack of a better name; also referred to as "target organ studies" or "special toxicity studies"), and mutagenicity studies. As one might predict, these categories reflect those found in guidelines issued by the FDA for the format and content of the toxicology section of an IND [22]. Reproductive toxicity studies would typically be included only if the early clinical development plans call for exposure of women of childbearing age. Recent initiatives to increases the representation of women in clinical trials and concerns about potential effects in males may make reproductive studies a more common component of future preclinical toxicology packages.

A. General Pharmacological Profiling

General pharmacology drug screening, also known variously as safety pharmacology, major organ systems toxicology, or regulatory pharmacology screening, is another component of the safety evaluation process [23]. These tests are often conducted very early in drug development, and therefore form an important foundation for the toxicological database. In addition to their importance in toxicological evaluation, these data have the added benefit of assisting drug discovery programs in the identification of more selective drug candidates and the potential to uncover unpredicted therapeutic indications. Although widely utilized within drug development research, there is less agreement between research groups on experimental model selection and study designs in general pharmacology than in other areas of safety evaluation. A tiered approach is sometimes taken, with results of primary screens dictating the selection of secondary screens. Recent efforts by the Pharmaceutical Manufacturers Association in the United States have brought representatives from different research groups together to learn from each other's experience; Japan has taken the regulatory initiative to issue preliminary guidelines for the conduct of general pharmacology studies. In addition, several European regulatory authorities have recently added safety pharmacology studies to the list of studies that should be done according to GLP. There is some agreement on the goals and the general approach to these evaluations. A discussion of these principles is fundamental to an understanding of preclinical drug safety assessment.

By concept, general pharmacological profiling is conducted to explore the pharmacological effects of an experimental drug beyond the intended therapeutic responses. As this description implies, these studies are typically carried out at doses at or near the therapeutic range, and not at overtly toxic doses [23]. This dose range is selected for greatest response detection sensitivity, since subtle responses may be overwhelmed or obscured by other toxicity at higher doses. Typically, doses are selected using data from in vivo and in vitro efficacy models. Drug efficacy is often quantified as ED50 and ED90 values, and multiplies of these may serve to define the range of general pharmacology test doses.

The exposure to test drug in general pharmacology studies is usually acute (single dose) in duration. This approach provides adequate response detection sensitivity while permitting a relatively rapid accumulation of data. Careful selection of the route of exposure and knowledge of pharmacokinetic properties in in vivo models can increase the validity of single-dose experiments.

It has been proposed that undesirable pharmacological responses may be described as fitting into one of two categories [24]. Type I responses are those effects that are a direct result of the primary pharmacological mechanism of action for the drug but are of no therapeutic value. An example of this type of response would be adverse cholinergic side effects caused by a cholinesterase inhibitor intended for use as an Alzheimer's disease therapy. Type II responses are due to extramechanistic or nonselective properties of the test drug. For example, it has been proposed that side effects such as cough and angioedema associated with angiotensin-converting enzyme (ACE) inhibitors may be due to the role of ACE in bradykinin and prostaglandin metabolism [25]. This is an example of a type II response because ACE catalyzes multiple pathways, not just the conversion of angiotensin I to angiotensin II that is responsible for therapeutic antihypertensive properties.

Classical paradigms from experimental pharmacology are typically employed by general pharmacology investigators in a systematic manner such that major organ systems are evaluated individually. Systems evaluated may include the central nervous systems (CNS), the cardiovascular system, the renal system, the gastrointestinal system, and the pulmonary system. The emphasis placed on any given system varies, depending on the research organization and the experimental drug in question. Accordingly, the current regulatory environment allows general pharmacology studies to be designed to fit organizational and project-based needs.

The data produced by these studies provide great insight into some of the fundamental properties of the test drug. Renal profiling is capable of evaluating drug effects on renal perfusion and urine formation, for example. Cardiovascular profiles may include physiological data such as drug effects on blood pressure or electrocardiograms. CNS profiling can often combine in vivo observational data such as drug-related behavioral changes with molecular level data such as competitive affinity for mammalian neurotransmitter receptors. Data from additional systems may include effects on gastrointestinal transit rates and smooth muscle function, or blood gases and respiratory physiology. Whatever the nature of the data produced, they are of great value to the toxicologist and should be incorporated into the evaluation of any adverse response detected in longer term studies.

B. Acute Toxicology

Acute toxicology has classically been thought of as studies to establish toxicity produced by single, relatively high dose in animal models. The typical study protocol involved administration of single doses at several different dose levels to groups of animals and monitoring responses over at least a 24-h period. Typically, the responses were limited to crude observational end points such as deaths, postural changes, or vocalization. The data tended to be summarized as an LD50 value, which is a mathematical value calculated from the midpoint on a dose–response curve where lethality would be predicted in approximately 50% of animals dosed (Fig. 1). The LD50 as a standalone piece of data is rapidly becoming outdated since it provides very little information on the nature of the toxicity observed or on the shape of the dose–response curve. In fact, at the recent International Conference on Harmonisation it was recommended that the LD50 determination be entirely abandoned. However, regulatory agencies in the United States and abroad still request acute lethality data.

The past tense is used above to describe "traditional" acute toxicology studies because modern study protocol refinements have greatly increased the volume of information obtained from acute studies, while the number of animals used for these studies has decreased. Lethality is still a valid observation, but it is no longer the central end point of interest. A number of articles and book chapters have been published recently describing modern approaches to acute toxicity testing [26–28]. Many of these authors offer dosing schemes that permit the evaluation of a wide range of doses while minimizing animal numbers. Typically, such dosing schemes follow an "up–down" design, where subsequent dose levels are determined by responses to initial doses, i.e., a dose that produced a marked adverse response such as convulsions would be followed by a lower dose to the next test group, while a dose that produced no response or a minimal response would be followed by a higher dose [28]. Another progressive dosing scheme is the "fixed-dose procedure" as described by van den Heuvel et al. [29]. In modern acute toxicity testing, comprehensive behavioral and activity observations are recorded according to onset, duration, and intensity. If lethality is observed, a necropsy is performed to establish the probable cause of death and to identify affected tissues [26].

During safety testing of experimental drugs, acute toxicity testing results are useful for establishing the dose range in which toxicity is observed and for identifying specific target organs and target systems of interest. This information is very helpful in the design and interpretation of longer term, multidose, animal toxicity studies.

C. Subchronic Toxicity Studies

Subchronic toxicity studies are the cornerstone of the preclinical safety data package. The outcome of these studies allows toxicity to be evaluated in a temporal sense relative to multidose kinetics. In practical terms, these studies usually determine the upper limits of dosing, in terms of both dose amount and duration, for early phase I trials in human subjects.

To clarify this review, the data collected from subchronic toxicity studies are divided into two categories: in-life observations and postmortem observations.

1. In-Life Observations

One goal of any toxicology study with living animals is to maximize the information obtained from each animal and thereby minimize the total number of animals needed for safety evaluation. This principle is most evident in preclinical toxicity studies. The number of individual data points collected in routine toxicology studies often runs into the thousands and represents a wealth of potential information. Many of these data are collected during the in-life phase of the study. This offers the toxicologist an opportunity to monitor responses as they happen, and to add supplemental, more directed tests when indicated. In this way, the design of a multidose toxicity study may evolve in response to the toxicities produced.

Clinical observations of the general appearance of test animals are made several times daily during the dosing period and therefore are the most frequently recorded in-life data. Behavioral responses such as activity level changes are noted, as are physical responses such as loose stools or salivation. Physical exams are also performed, to evaluate skin and muscle tone, pupillary response, capillary refill, and other clinical end points. These data can be very sensitive indicators of certain types of toxicity, such as CNS effects. Food consumption is also commonly monitored in preclinical safety studies; these data also can be a very sensitive indicator of the general condition of test animals. Body weights are obtained at regular intervals, for correct dosage calculations and as a potential indicator of toxicity. Vital signs are monitored regularly, including but not limited to heart rate, respiratory (ventilation) rate, body temperature, and blood pressure. Electrocardiograms are commonly obtained in large animal studies to assist in the diagnosis of cardiovascular toxicity. All of these clinical data are reviewed by the toxicologist, who is looking for recognizable changes and patterns, much like a physician evaluates a routine physical exam.

Clinical pathology tests are useful diagnostic tools at the toxicologist's disposal. Extensive clinical chemistry, hematology, and urinalysis data are collected prestudy to establish baseline values, and then at regular intervals during the dosing period. It is important that the toxicologist understand the proper interpretation of each test result, and that the meaning of results in different species also be appreciated. This is because many of the marker substances measured in clinical chemistry and urinalysis are present at different levels in different species, and the magnitude of change in response to drug exposure may also be species-dependent. For example, γ-glutamyl transpeptidase (GGT) is found in biliary cells of all species used in toxicology studies and in humans, although it is present at very different amounts in different species. This difference may be demonstrated by phenobarbital administration at high doses, which will produce serum GGT elevations in rabbit (which have relatively high liver GGT, like humans) but will not change serum GGT levels in rat [30].

Blood samples for clinical chemistry and hematology testing are usually obtained from large animals by venipuncture of a peripheral vein, while samples are usually obtained from the retro-orbital sinus of smaller species. Indwelling catheters are sometimes used if more frequent samples are needed. The end points selected for serum chemistry analysis usually include a wide variety of tests to help in the detection of a variety of potential target organ toxicities, metabolic toxicities, and other drug-induced responses. Serum electrolyte levels, such as sodium, potassium, calcium, and chloride, are routinely measured. Serum enzyme activities such as alkaline phosphatase, serum transaminases, creatine phosphokinase, GGT, 5'-nucleotidase, and ornithine carbamyl-transferase are also often determined. Additional indicators of biliary function including total/direct bilirubin, and serum bile acids may be measured. Indicators of renal function, such as blood urea nitrogen and creatinine levels, and of pancreatic function, such as serum glucose and amylase activity, are commonly included. Serum lipids such as cholesterol and triglycerides may be measured as well. Some or all of these tests may be included in any given study, depending on the goals of the study and the nature of the test drug. Many additional tests are at the toxicologist's disposal to aid in the accurate diagnosis of toxic responses. A very complete text on the subject of clinical chemistry testing of laboratory animals was recently published [31].

Routine hematology evaluations are also performed during toxicology studies, and are very useful for the detection of toxicity to the elements of the blood and the blood-forming organs. A complete blood count (CBC) is usually performed, including white cell count, platelet count, red cell count, hematocrit, hemoglobin content, and cell volume data. Additional values such as mean red cell hemoglobin may be calculated from these data. Functional analysis of coagulation is often performed, since blood clotting can be affected by many chemicals.

The value of comprehensive urinalysis in preclinical safety studies is sometimes questioned due to the difficulty of collecting an accurate, clean, and complete urine sample [32]. Nevertheless, important data may be obtained if precautions are taken during collection to limit sample contamination and loss. A simple urinalysis screen for use in animal safety studies may include measurement of urine pH, specific gravity, and volume, and may also include qualitative screening for glucose, blood, ketones, and bilirubin. Urinary sediment analysis may also be revealing. If clinical chemistry or urinalysis screening data indicate that the kidney may be a target organ, better urine samples may be obtained for more complete analysis by using specially designed metabolism cages for small animals, or by catheterization of the bladder of larger animals. Fecal analysis may also be performed, if indicated by study design and goals, or by clinical signs.

2. Postmortem Observations

Extensive postmortem examination of tissues from study animals is a key component of any standard toxicology study design. These data allow the pathologist/toxicologist to pinpoint target tissues and target cell populations within target tissues based on physical evidence. In addition, histochemical staining techniques can reveal subcellular physical and biochemical changes caused by test drug administration [33].

Complete postmortem exams are conducted by certified veterinary pathologists and include both gross evaluation of tissues at necropsy and microscopic examination of stained tissue sections. A selected group of major organs are weighed at necropsy for drug-induced changes. Tissues weighed may include such organs as liver, kidneys, testes, heart, brain, and adrenals. Organ weights may be expressed as raw weight or as a fraction of body weight. Organ weights may also be expressed as a ratio to brain weight, since brain weights tend to be stable compared to body weights.

Microscopic examination of tissues is a laborious, time-consuming process. The number of microscope slides produced in a single study may number in the thousands. However, the results more than justify the effort invested. A great deal of the special value of animal toxicology studies in the safety assessment process is due to the availability of histopathology data, i.e., data that are unavailable or minimal in other categories of preclinical and clinical safety studies. A common approach to reviewing tissues under the microscope is to examine a full range of tissues from control and high-dose animals first. Control animals are examined first to establish baseline lesion incidence, if any, while high-dose slides are examined because they are most likely to reveal drug-induced changes if any are present. Any tissues that have treatment-related lesions are then also examined at the lower dose levels, as well as any tissues with grossly apparent lesions, or any other tissues indicated as potential targets for toxicity by in-life results and/or historical data from the same or similar test drugs. Special histochemical staining may be requested by the pathologist to clarify subtle changes. Electron microscopy may also be used to visualize samples at the ultrastructural level.

D. Genetic Toxicology

Genetic toxicology testing, as the name implies, is concerned with identifying test drugs with genotoxic activity in various in vitro and in vivo test systems. These tests are used exclusively for the evaluation of mutagenic potential. It is generally believed that genotoxic or mutagenic compounds are likely to also be carcinogenic, although the value of these tests for predicting the outcome of chronic carcinogenicity bioassays in animals has been questioned [34]. The predictive value of genotoxicity testing relative to human cancer is even less well understood. It has been observed that the majority of known human carcinogens are genotoxic, although such associative evidence may be of little predictive value [35].

Short-term genetic toxicology tests generally are designed to detect mutations at the nucleotide level (gene or point mutations) or mutations at the chromosome level (chromosomal aberrations). Common tests employed in the detection of gene mutations include the Ames bacterial reverse mutation assay and the mammalian cell gene mutation assay. Tests used for the detection of chromosomal aberrations include the in vitro cytogenetics test which may be done using human lymphocytes, the mouse micronucleus test which looks for DNA fragments in mouse bone marrow cells, and the unscheduled DNA synthesis test which measures the inclusion of radiolabeled thymidine into drug-treated cells. Many other tests have been developed that allow further characterization of the precise type of genetic damage induced. A more in-depth review of this fascinating area is beyond the scope of this chapter; however, many excellent reviews of the subject have been published [36–38].

E. Special/Mechanistic Studies

Another, more loosely defined category of preclinical toxicology studies is special and mechanistic studies. Special toxicology studies are those studies that are deemed necessary because of special circumstances or characteristics associated with the test drug. For example, a drug that is to be given as a suppository may require rectal irritation studies, or a drug to be applied topically may require pharmacokinetic studies to determine the amount of absorption through the skin. Drugs intended for parenteral administration generally require irritation studies as well as blood compatibility studies. The pharmacological properties of a test drug may also determine the need for special studies. Drugs that are identical to endogenous substances and drugs intended for AIDS or cancer therapy, all very active areas of pharmaceutical research, typically follow an abbreviated preclinical safety evaluation program [39–41]. In addition, the intended patient population for a new drug may determine the design of the preclinical toxicology program. With cancer and AIDS therapies in particular, the special needs of the patient population are a prime consideration because the potential benefits of an experimental drug greatly increase the level of potential risk that is acceptable. Moving these types of drugs to the clinic more quickly has allowed more patients timely access to experimental therapies while minimizing unacceptable toxicity [42].

The other type of toxicology study in this category is the directed mechanistic study. The tremendous explosion of knowledge and information in recent years in fields such as molecular biology and immunology has provided exciting new techniques useful for describing and explaining the causes of toxicity. The benefits of mechanistic studies are many, to the general science of toxicology, to the public health by continuing development of drugs that would have otherwise been considered too toxic, and to the sponsor of a new drug. Mechanistic studies could correctly identify a species-specific toxicity and therefore more accurately predict the response in humans. This appears to be the case with peroxisome proliferators such as clofibrate, which have been associated with hepatocellular carcinoma in rodents but not in humans [43]. Mechanistic studies also have the potential to reveal better ways to clinically monitor and treat known toxicities. The potential types and uses of mechanistic studies are as varied as the types of drugs that are being tested. It is sufficient to state that any serious toxicity detected in routine studies should be evaluated thoroughly in directed, mechanism-based studies before human subjects are exposed to the test drug.

V. DATA ANALYSIS AND INTERPRETATION

As indicated by the above discussion, the database created in a routine preclinical toxicology package is enormous by any standards. The organization, interpretation, integration, and summation of these data are the responsibility of the toxicologist. To adequately review all of the information collected, the toxicologist draws on a working understanding of pharmacology, physiology, biochemistry, pathology, pharmacokinetics, and other fields within the medical sciences.

Interpretation of toxicology data is a complex process, with input from many support professionals such as pathologists, pharmacokinetics/drug metabolism experts, clinical veterinarians, and others.

The data analysis process may best be understood as proceeding on three levels, namely, the individual animal level, the study level, and the risk assessment level. These three levels of analysis incorporate the three main tasks of experimental toxicology as described by Zbinden: (a) description of the spectrum of toxicity via dose–response relationships; (b) extrapolation of these data to predict adverse effects in other species; and (c) prediction of safe exposure conditions in other species, usually humans [44].

The individual animal level is where the actual diagnoses of toxic responses are made. Drug-induced responses are often first detected by clinical evaluation, via either changes in clinical pathology values, altered behavior or vital signs, or other clinically detectable changes. These clinical data are then compared to pathology results and plasma drug concentration data on an animal-by-animal basis to support or verify the diagnosis. Diagnoses at this level provide critical information about the onset, severity, and duration of toxic responses.

Even though animals used in toxicology studies are usually bred specifically for use in biomedical research, there is considerable interindividual variation in response rates, which may vary greatly in a single-dose group. By integration of a variety of individual data such as hematology, histopathology, and plasma drug concentrations, the investigator may be able to identify the reason why a given animal responded while other animals in the same dose group responded less or not at all. Often individual variation of this type is explained by plasma drug concentration data, such that a correlation can be established between drug level and degree of response within a dose group. It is not unusual for one sex to be more sensitive than the other to a test drug due to gender-dependent kinetic differences. These examples underscore once more the important role of adequate plasma drug concentration data in the safety assessment process.

Data interpretation at the study level is primarily concerned with comparing drug-induced toxic responses between dose groups. If responses have been observed and doses correctly chosen, a dose–response relationship may be constructed for each toxic end point. Establishing a dose–response within a study is the first step in the risk assessment process. Unlike pharmacologists, who tend to be more interested in the middle of dose–response curves, toxicologists tend to be more concerned with the upper and lower limits of the curves (Fig. 1). The upper end of the curve provides information about dose-limiting toxicity and therefore is useful information for the selection of high doses for subsequent studies. The upper range of the curve can also help determine if a toxicity is progressive with time, such that a longer duration of a constant dose produces an increased toxic response. Progressive toxicity often suggests that the toxic form of the test drug is accumulating in the blood or in a target tissue. Progressive toxicity can also suggest that the toxicity produced by a test drug is interfering with its metabolism or elimination.

The lower end of the dose–response curve defines doses where toxicity is not produced. As stated earlier, it is desirable in toxicology studies to have at least one dose level that produces no evidence of toxicity. This is the no-effect level (NOEL), which is more properly described as the "no observed adverse effect level" (NOAEL). Once the NOAEL dose level is established in the most sensitive species used in multiple-dose toxicity studies, the upper limits of initial clinical doses for use in phase I safety studies may be determined. Generally, clinical dosing begins at a small fraction of the NOAEL from animal studies, although the exact multiple is determined by the nature of the toxicity observed, the therapeutic drug class, route and exposure conditions, and the human subject population to be exposed. Depending on the characteristics of the test compound, it may be useful for the safety range between human subjects and animals to be defined by relative plasma drug concentrations when dealing with systemic toxicity of test material. Concentration-based multiples have the advantage of providing a means for comparison between species; however, the predictive value of this approach is questionable [45]. Nevertheless, plasma concentration vs. response curves generally represent the relationship between exposure and systemic responses more accurately than dose vs. response curves. For this reason, the importance of plasma concentration data in toxicology studies is evident [46,47].

The slope of the central, linear portion of dose–response curves provides information on the toxicity dose range, or the distance between safe doses and toxic doses. A very steep slope indicates that there is relatively little difference between toxic and nontoxic doses, as is seen with drugs such as digitalis. Administration of these type of drugs must be monitored carefully to avoid adverse effects.

Only after toxicity has been evaluated on an individual animal and a toxicology study level can the real process of risk assessment begin. As discussed above, the major portion of an IND is in fact a risk assessment, in which all available preclinical data are presented and reviewed to predict any potential risk to human subjects from test drug exposure. There are two primary challenges to the toxicologist in this data review process. First is the complete integration of relevant data from a variety of test models, species, and systems into a single comprehensive statement on the toxicity(s) produced by the test compound. This process is the essence of toxicology, in which data of many types from diverse sources are evaluated for common themes. A toxicologist must draw on all of his or her training, experience, and intuition to piece together the responses observed and their underlying causes.

The second major challenge in the risk assessment process is the extrapolation of safety data, both between different animal test species and from these species to humans [48,57]. The predictive value of animal data in toxicology is only as good as the skill of the persons evaluating the data [58]. Without a thorough understanding of the inherent differences and unique characteristics of the test species used, the relevance of animal data to humans cannot be established [49,54,56]. Interspecies extrapolation has been one of the most difficult challenges facing toxicologists for decades. Historical data collected in multiple animal species show that acute and subchronic toxicity such as hepatotoxicity and nephrotoxicity are somewhat predictable (30%) from one animal species to another [50]. The predictive value between animal species is probably much higher when the parent drug is the primary toxicant and when plasma drug concentrations are comparable between species, although the database to support this assertion is lacking.

The ability of toxicology studies to detect responses with sensitivity and to predict the outcome of human exposure is at least in part dependent on the nature of the toxic effect observed. For example, gastrointestinal side effects such as emesis are quite predictable in humans based on animal responses; however, CNS effects such as lightheadedness or euphoria are less well predicted. Animal studies are often also able to predict adverse effects due to overexpression of pharmacological effects. It is apparent from the general infrequency of unexpected marked toxicity produced in phase I clinical studies that animal safety studies are able to predict acute and short-term adverse responses in humans with some degree of success [51,52]. This observation has been supported by a retrospective examination of the available database, although there is no way of knowing what the human response would have been to drugs that were discontinued due to animal toxicity prior to phase I studies. The predictive value of animal studies for chronic toxicities is more difficult to assess. Convincing data have been presented to show that little additional information is gained from toxicology studies of greater than 6 months duration [53]. Indeed, one proposal from the recent International Harmonisation Conference was to evaluate the need for studies beyond 6 months on a case-by-case basis. Carcinogenicity studies are routinely conducted with drugs intended for chronic use, although the predictive value of these studies is unclear when high doses are used [55]. Much has been written about the predictive value of animal studies, and the issue is far from resolved. One thing is certain: the future gains in understanding the kinetic, metabolic, biochemical, and physiological differences between animals and humans will permit more rational toxicology study design and interpretation, as well as contribute to the risk assessment process.

VI. FUTURE TRENDS

It has been said that toxicology is a science without a scientific basis, that it is based on assumptions that are inaccurate or poorly defined [52]. Criticisms such as these are short-sighted, and underestimate the purpose and utility of toxicology. Although toxic agents and responses have been studied for centuries, much of what we know as toxicology today has been created in recent years by public pressure for safe products and by governments seeking to regulate and control therapeutic drugs. This is quite unlike other sciences, which have been allowed to evolve naturally from firm scientific foundations. The practice of regulatory toxicology is also unusual as a science in that toxicologists are repeatedly asked to demonstrate a negative, i.e., to demonstrate "safety" or that toxicity is not present. Toxicologists have struggled to meet these societal and legal demands, perhaps to the detriment of scientific progress.

Today we can observe numerous examples of the science of toxicology beginning to catch up to its applications. Toxicology currently functions more as a true science, as toxicologists spend more time explaining and understanding the causes of toxicity and less time reporting limited "observational" data. The current international efforts to harmonize regulatory requirements for toxicology studies offer the promise of a more rational approach to preclinical safety assessment. Many countries have expressed an interest in joining in this effort. Numerous workshops and symposia addressing the need for more and better pharmacokinetic information from toxicology studies are changing the way these data are collected. The FDA is in the process of evaluating methods of assessing the potential behavioral and neurotoxicity of drugs. Guidelines for behavioral assessment are already in place for compounds regulated by the Environmental Protection Agency. The desire to reduce the use of laboratory animals in toxicology coupled with the search for faster, cheaper, and more accurate predictors of toxicity has greatly expanded the number of valid alternative testing strategies in recent years [59]. Strains of laboratory animals that have been altered genetically to express useful traits are already in use; more will certainly follow. Although computer-based simulations of all but the most rudimentary biological processes are still a long way off, complex physiology-based kinetic models can now be computer-manipulated with relative ease.

One thing is certain: toxicology will continue to evolve rapidly. The preclinical safety evaluation of drugs in the next century will likely produce data of much greater relevance and predictive value, but the future process may bear little resemblance to current practices.

REFERENCES

1. Worldwide pharmaceutical R&D expenditure estimated at $214bn for 1990. *CMR News.* 1991;9(3):1–3.
2. Grabowski H. Pharmaceutical research and development: returns and risk. Centres for Medicines Research Annual Lecture, July 1991.
3. Pharmaceutical manufacturers association (PMA) firms: allocation of research and development (R&D) budget (F). *Scrip.* Dec. 03, 1990;14.

4. 21 CFR 1. Subpart B—Investigational New Drug Application (4–1–88 Edition) Section 312.20–312.55.
5. Golightly LK, Smolinske SS, Bennett ML, Sutherland EW, Rumack BH. Pharmaceutical excipients: adverse effects associated with inactive ingredients in drug products (Part 1). *Med Toxicol.* 1988;3:128–165.
6. Golightly LK, Smolinske SS, Bennett ML, Sutherland EW, Rumack BH. Pharmaceutical excipients: adverse effects associated with inactive ingredients in drug products (Part II). *Med Toxicol.* 1988;3:209–240.
7. Scheuplein RJ, Shoaf SE, Brown RN. Role of pharmacokinetics in safety evaluation and regulatory considerations. *Ann Rev Pharmacol Toxicol.* 1990;30:197–218.
8. Smith DA. Species differences in metabolism and pharmacokinetics: are we close to an understanding? *Drug Metab Rev.* 1991;23(3&4):355–373.
9. Monro AM. Interspecies comparisons in toxicology: the utility and futility of plasma concentrations of the test substance. *Reg Toxicol Pharmacol.* 1990;12: 137–160.
10. Peck CC, Barr WH, Benet LZ, et al. Opportunities for integration of pharmacokinetics, pharmacodynamics, and toxicokinetics in rational drug development. *Clin Pharmacol Ther.* 1992;51(4):465–473.
11. Lu FC. Safety assessment of chemicals with threshold effects. *Reg Toxicol Pharmacol.* 1985;5:460–464.
12. Gibaldi M, Perrier D. *Pharmacokinetics* (vol 15 in the Drugs and the Pharmaceutical Sciences Series), New York: Marcel Dekker; 1982.
13. Welling P, Tse FL. *Pharmacokinetics: Regulatory, Industrial, Academic Perspectives* (vol 33 in the Drugs and the Pharmaceutical Sciences Series), New York: Marcel Dekker; 1988.
14. Food and Drug Administration. Toxicological principles for the safety assessment of direct food additives and color additives used in food. Report by the US FDA; 1982.
15. 21 CFR 58. Good Laboratory Practices for Nonclinical Laboratory Studies 1983.
16. Calabrese EJ. Suitability of animal models for predictive toxicology: theoretical and practical considerations. *Drug Metab Rev.* 1984;15(3):505–523.
17. Smith RL. The role of metabolism and disposition studies in the safety assessment of pharmaceuticals. *Xenobiotica.* 1988 18(1 Supp.):89–96.
18. Omaye ST. Effects of diet on toxicity testing. *Fed Proc.* 1986;45(2):133–135.
19. Lang CM, Vesell ES. Environmental and genetic factors affecting laboratory animals: impact on biomedical research. *Fed Proc.* 1976 35:1123–1131.
20. Council Recommendation (83/571/EEC) Annex I-Repeated Dose Toxicity. *Official Journal of the European Communities.* 1983;332:12–17.
21. Toxicity Test Guideline. Pharmaceutical Affairs Bureau, Ministry of Health and Welfare, Japan, 1984.
22. Guideline for the format and content of the nonclinical pharmacology/toxicology section of an application. US Department of Health and Human Services, Public Health Service, Food and Drug Administration, 1988.
23. Weissinger J. Nonclinical pharmacologic and toxicologic considerations for evaluating biologic products. *Reg Toxicol Pharmacol.* 1989;(10):255–263.

24. Williams PD. The role of pharmacological profiling in safety assessments. *Reg Toxicol Pharmacol*. 1990;(12):238–252.

25. Swartz SL, Williams GH, Hollenberg NK, Moore TJ, Dluhyu RG. Converting enzyme inhibition in essential hypertension: the hypotensive effect does not reflect only reduced engiotension II formation. *Hypertension*. 1979;1:106–111.

26. Elsberry DD. Screening approaches for acute and subacute toxicity studies. In: Lloyd WE. ed. *Safety Evaluation of Drugs and Chemicals*. New York: Hemisphere;1986:145–150.

27. Sutton TJ, Reilly LM. Variable group size can further reduce animal usage in acute toxicity tests. *Arch Toxicol*. 1991;65:260–261.

28. Yam J, Reer PJ, Bruce RD. Comparison of the up-and-down method and the fixed-dose procedure for acute oral toxicity testing. *Fd Chem Toxicol*. 1991;29(4): 259–263.

29. van den Heuvel MJ, Clark DG, Fielder RJ, et al. The international validation of a fixed-dose procedure as an alternative to the classical LD_{50} test. *Fd Chem Toxicol*. 1990;28:469–482.

30. Sulakhe SJ, Lautt WW. The activity of hepatic gamma glutamyl transpeptidase in various animal species. *Comp Biochem Physiol*. 1985: 82B:263–264.

31. Loeb WF, Quimby FW. eds. *The Clinical Chemistry of Laboratory Animals*. New York: Pergamon Press; 1989.

32. Evans GO, Parsons CE. Potential errors in the measurement of total protein in rat urine using test strips. *Lab Animals*. 1986;20:27–31.

33. Ettlin RA, Oberholzer M, Perentes E, Ryffel B, Kolopp M, Qureshi SR. A brief review of modern toxicologic pathology in regulatory and explanatory toxicity studies of chemicals. *Arch Toxicol*. 1991;65:445–453.

34. Mason JM, Langenbach R, Shelby MD, Zeiger E, Tennant RW. Ability of short-term tests to predict carcinogenesis in rodents. *Ann Ref Pharmacol Toxicol*. 1990;30:149–168.

35. Shelby MD. The genetic toxicity of human carcinogens and its implications. *Mutation Res*. 1988;204:3–15.

36. Environmental Protection Agency. EPA guidelines for mutagenicity risk assessment. *Fed Reg*. 1986;51:34006–34012.

37. Tennant RW, Margolin BH, Shelby MD, et al. Prediction of chemical carcinogenicity in rodents from *in vitro* genetic toxicity assays. *Science*. 1987;236:933–941.

38. Brusick DJ. *Principles of Genetic Toxicology*. New York: Plenum Press; 1980.

39. Giss HE. ed. *Preclinical Safety of Biotechnology Products Intended for Human Use*. New York: Alan R. Liss; 1987.

40. Weissinger J. Nonclinical pharmacologic and toxicologic considerations for evaluating biologic products. *Reg Toxicol Pharmacol*. 1989;10:255–263.

41. Teelmann K, Hohbach C, Lehmann H. The International Working Group. Preclinical safety testing of species-specific proteins produced with recombinant DNA techniques. *Arch Toxicol*. 1986;59:195–200.

42. Collins JM, Grieshaber CK, Cabner BA. Pharmacologically guided phase I clinical trials based upon preclinical drug development. *J Nat Cancer Inst*. 1990;82(16):1321–1326.

43. Lock EA, Mitchell AM, Elcombe CR. Biochemical mechanisms of induction of hepatic peroxisome proliferation. *Ann Rev Pharmacol Toxicol.* 1989;29:145–163.
44. Zbinden G. Predictive value of animal studies in toxicology. *Reg Toxicol Pharmacol.* 1991;14:167–177.
45. Watanabe PG, Schumann AM, Reitz RH. Toxicokinetics in the evaluation of toxicity data. *Reg Toxicol Pharmacol.* 1988;8:408–413.
46. Eason CT, Bonner FW, Parke DV. The importance of pharmacokinetic and receptor studies in drug safety evaluation. *Reg Toxicol Pharmacol.* 1990;11:288–307.
47. Davies DS. An introduction to metabolic and kinetic aspects of toxicological studies. *Xenobiotica.* 1988;18(1):3–7.
48. Lumley CE, Walker SR. eds. *Animal Toxicity Studies: Their Relevance for Man.* Lancaster UK: Quay; 1990.
49. Voisin EM, Ruthsatz M, Collins JM, Hoyle PC. Extrapolation of animal toxicity to humans: interspecies comparisons in drug development. *Reg Toxicol Pharmacol.* 1990;12:107–116.
50. Morton D. Expectations from animal studies. In: Lumley CE, Walker SR. eds. *Animal Toxicity Studies: Their Relevance for Man.* Lancaster, UK: Quay; 1990: 3–14.
51. Lumley CE. Clinical toxicity: Could it have been predicted? Pre-marketing experience. In: Lumely CE, Walker SR. eds. *Animal Toxicity Studies: Their Relevance for Man.* Lancaster, UK: Quay; 1990:49–56.
52. Heywood R. Clinical toxicity: Could it have been predicted? Post-marketing experience. In: Lumley CE, Walker SR. eds. *Animal Toxicity Studies: Their Relevance for Man.* Lancaster, UK: Quay; 1990:57–70.
53. Lumley CE, Walker SR. A critical appraisal of the duration of chronic animal toxicity studies. *Reg Toxicol Pharmacol.* 1986;6:66–72.
54. Schmidt-Nielsen B. Research animals in experimental medicine. *Exp Biol Med.* 1982;7:46–55.
55. Schach von Wittenau M. Strengths and weaknesses of long-term bioassays. *Reg Toxicol Pharmacol.* 1987;7:113–119.
56. Smith CC. Animal studies: How well do they predict xenobiotic metabolism in humans? In: Lloyd WE, ed. *Safety Evaluation of Drugs and Chemicals.* New York: Hemisphere; 1986:83–125.
57. Vocci F, Farber T. Extrapolation of animal toxicity data to man. *Reg Toxicol Pharmacol.* 1988;8:389–398.
58. Smith CG. Past, current and future safety and efficacy trends in the drug industry. *Reg Toxicol Pharmacol.* 1985;5:241–254.
59. Mehlman MA. ed. *Benchmarks: Alternative Methods in Toxicology.* Princeton, NJ: Princeton Scientific; 1989.

2

Adverse Drug Events in Clinical Trials

Deborah S. Kirby

Pfizer Inc.
Groton, Connecticut

I. INTRODUCTION

Drug safety concerns are of paramount importance in both therapeutic and diagnostic medicine. Historically, this concern probably predates even the Hippocratic Oath, which states that to "do no harm" is a primary goal of the physician. Unfortunately, adverse events from drugs will occur as long as there are drugs to treat patients, though many adverse drug events are predictable and preventable. Drug safety issues assume even greater significance in clinical trials of investigational medications. This chapter begins with a discussion of adverse drug events in general and continues by focusing on their occurrence and management in clinical trials.

II. DEFINITION OF AN ADVERSE DRUG EVENT (ADVERSE DRUG REACTION)

There are multiple definitions for an adverse drug event, though it is generally defined as an undesired effect related to therapy with a certain medication. The World Health Organization [1] defines adverse drug events as

> any noxious or unintended response to a drug that occurs at doses usually used for prophylaxis, diagnosis, or therapy of disease or for the modification of psychological function.

Some definitions differentiate adverse events resulting from drug abuse, over-dosage, or withdrawal. The U.S. Food and Drug Administration (FDA) [2,3] broadens the definition of an adverse drug event to

> any adverse event associated with the use of a drug in humans, whether or not considered drug related, including the following: an adverse event occurring in the course of the use of a drug product in professional practice; an adverse event occurring from drug overdose, whether accidental or intentional; an adverse event occurring from drug abuse; an adverse event occurring from drug withdrawal; any significant failure of expected pharmacologic action.

The FDA also describes adverse drug events resulting from interactions between drugs as pharmacological responses that cannot be explained by the action of a single drug but rather two or more drugs acting simultaneously. Other definitions of adverse drug events differentiate drug interactions, treatment failures, errors, noncompliance, overdosage, drug abuse, drug withdrawal syndromes, and experimental therapy [1]. The FDA also categorizes adverse drug events as expected or unexpected; an expected event is already described in the labeling for the drug and an unexpected event is not. These categories, expected and unexpected, conceptually correlate with another common subdivision of adverse drug events into type A and B events.

A. Type A Adverse Drug Events

The majority of adverse drug events are type A ("augmented") or type I events, which are predictable, dose-related effects arising from the pharmacological actions of a drug [1,4–6]. An example is the excessive pharmacological effect of a medication dosage that exceeds a particular patient's tolerance threshold for that medication. Dose reduction often easily reverses the adverse drug event. Susceptibility to type A adverse drug events is modified by differences in individual metabolism (pharmacokinetics) and tissue response to certain drug levels (pharmacodynamics). Susceptibility depends on genetic factors, intercurrent illnesses, and concomitant medication usage. Animal models can usually be developed to reflect this type of adverse effect [7].

B. Type B Adverse Drug Events

Type B ("bizarre") or type II adverse drug events are idiosyncratic, unpredictable effects that often appear unrelated to the dosage or pharmacological activity of the inciting drug [1,4–6]. Though relatively rare, these events comprise many of the more serious adverse drug events. Type B adverse drug events do not usually improve with dose reduction and are more difficult to separate from underlying disease. Because these events are rare and atypical, it is difficult to recognize or avoid them. In fact, the ability of a drug to cause a relatively rate type B side effect may only be seen after the drug has been available for several years and used by a large number of patients. These side effects probably occur in a genetically susceptible subpopulation [1,7,8]. Examples of these adverse drug events include inordinate susceptibility to a drug's pharmacological activity, drug allergy, and other idiosyncratic events. It is difficult to develop a pertinent animal model because of the rarity and unpredictability of these events.

III. RECOGNITION OF AN ADVERSE DRUG EVENT

Adverse drug events may be difficult to recognize if they are nonspecific because they may be confused with intercurrent illnesses, newly emergent illnesses, or background symptoms. A drug may set off a cascade of events resulting in an adverse event whose connection to the initiating drug may be almost impossible to recognize. The subconscious preconceptions of evaluators will also affect the recognition of adverse drug events. Because of these difficulties, many adverse drug events probably go unrecognized [9]. Criteria have been established to causally associate an adverse event with a medication, e.g., the association should be consistent and reproducible, the association should be strong (generally showing a dose response), the association should be specific (likelihood of drug causation decreases if the disorder occurs frequently in other conditions), there should be a reasonable temporal relationship, and it should be plausible according to the known facts [4,10,11]. Clearly, then, it is simpler to link type A than type B adverse drug events to a medication.

In clinical trials, especially early in development, the clinician is less likely to know the typical side effect profile of the investigational medication. If the new drug belongs to a class of drugs that is already represented on the market, it is reasonable to be vigilant for side effects similar to those of the marketed drug(s). For investigational drugs unrelated to marketed drugs, prediction is more difficult. It is especially difficult to identify idiosyncratic events because of their rarity. Although common side effects are easily elicited even in fairly small clinical trials, a rare adverse drug event will probably not be found during the drug development process, even if as many as 10,000 patients are treated during that time. As stated previously, it is not unusual for rare adverse drug events to be unrecognized until the postmarketing period.

A. Incidence of Adverse Drug Events

The incidence of adverse drug events has been ascertained in many studies and varies from a few percent up to 40% or more [1,12]. Unfortunately, it is difficult to compare the results of available studies because of variability in the definition of an adverse drug event, the diagnostic criteria for assigning causality to the drug in question, the inclusion or exclusion of very mild events or of indeterminate events, the nature of the study (e.g., prospective or retrospective), the use or avoidance of checklists, the patient population assessed, and other factors. Standardized criteria and algorithms have been developed to assess the relationship between an adverse event and a drug in question [10–12], but some of these algorithms can be cumbersome to apply.

When adverse drug events are ascertained via spontaneous reporting systems, it is important to note that reporting is higher for drugs approved recently. For example, the reporting rate during the second year after approval is about five times greater than that during the fifth year after approval [13]. The FDA takes this into account when it monitors adverse drug events, watching for certain deviations from the norm.

B. Risk Factors for Adverse Drug Events

Certain factors predict an increased risk for adverse drug events. Several studies have shown that the risk increases with the number of concomitant medications, the number of active medical problems, and a previous history of an adverse drug event. Concomitant medications or other active medical problems may make a target organ more susceptible to drug-related effects. For example, a drug that affects the ability of the bladder to empty itself is much more likely to cause a problem in a male patient who already has partial urinary obstruction from an enlarged prostate gland. There is also evidence that patients who are cognitively impaired, patients who frequently self-medicate with over-the-counter medications, and patients with more than one prescribing physician are at higher risk for adverse drug events.

The effect of increasing age on the incidence of adverse drug events has been debated [9,12,14,15]. Certainly there are changes with age that could increase susceptibility to adverse drug events. Age-related declines in renal function could result in slower elimination of drugs cleared by the kidney. Changes in liver metabolism with age are less predictable, and some metabolic processes may be decreased while others are influenced less. There may be changes in receptor sensitivity. Increases in body fat, associated with decreases in water fraction and lean body mass, can change the volume of distribution of drugs, resulting in increased half-life or higher maximum plasma concentrations of some drugs. Decreases of serum albumin with age can cause an increase in the free fraction of drugs that are highly protein-bound.

More recent studies have suggested that age is not an independent variable. It appears that the higher incidence of adverse drug events in elderly patients is explained by their greater number of active medical problems and by their greater use of medications as a result. Although adults aged 65 or older compose 11–12% of the U.S. population, they utilize up to a third of all medications. Of these prescriptions, about 40% are used by patients taking 3–12 prescriptions. In addition, 80% of the elderly have at least one chronic medical condition and over 50% have two or more [9]. The elderly are also more likely to have cognitive impairment, a risk factor for adverse drug events. In summary, many studies and surveys have found that adverse drug events are more common in the elderly, and the incidence correlates primarily with the number of disease states and the number of other drugs taken.

C. "Index of Suspicion"

The key to recognizing an adverse drug event is to have a high index of suspicion, always considering possible effects of drugs in the differential diagnosis of any sign or symptom where the etiology is not clear [16]. Knowledge of the patient's other illnesses, and the symptoms or complications related to them, is important. The physician should consider whether these illnesses could affect the pharmacokinetics or pharmacodynamics of the drug, especially through altered renal or liver function. The current incidence of background illnesses in the community should be ascertained and the incidence of background symptoms considered. The suspect drug history should be scrutinized, including duration of therapy, recent dosing changes, mode of administration, addition or deletion of concomitant medications that could interact with the drug, and the common pattern of adverse events associated with the drug.

In clinical trials, a high index of suspicion that the investigational drug could be responsible for emerging signs and symptoms is even more important because the side effect profile of the drug may not be well characterized. If another cause of an adverse event is definitely established, the adverse event is classified as an unrelated side effect or an intercurrent illness. Otherwise, it is classified as possibly or probably related to the study medication.

D. "Background" Signs and Symptoms

Careful health examination in a population reveals variations from the baseline or normal ranges 5–15% of the time [1,17]. Mild symptoms are common, such as anorexia, irritability, fatigue, altered sleep, and constipation. In one study, the 20 symptoms most commonly associated with antihypertensives were elicited from both the treated and control groups, and only two of these symptoms were more common in the treated group [1]. In another study that involved a 2-week follow-up of healthy postmenopausal women, 29% complained of five or more symptoms, 57% complained of one to four symptoms, and only 14% reported no symptoms. Frequent complaints were lack of energy, feeling "blue," headaches, and aches or stiffness of the joints. Less common symptoms were dizziness, cough, cold sweats, sore throat, and loss of appetite [1].

In double blind studies, the incidence of side effects in the placebo group varies in published reports from <1% to as much as 60%, and the side effect profile for placebo tends to assume a similar form to the side effect profile for the active medication. This suggests that preexisting or emergent conditions—background signs, symptoms, and minor illnesses—which might otherwise have gone unnoticed are uncovered and regarded as side effects. It is important to recognize these background signs and symptoms because many of them will be attributed to the study medication during a clinical trial. The true relationship between an adverse event and the drug may only become clear, especially for common and often relatively minor side effects, when the frequency of occurrence of the adverse event is tabulated and compared between treatment groups.

E.   Role of Drug Interactions

Drugs may act together to additively or synergistically cause either adverse or beneficial events. Beneficial drug interactions should be exploited therapeutically, such as the use of probenecid to increase blood levels of concomitantly administered penicillin. Other drug interactions lead to reduced efficacy or other adverse events. Adverse drug interactions represent up to a quarter of all adverse drug events, especially when alcohol is included, and 90% of adverse drug interactions are due to cumulative effects on vulnerable organ systems [4]. Less commonly, one drug may alter the metabolism and elimination of another drug, resulting in either increased or decreased therapeutic effects from the other drug. These interactions are more common for drugs with narrow therapeutic windows, high plasma protein binding, and toxic metabolites. Genetic differences in drug metabolism probably play a role in individual susceptibility, though an understanding of some of the metabolic pathways involved does not always lead to the ability to predict drug interactions because conflicting effects on metabolism may occur. Other factors that may affect drug interactions include the sequence in which the medications are administered, route and time of administration, duration of therapy, and dosages [4,16].

Because the potential drug interactions for a new compound are generally unknown, a new drug should first be introduced in a population that is not on concomitant medications. As development of the compound progresses, the therapeutic and toxic effects of the new medication should be compared in patients both with and without concomitant drug therapy. If predictions can be made based on the compound's characteristics, drug interaction studies should be completed with medications that are more likely to interact with the compound. For example, a compound with high protein binding is likely to participate in interactions with drugs that compete for protein binding, and a compound that can induce hepatic enzymes often affects the clearance of drugs that are metabolized by the liver.

IV. HANDLING OF ADVERSE DRUG EVENTS IN CLINICAL TRIALS

A. Prediction and Prevention of Adverse Drug Events

The first step toward recognizing adverse drug events in clinical trials is to form some predictions regarding the types of adverse events it would be reasonable to expect. Common adverse events such as gastrointestinal disturbances and rashes should be expected in at least some patients for all drugs. Some adverse events are more likely with certain categories of drugs and therefore can be anticipated when testing a new drug. These "expected" adverse drug events are often of the type A variety. For example, antihypertensives may lower the blood pressure excessively in the standing position and cause lightheadedness when the patient is standing (postural hypotension) by exaggeration of the therapeutic effect of lowering the blood pressure.

The length of drug administration is pertinent because some adverse drug events are much more common early in therapy, such as hypersensitivity events. Some medications also cause adverse events to which patient tolerance will develop as treatment is continued. For example, patients may develop excessive hypotension when certain blood pressure medications are first administered, but the effect abates even though the same dosage is continued. Conversely, other medications cause adverse events later in therapy as the drug accumulates over time [1].

Understanding the pharmacokinetics of a drug helps predict the potential for adverse drug events, especially type A events. Drugs with long half-lives may be more likely to cause side effects, especially if dosage adjustments are not made to account for accumulation. The primary route of drug elimination may predict populations at higher risk of drug accumulation. For example, a drug eliminated primarily by the kidney may accumulate in patients with inadequate renal function, or a drug metabolized primarily by the liver may accumulate in patients with liver disease. Compound-specific knowledge of the body's handling of the drug and of conditions that can affect the body's ability to eliminate the drug are also helpful in predicting patients at high risk for adverse drug events. Knowledge of the mechanism of action of a drug is also useful in predicting which drug interactions are most likely to occur.

Although animal models may be used to predict potential adverse drug events in humans, animal models are often not helpful because the genetic differences between species are so great that the mechanisms of toxicity can be different [4,18,19]. Even strains within one animal species may show important differences. Therefore, more than one animal species is generally tested. Some adverse events are difficult to detect in animal models, such as central nervous system effects. It is also difficult to provide good animal models for immunologically mediated adverse events.

Prevention of adverse drug events is facilitated by identification of populations at risk. When selecting patients for clinical drug trials, especially early in the development process, it is wise to use screening procedures to identify patients at high risk for certain side effects. This includes patients with abnormal laboratory tests or active intercurrent illnesses, or a history of certain adverse drug events, especially more serious adverse events or adverse events from drugs that are similar to the investigational drug. When a compound is first tested in humans, it is important to select as healthy a study population as possible to reduce the possibility that a side effect or laboratory abnormality could be caused by an intercurrent or underlying illness. As the side effects of the compound become better defined, the entrance criteria can be a little less strict and the clinical trial can more closely match the real-life situation.

Clinical trial screening procedures should generally include a complete medical history and physical examination, basic safety laboratory tests (complete blood count, urinalysis, serum chemistry panel), and some questions tailored to identify patients who could pose specific risks. For example, patients entering studies of nonsteroidal anti-inflammatory drugs (NSAIDs) should always be asked if they have an allergy to any other NSAIDs, including aspirin. Patients selected for a drug study should be capable of following dosing instructions, willing to return for follow-up visits, and willing to return for extra safety-related testing if indicated. Instructions for taking the study drug should be very clear, and the study should be well supervised.

B.   Detection and Follow-Up of Adverse Drug Events

The screening visit for a clinical trial is generally done about a week before administration of study drug [18,20]. When drug therapy is begun at the baseline visit, safety testing should be repeated, and periodic safety assessments should be made throughout the study. These safety assessments will be more frequent earlier in the study, and clinical trials of drugs that are early in development will be shorter with more intensive and more frequent safety monitoring. After the baseline visit, it is reasonable to repeat safety testing at 24 and/or 72 hr (in earlier trials), 1 week, 2 weeks, 1 month, and then at monthly intervals through 6 months. Follow-up beyond 6 months could occur every 3 months for up to 2 years, and then potentially occur less frequently after the 2-year time point. In addition to laboratory monitoring, these visits should include assessment of any new signs or symptoms. Patients may be assessed with a checklist, though checklists are associated with an increased reporting of very minor side effects. Alternatively, patients may spontaneously report any problems that they have noted since the last visit.

If an adverse event occurs in a clinical trial, the first course of action is to confirm it and document its extent and severity. A decision must be made whether to immediately withdraw or reduce the dose of the investigational drug, at least temporarily, depending on the severity and time course of the adverse event. Once the adverse event is confirmed, a history and physical examination should be performed; a more serious adverse event requires an especially meticulous and thorough approach. The history should include details of all concomitant medication use, including over-the-counter preparations. If the drug is not discontinued, close monitoring is indicated, varying with the severity of the adverse event, and the benefits of continuing therapy with the investigational drug must be weighed with the possible risks to the patient on an ongoing basis. Because most adverse drug events are mild, study drug often does not need to be withdrawn although dose reduction may be necessary. However, mild symptoms or laboratory abnormalities may necessitate drug withdrawal if they worsen progressively during follow-up. First and foremost, maintenance of the patient's health and safety should be the overriding consideration in evaluation, treatment, and follow-up of adverse events.

Any patient who develops an adverse event during a clinical trial must be followed until the event resolves or becomes insignificant. The time course of an adverse drug event may clarify its etiology. If the study drug was withdrawn, a drug-related adverse event will usually resolve. If the study drug dosage was reduced, a related event will usually resolve or improve. If the problem clearly disappears without any change in the medication dosage, causation by the study drug is less likely. If the adverse event is clearly identified to be not drug-related, the investigator and sponsor may agree at some point that follow-up will no longer be monitored by the sponsor, though the clinician will continue to monitor and treat the condition. All phone logs and records regarding attempts to contact patients for safety follow-up should be documented in the patient chart and study records, especially if difficulty is encountered in getting the patient to return for follow-up visits. If the site is not making adequate efforts to follow adverse events, payments to the site should be withheld until all follow-up is complete [17].

Significant adverse events that are clearly not related to the study drug must be considered on an individual basis. For example, a patient could be severely injured in a car accident. In such a case, termination or continuation of the patient in the study would depend on a variety of factors, including time course of the patient's participation, length of the clinical trial, length of time study drug may need to be temporarily discontinued during the adverse event, and any effect the event could have on the benefit/risk ratio for continuing the patient in the study.

C. Breaking Double-Blind Codes

In double-blind clinical trials, it is almost never necessary or appropriate to break the code indicating which medication the patient is receiving [17]. The decision to discontinue the medication after an adverse drug event should be made without knowledge of the patient's treatment group—study drug, active comparator, or placebo. Evaluation and treatment of an adverse event can be undertaken in most cases without knowing the identity of the study drug. The investigator's final assessment as to study drug causality of the adverse event should also be made without knowledge of the patient's treatment group. Otherwise, the temptation exists to follow treatment groups differently or to assign side effects as not related to study drug therapy if the patient was taking placebo.

Breaking the code is necessary only when it serves a valid clinical purpose. A valid reason to break a code exists when one of the agents being studied is needed for the patient's therapy after the study drug is discontinued, especially if the therapy is for a life-threatening condition that has nonexistent or inferior alternative therapy. In rare cases, an overdose may necessitate breaking the double-blind code. It is important to remember that breaking the double blind code almost inevitably leads to some bias in evaluation, attribution, and follow-up of adverse events.

D.   Reporting Responsibilities

For any clinical trial, the research team or sponsor must have a mechanism in place to collect accurate data on adverse events. Reporting requirements have been mandated by the FDA [2,3,21]. The reporting time period is defined according to whether the adverse event is serious or not, expected or unexpected, and drug-related or not. The institutional review board (IRB) that approved the research project should be notified of any serious adverse events, and the research site should be aware of the IRB's reporting requirements for less serious adverse events.

E.   Dechallenge and Rechallenge

Discontinuation of a drug that may have caused an adverse event is sometimes referred to as dechallenge [4]. Although the adverse drug event will usually resolve with dechallenge, there can be misleading circumstances. If the adverse event was actually caused by an intercurrent illness that then resolved or by some background symptom, dechallenge will be associated with resolution of the adverse event even though the study drug did not cause the event. Also, an adverse drug event may not disappear rapidly if the medication has a long duration of action, if drug metabolites have a long duration of action, or if structural damage has occurred. Therefore, dechallenge alone may not determine whether the adverse event was related to the suspect drug.

Rechallenge is the process of reinstituting therapy with a medication that was previously discontinued because of an adverse event. The purpose of rechallenge is usually twofold. First, it provides the patient another opportunity to take a medication if it had a therapeutic benefit. This is more important if the therapeutic benefit is proven and substantial, or if alternative treatments are inferior, scarce, or nonexistent. Second, it is one of the most obvious ways to confirm drug etiology of the adverse event for which the drug was withdrawn. Unfortunately, there are many false-positive and negative responses with rechallenge. For example, the drug may have precipitated the adverse event by interacting with an unrecognized intercurrent illness that subsequently resolved. In this case, rechallenge will not cause the adverse drug event to recur, even if the drug was partly responsible.

Because patient safety is the paramount concern, rechallenge is probably only justified when it is of vital importance to the patient that the relationship of the drug to the adverse event be established beyond doubt. The risk of rechallenge should be determined taking into consideration the severity of the adverse event. If rechallenge is planned, proper approval and understanding of the risks involved are required. The risks of rechallenge must be carefully explained to the patient, including a discussion of alternative therapies. The patient must then sign a special consent form reflecting the risks and benefits of rechallenge. Before rechallenge with the suspect medication, it is important for the adverse event to resolve. If the adverse event was an abnormal laboratory test, then the lab test(s) should be normal on two occasions about 2 weeks apart before rechallenge is undertaken. Single-dose rechallenge may be indicated before the drug is started on an ongoing basis. In this case, a single dose is given and safety monitoring is done periodically over the following few days. If the result is satisfactory, drug can be started on an ongoing basis. When rechallenge is done, the lowest dose of the drug should probably be used. Extra safety monitoring is indicated initially and at any time the drug dosage is increased. If the abnormality recurs, the drug should be discontinued. As always, the benefit/risk ratio for the patient should guide details in each individual case.

V. SUMMARY

Over the past 10–15 years, society has become increasingly preoccupied with medication safety issues [4]. This may reflect an increasingly widespread concern with the rights and protection of the consumer and with environmental concerns. However, it is not generally recognized by the lay public or the press that approval of a drug does not imply safety. First, it is unrealistic to ever assume that any medication is entirely safe. Therefore, medication safety is a relative balance of benefits and risks. Second, rare side effects are usually not recognized until a drug has been approved and in use for several years. Therefore, the final test of safety is a drug's record in clinical practice over many years. This emphasizes the importance of postmarketing adverse drug event reporting and leaves open the possibility for extremely rare adverse drug events to be recognized even years into marketing.

There is an interesting recent trend to approve new medications more quickly. The benefit would be the earlier availability of potentially valuable medications to the public, but there would also be earlier exposure of the public to potential risks from new medicines whose safety and possibly even efficacy profiles are not yet fully known. It is easier to justify earlier approval for medications that treat either terminal conditions or severe conditions with few or nonexistent alternative therapies.

Ultimately, the therapeutic use of any drug, approved or investigational, must be based on the individual benefit/risk ratio for each patient, as determined by the physician. Where the benefit/risk ratio does not clearly chart a course, the physician and patient should make a decision together. Assessment of the benefit/risk ratio will never be correct in every case, but it will be as meaningful and accurate as possible when complete information is available to the physician concerning the severity and prognosis of the patient's illness, the alternative treatments available, the potential therapeutic benefit of the proposed treatment, and the potential risks of the treatment to the patient.

REFERENCES

1. Lamy PP. Adverse drug effects. *Clin Geriatr Med.* 1990;6:293–307.
2. Jones LL, ed. Records and reports concerning adverse drug experiences on marketed prescription drugs for human use without approved new drug applications. *Fed Register.* 21; CFR. 1991;310.305, 22–25.
3. Jones LL, ed. Postmarketing Reporting of Adverse Drug Experiences. *Fed Register.* 21; CFR. 1991;314.80, 108–111.
4. Folb Pl. *The Safety of Medicines.* Berlin: Springer-Verlag; 1980.
5. Blaiss MS, deShazo RD. Drug allergy. *Pediatr Clin North Am.* 1988;35:1131–1147.
6. Rawlins MD, Thompson JW. Pathogenesis of adverse drug reactions. In: Davis DM, ed. *Textbook of Adverse Drug Reactions.* Oxford: Oxford University Press; 1981, 11–34.
7. Yacobi A, Skelly JP, Batra VK, eds. *Toxicokinetics and New Drug Development.* New York: Pergamon Press; 1989.
8. Neuberger J. Drug-induced jaundice. *Baillieres Clin Gastroenterol.* 1989;3:447–466.
9. Kleinfeld M, Corcoran AJ. Medicating the elderly. *Comprehens Ther.* 1988;14:14–23.
10. Kramer MS, Leventhal JM, Hutchinson TA, Feinstein AR. An algorithm for the operational assessment of adverse drug reactions. *JAMA.* 1979;242:623–632.
11. Naranjo CA, Busto U, Sellers EM, Sandor P, Ruiz I, Roberts EA, et al. A method for estimating the probability of adverse drug reactions. *Clin Pharmacol Ther.* 1981;30:239–245.
12. Hutchinson TA, Flegel KM, Kramer MS, Leduc DG, Kong HHP. Frequency,

severity and risk factors for adverse drug reactions in adult out-patients: a prospective study. *Chron Dis.* 1986;39:533–542.

13. Paulus HE. FDA Arthritis Advisory Committee Meeting: postmarketing surveillance of nonsteroidal antiinflammatory drugs. *Arth Rheum.* 1985;28:1168–1169.

14. Everitt DE, Avorn J. Drug prescribing for the elderly. *Arch Intern Med.* 1986;146:2393–2386.

15. Gurwitz JH, Avorn J. The ambiguous relation between aging and adverse drug reactions. *Ann Intern Med.* 1991;114:956–966.

16. Brodie MJ, Feely J. Adverse drug interactions. *Br Med J.* 1988;296:845–9.

17. Iber FL, Riley WA, Murray PJ. *Conducting Clinical Trials.* New York: Plenum; 1987.

18. Davidson CS, Leevy CM, Chamberlayne EC, eds. Guidelines for Detection of Hepatotoxicity Due to Drugs and Chemicals. National Institutes of Health (NIH Publication No. 79-313), 1979.

19. Dollery CT. The risk identified from clinical trials. In: Walker SR, Asscher AW, eds. *Medicines and Risk/Benefit Decisions.* Lancaster, UK: MTP Press Ltd; 1987:57–65.

20. Food and Drug Administration: General Considerations for the Clinical Evaluation of Drugs (FDA 77-3040). Rockville, MD. 1977.

21. Food and Drug Administration: Draft Guideline for Postmarketing Reporting of Adverse Drug Reactions (Docket No 85D-0249). Rockville, MD: Division of Drug and Biological Products, Experience Center for Drugs and Biologics; 1985.

3

Laboratory Testing in Clinical Trials

Deborah S. Kirby

Pfizer Inc.
Groton, Connecticut

I. INTRODUCTION

An important part of safety assessment of patients, either in medical practice or in clinical trials, is laboratory testing. The patient's blood and urine are commonly examined for specific components and the results compared to normal ranges devised from population studies. The cellular components of blood are examined in the complete blood count. The noncellular portion of blood is examined for electrolyte, enzyme, and protein constituents that predict the function and health of various bodily organs. The urine is examined for its appearance, physical properties, and the presence of abnormal cellular and noncellular elements. In this chapter, common laboratory tests and their interpretation will be discussed [1,2]. Rather than an exhaustive discussion of potential abnormalities, the meaning of common abnormalities will be emphasized to provide a basic understanding of the laboratory tests and their usefulness in both clinical practice and clinical drug trials.

II. INTERPRETATION OF LABORATORY TESTS
IN CLINICAL TRIALS

Each laboratory test requires a certain sample type, and the sample type will dictate the type of collection tube that is required. Blood tests can be run on whole blood, plasma, serum, or on cellular components of blood. Serum and plasma are used most commonly. Serum is the portion of blood remaining after the cells have clotted and been removed. Therefore, serum does not contain fibrinogen and other factors involved in the clotting process. Plasma is the protein-rich fluid portion of blood from which only cells have been removed. To collect plasma, clotting must be prevented and the cells must be separated out.

The units used for reporting test results must be noted because more than one system of units may be in use for a specific laboratory test. For example, a result could be reported in mg/dl or in mmol/L. The normal ranges listed in the following sections are approximate; in specific instances, the normal range for the testing laboratory should be used.

A. Complete Blood Count

The noncellular protein-rich plasma composes about 50–55% of the total blood volume. Conversely, about 45% of the blood volume is taken up by red blood cells and an additional few percent by white blood cells and platelets. Measurement of the cellular components of blood is done with the complete blood count (CBC). The primary components of the CBC—the hemoglobin, hematocrit, and white blood cell count—are probably the most commonly ordered tests in clinical practice. Monitoring of the CBC is essential in clinical drug trials because changes in the parameters are fairly common indicators of various drug toxicities as well as of many illnesses. When abnormalities occur in one of the parameters, it is important to look at the other parameters to see if they are involved. Patterns of involvement can suggest the etiology. For example, a simultaneous drop in hemoglobin, white blood cell count, and platelet count should suggest a production problem in the bone marrow, whereas an isolated drop in hemoglobin should suggest the possibility of gastrointestinal bleeding. The quantitative portions of the CBC are often performed with automated counters. In addition, a "peripheral smear" is made from a drop of blood and viewed under the microscope for qualitative abnormalities, which generally will reflect abnormalities detected with the quantitative measures.

1. Red Blood Cell Measurements

The red blood cells, or erythrocytes, are the blood cells responsible for carrying oxygen from the lungs to all parts of the body. When mature, these cells lose their nuclei and have a doughnut-shaped appearance by microscopy. Each erythrocyte contains hemoglobin, the component that actually attaches and carries most of the oxygen molecules. The two most common measures of erythrocytes are the hematocrit and the hemoglobin. The hematocrit is a measure of the fraction of the blood volume that is taken up by erythrocytes expressed in ml/100 ml whole blood. The hemoglobin is a measure of the amount of hemoglobin in the erythrocytes expressed in g/100 ml. The results should correlate, with the hematocrit being roughly three times the numeric value of the hemoglobin. An additional measurement, the erythrocyte count, is expressed as million cells per mm^3; it is less useful because it does not take cell size into account and can therefore be misleading.

Several other erythrocyte measurements are useful as well. These are the red cell indices, which can be derived by calculation from other measurements although the mean corpuscular volume, described below, can be measured directly with the currently available automated counters. The mean corpuscular volume (MCV) can be obtained by dividing the hematocrit by the erythrocyte count. It is a measure of the average size of an individual erythrocyte in μm^3. The mean corpuscular hemoglobin concentration (MCHC) can be obtained by dividing the hemoglobin by the hematocrit. It is a measure of the amount of hemoglobin in an individual erythrocyte expressed as a percentage. The mean corpuscular hemoglobin (MCH) can be obtained by dividing the hemoglobin by the erythrocyte count. Frequently expressed in pg, this value is less useful than the MCV and MCHC. The red cell indices, especially the MCV, can give supplemental information that make the hemoglobin or hematocrit result more meaningful.

In addition to all the quantitative values, the erythrocytes are qualitatively evaluated on the peripheral smear. This assessment describes cellular size, shape, and abnormalities. For example, erythrocytes that are larger than normal and contain some blue as well as red color (polychromatophilia) are usually immature erythrocytes. An increase in immature erythrocytes, or reticulocytes, suggests hemorrhage or hemolysis. Erythrocytes shaped like little targets occur in certain blood disorders, and sickle-shaped cells are the hallmark of sickle cell anemia. Portions of malarial or babesiosal parasites may be seen in erythrocytes. Severely distorted erythrocytes may be seen if mechanical damage to the cells occurs, such as in some patients with artificial heart valves.

Polycythemia, an abnormally high hemoglobin and hematocrit, may be caused by the primary disorder polycythemia vera but is more commonly secondary to hypoxia—lack of appropriate oxygen supply to body tissues—induced by a wide variety of conditions. Polycythemia has clinical significance when the hemoglobin climbs above 18–20 g/dl because it causes increased blood viscosity. The resulting sluggish flow of blood through the vessels can lead to ischemic events or thrombosis. Low hemoglobin, or anemia, also has a multitude of causes. Severe anemia, in contrast to polycythemia, causes a drop in the blood viscosity to as low as 1.5 times that of water rather than the normal value of about 3. This reduces the resistance to blood flow in the peripheral vessels so that much greater quantities of blood return to the heart than is normal. Hypoxia from diminished transport of oxygen causes dilatation (widening) of tissue vessels, further increasing blood return to the heart. The result is a large increase in cardiac output and cardiac work as the blood volume circulates much more rapidly than normal. Adding the increased workload of the heart to the tissue hypoxia may add up to myocardial ischemia or high-output heart failure. Although these general effects of anemia are usually the most significant, anemia may also be associated with specific symptoms related to the underlying cause.

In general, anemias can be classified as those due to decreased production or due to enhanced destruction of erythrocytes. The anemias of decreased production are probably more common, and the MCV is especially useful in helping to determine their etiology. When the MCV is low, corresponding to abnormally small erythrocytes under the microscope, the patient is said to have a microcytic anemia. The classic microcytic anemia of decreased production is iron deficiency anemia, which is usually caused by blood loss. Any medication that can cause blood loss should be suspect in a patient who has iron deficiency anemia. Another microcytic anemia is sideroblastic anemia, named for the characteristic abnormal erythrocytes called ringed sideroblasts. Medications that produce abnormalities in pyridoxine metabolism or heme synthesis can cause sideroblastic anemia. Sideroblastic anemia may also be a preleukemic condition with associated abnormalities in other blood cells. Microcytic anemia is also caused by some congenital disorders, most classically thalassemia.

When anemia is associated with an elevated MCV, corresponding to abnormally large erythrocytes under the microscope, the patient is said to have a macrocytic anemia. The classic macrocytic anemias, most commonly caused by folic acid or vitamin B_{12} deficiency, are referred to as megaloblastic anemias because of their characteristic macrocytic erythrocytes, hyperlobulated neutrophils, and bizarre, misshapen platelets. Megaloblastic anemia may be associated with decreased white blood cells and platelets, and abnormally increased serum unconjugated bilirubin from the breakdown of erythrocytes in the bone marrow that occurs in megaloblastic anemias. B_{12} deficiency megaloblastic anemia usually results from the failure to absorb vitamin B_{12} properly that occurs in pernicious anemia, total gastrectomy, and significant intestinal malabsorption. Folate deficiency megaloblastic anemia may be caused by lack of dietary folate or it may be secondary to drugs that interfere with folate metabolism such as methotrexate or trimethoprim. Drugs which impair DNA metabolism may also cause megaloblastic anemia. For example, megaloblastic anemia is the major toxicity of zidovudine (AZT), a drug used in the treatment of acquired immune deficiency syndrome (AIDS). Causes of megaloblastic anemia may be additive. For example, a patient with borderline dietary intake of folic acid may develop an acute megaloblastic state if given drugs that interfere with folate metabolism.

When anemia is associated with a normal MCV, the patient is said to have a normocytic anemia. If the erythrocyte hemoglobin concentration (MCHC) is also normal, the anemia is further classified as normochromic. An extremely common normocytic, normochromic anemia is anemia of chronic disease, which occurs in patients who have had an underlying inflammatory illness or advanced malignancy for more than a month. Although anemia of chronic disease is usually normochromic, it may be microcytic. Anemia of chronic disease is associated with a defect in the ability to utilize iron to synthesize hemoglobin.

The classic anemia of increased destruction of erythrocytes is hemolytic anemia, which results when erythrocytes are destroyed, or lysed, after their release from the bone marrow. Significant hemolysis usually causes a normocytic or macrocytic anemia because the compensatory increase in erythrocyte production causes an increase in circulating reticulocytes, which are larger than mature erythrocytes. The hemolysis usually occurs in the spleen rather than in the circulation itself. The highly porous capillaries of the spleen allow whole erythrocytes to pass out of the capillaries into the substance, or cords, of the red pulp of the spleen. The erythrocytes then gradually squeeze through the trabecular meshwork of the cords and return through the endothelial wall of the venous sinuses into circulation. As they pass through the substance of the spleen, old and abnormal cells are ingested by phagocytic cells.

Hemolytic anemia may be caused by medications via several different mechanisms. A drug may induce formation of antibodies that attach to erthrocyte surfaces or circulate in the peripheral blood. These antibodies may then result in immunological attack on the erythrocytes as though they were foreign agents. Another cause of drug-induced hemolysis is a variety of inherited abnormalities in erythrocyte glycolytic enzymes. Abnormalities in the main metabolic pathway, the anaerobic Embden–Meyerhof pathway, usually result in congenital hemolytic anemia. Abnormalities of the hexose monophosphate shunt, responsible for about 10% of the erythrocyte's glycolytic activity, usually cause hemolysis only after oxidant exposure. In addition to oxidant drugs like sulfa drugs, antimalarials, and nitrofurantoin, hemolysis can be initiated by other events such as viral and bacterial infections. The most common deficiency of the hexose monophosphate shunt is deficiency of glucose-6-phosphodiesterase (G6PD). Because the G6PD gene is on the X chromosome, females are generally unaffected carriers and males who inherit the gene on their X chromosome have the hemolytic condition. When hemolysis occurs in these individuals, it usually is limited to the older population of erythrocytes because they have less G6PD activity than younger cells. There are more than 250 variants of G6PD deficiency affecting millions of individuals, including one variant that affects up to 15% of the U.S. black population.

Abnormal erythrocyte tests at the screening visit of a clinical trial must be evaluated to determine whether the patient should be excluded from the trial. If the primary disease targeted by the clinical trial can cause polycythemia or anemia, more leeway is often necessary in entrance hemoglobin values. In any clinical trial of a drug with oxidant potential that includes a significant number of black male subjects, testing for G6PD activity in susceptible populations may be indicated.

During the course of a clinical trial, one of the most common abnormalities encountered is a dropping hemoglobin and hematocrit. Iron deficiency should be sought because it usually indicates chronic blood loss. Iron deficiency results in typical findings of anemia, microcytosis (low MCV), and hypochromia (low MCHC). Acute blood loss may result in a normochromic, normocytic anemia, although the abnormalities of iron deficiency may develop in the weeks after a significant bleeding episode. It is important to rule out blood loss first because it may be caused by serious lesions such as bleeding peptic ulcers or cancers of the gastrointestinal tract (especially colon). Another common cause of chronic blood loss is excess menstrual bleeding in younger women. It is not unusual to find more than one cause contributing to an anemia. For example, patients with chronic inflammatory disease may become anemic more quickly from mild ongoing blood loss during a clinical trial because they cannot make erythrocytes fast enough to maintain a normal hemoglobin.

If a newly developed anemia is associated with other hematological abnormalities, it is imperative to consider bone marrow disorders. For example, sudden drops in hemoglobin, white cell count, and platelet count may presage the development of aplastic anemia, which occurs when the bone marrow fails to function in producing blood elements. This is one of the most serious idiosyncratic hematological conditions that has been associated with drug therapy, and it may be irreversible.

2.   White Blood Cell Measurements

The second major cellular element of the blood is the white blood cell, or leukocyte. These nucleated cells derive from two major cell lines, the myelocytic (myelogenous) cells and the lymphocytic (lymphogenous) cells. The myelocytic cells are formed only in the bone marrow, whereas the lymphocytic cells are formed mainly in the lymphogenous organs—the lymph glands, spleen, thymus, tonsils, and lymphoid tissue in the bone marrow and gastrointestinal tract. The functions of leukocytes are to engulf and destroy foreign agents that enter the body, and to form antibodies or sensitized lymphocytes that can result in removal or destruction of the foreign agents. Leukocytes are stored in the bone marrow and lymphatic tissue until needed. For example, about a 6-day supply of granulocytes is stored in the bone marrow. The leukocytes are released in response to, and frequently are specifically attracted to, areas of inflammation.

The normal leukocyte count or "white count" is about 7000 leukocytes/mm^3 (μl) of blood. Because relative percentages as well as absolute amounts of different cell types are important, the leukocyte count usually includes a "differential." The differential is the percentage of different types of leukocytes present in a representative sample of the patient's blood. For example, a typical result would be about 62% neutrophils, about 30% lymphocytes, about 5.3% monocytes, about 2.3% eosinophils, and about 0.4% basophils. An elevated leukocyte count is called leukocytosis and a decreased leukocyte count is called leukopenia. An elevation or decrease in any of the specific leukocyte types is indicated by the respective suffix -*philia* or -*penia*. For example, an excess of neutrophils is neutrophilia and a dirth of neutrophils is neutropenia.

The most numerous leukocytes are the polymorphonuclear cells, named because of their lobulated nuclei. These myelocytic cells are also called granulocytes because of their cytoplasmic granules. Each type of granulocyte is named according to the staining characteristics of its cytoplasmic granules as neutrophils (polymorphonuclear neutrophils), eosinophils (polymorphonuclear eosinophils), or basophils (polymorphonuclear basophils). The normal life span of granulocytes once released from the bone marrow is about 4–8 hr circulating in the blood and another 4–5 days in the tissues. During an infection, their life span may be shortened. Another type of myelocytic leukocyte is the monocyte. The monocytes live 10–20 hr in the blood before moving into the tissues, where they develop into tissue macrophages that can live for months to years unless destroyed in the line of duty. The primary lymphocytic cells, or lymphocytes, are the second most numerous leukocyte in the peripheral blood. Plasma cells, formed from one type of lymphocyte, are occasionally seen in the peripheral blood.

Neutrophils   These normally compose half to three fourths of the circulating leukocytes. A normal absolute neutrophil count ranges from about 3000 to 5800/mm^3. Neutropenia is defined as an absolute neutrophil count less than 2000/mm^3; counts from 1000 to 2000 are considered to be mild neutropenia and counts from 500 to 1000 to be moderate neutropenia. Severe neutropenia, or agranulocytosis, is defined as a neutrophil count less than 500/mm^3. Because neutrophils play a major role in the body's system for fighting infectious and toxic agents, the risk of infection increases when the absolute neutrophil count falls below 1000/mm^3, and most patients with a neutrophil count less than 100/mm^3 develop infection. Immature neutrophils are called "band cells" because their nucleus looks like a curved band rather than being multilobulated. A small percentage of these cells is normal (1–2%), but a large percentage suggests abnormalities such as severe stress reaction, severe infection, or leukemia. In these conditions, cells that are even more immature than band cells may be seen in the peripheral smear.

Neutrophil counts show wide racial variations. Blacks and Yemenite Jews with so-called ethnic neutropenia or chronic benign neutropenia commonly have neutrophil counts of 1000–2000 mm^3 or less, though they usually do not have an increased incidence of infections. Pseudoneutropenia may occur with malnutrition and anorexia nervosa. The neutrophil counts in patients with both chronic benign neutropenia and pseudoneutropenia rise normally when the body is challenged with an infection or other stressful event. Artifactitious neutropenia can result with automated counts if cells are fragile from chemotherapy or clumped by the excessive plasma proteins present in some conditions.

Like erythrocytes and other leukocytes, neutrophil counts will drop if either neutrophil production or survival time is decreased, although both mechanisms are often implicated. Neutropenia of decreased production is most commonly due to dose-related bone marrow suppression from many of the drugs used to treat cancer. These type A adverse drug events are probably the most frequent cause of severe neutropenia in the United States. Drug interactions can also lead to bone marrow suppression; an example is the additive folic acid antagonism resulting from concurrent use of methotrexate and trimethoprim-sulfamethoxazole. Idiosyncratic neutropenia of decreased production may be an isolated syndrome or part of a generalized bone marrow failure syndrome such as aplastic anemia. Immunological destruction of bone marrow neutrophil precursors will result in decreased production of neutrophils, and immunological destruction of a pluripotential bone marrow stem cell can affect multiple cell lines.

Neutropenia from increased neutrophil destruction is most common in severe overwhelming infections where the body is unable to keep pace with the demand for neutrophils. Foreign agents, including drugs and infectious agents, may induce immunological effects that result in specific destruction of neutrophils. An enlarged spleen also contributes to neutropenia as well as to drops in platelet counts because it will "sequester" these leukocytes and platelets as well as destroy a larger number than usual.

Significant neutropenia occurring during the course of a drug study merits immediate attention. It is safest to assume that the study drug is the cause until another cause can be established. Depending on the severity of the abnormality and the time course in relationship to other symptoms and other medication use, it is often desirable to temporarily discontinue the study drug therapy until a white count and differential can be repeated and a search begun for other causes of neutropenia. If the neutropenia develops gradually, it is wise to discontinue the suspect drug if the neutrophil count drops under $2000/mm^3$. Drug-induced neutropenia usually resolves rapidly once the offending compound has been withdrawn, though hospitalization may be required if the patient is acutely ill.

Neutropenia developing during a clinical trial may prove to be unrelated to the study drug. Neutropenia may be chronically associated with an underlying disorder, such as rheumatoid arthritis or lupus, that may even be the primary disorder studied in the clinical trial. Viral infections may transiently cause neutropenia, as can other acute disease states. In such states, there will usually be a spectrum of symptoms related to the acute disease, such as the infectious symptoms of overwhelming bacterial or mycobacterial (tuberculosis) infection. In addition to infectious agents, other causes of neutropenia that should be considered are anaphylactic shock, radiation injury to the bone marrow, and hematological diseases such as pernicious anemia, leukemia, and aplastic anemia.

Neutropenia itself may result in nonspecific symptoms such as fatigue, mouth sores, sore throat, dysphagia, and other constitutional symptoms. Fever may presage sepsis, and organ system complaints may be clues to a site of infection, although infections may be hard to localize because the neutropenia results in reduced local inflammatory signs. If the bone marrow stops making neutrophils and other leukocytes, within 2 days ulcers may appear in the mouth and colon as the bacteria that are normally symbiotically present begin to penetrate the tissue. The patient may also develop secondary infections in the respiratory system, urinary tract, or various other sites. Bacteria from sites of tissue penetration then rapidly spread to the blood and other tissues. Without treatment, death often occurs within 3–6 days after acute total leukopenia.

Neutrophilia is the most common cause of leukocytosis, and it arises in conditions involving inflammation and/or stress. Neutrophilia may be acute or chronic depending on the underlying cause. Acute neutrophilia is characteristic of such states as infection, poisoning, hemorrhage, hemolysis, acute leukemia, and tissue death from myocardial infarction and severe burns. Neutrophilia may occur within a few hours after the onset of severe inflammation. The number of neutrophils may increase as much as four to five times, up to $15,000-25,000/\text{mm}^3$. When the total leukocyte count, including neutrophils, is over $25,000-50,000/\text{mm}^3$, the leukocytosis is called a leukemoid reaction. Chronic neutrophilia is seen with rheumatoid arthritis, with some of the chronic myelocytic leukemias, and with the administration of corticosteroids.

An elevated neutrophil/leukocyte count in itself does not usually cause problems unless it is extremely high. When counts rise above 100,000, especially with some types of leukocytes, symptoms may occur due to the leukocytosis itself. Symptoms of extreme leukocytosis include those of high blood viscosity and leukostasis syndromes such as hypoxia.

Eosinophils   These are granulocytes with characteristic red cytoplasmic granules. The number in the peripheral blood is about $50-250/\text{mm}^3$, composing about 1–3% of all the circulating leukocytes. Eosinophils are relatively weak phagocytes, but they can attach to and kill parasites. This may be the reason they are often produced in very large numbers in patients with parasitic infections. Eosinophils also collect in tissues undergoing allergic reactions, where they may play a role in reducing inflammation and removing allergen–antibody complexes.

Eosinopenia, or a reduced eosinophil count, is common with glucocorticoid treatment and may also occur with stress or infection. Conversely, eosinophilia is a blood eosinophil count greater than about $250-500/\text{mm}^3$. Parasitic infestations often cause eosinophilia when tissue invasion has occurred, and allergic diseases commonly associated with eosinophilia include asthma, hay fever, and urticaria. Isolated eosinophilia as the only presentation of drug allergy has been associated with many medications. Eosinophilia may also be seen in chronic leukemias, tumors, poisoning, inflammatory bowel disease, inflammation of the blood vessels (vasculitis), and sarcoidosis. Improperly stained neutrophils may appear to be eosinophils.

Basophils   These are granulocytes whose large cytoplasmic granules stain with a blue appearance. The number in the peripheral blood is relatively low, about 50–250/mm^3, representing only about 0–1% of circulating leukocytes. Basophils are very similar to the large tissue cells called mast cells, which are located immediately outside many of the body capillaries. Both types of cells are important in immediate hypersensitivity reactions because immunoglobulin E (IgE) can attach directly to mast cells and basophils. When a foreign antigen reacts with the IgE antibody, the mast cell or basophil may rupture and degranulate, releasing histamine and other mediators that cause the vascular and tissue reactions characteristic of immediate hypersensitivity.

Basopenia, a decreased basophil count, may not be noted because of the small number of basophils present under normal conditions. Basopenia may be secondary to glucocorticoid therapy, acute infection, and pregnancy; its clinical significance is usually low. Conversely, basophilia may occur in viral infections, hypothyroidism, kidney disease, and after splenectomy. More significantly, it may be the sign of an underlying granulocytic malignancy such as myelocytic leukemia or Hodgkin's disease. A normal absolute basophil count with a high relative count occurs when basophil counts are normal but other leukocytes are decreased. Therefore, an increased percentage of basophils in the differential count may be a sign of impending neutropenia.

Monocytes   These are myelocytic cells with a round or oval nucleus that do not have the characteristic granules associated with the polymorphonuclear cells. The number in the peripheral blood is about 300–500/mm^3, composing about 3–7% of the circulating leukocytes. The life cycle of monocytes leads them to eventually migrate to the tissue and become macrophages, which are important in the phagocytosis of foreign material.

Monocytopenia occurs with acute infections, stress, glucocorticoid administration, and acute myelocytic leukemia. Conversely, monocytosis can be caused by leukemia, protozoal (e.g., malaria) and rickettsial (e.g., Rocky Mountain spotted fever) infections, bacterial and mycobacterial infections (tuberculosis), chronic inflammatory bowel disease, sarcoidosis, and collagen diseases such as lupus. Monocytosis may also occur in the recovery phase after leukopenia because the monocytes may recover more quickly than other leukocytes.

Lymphocytes   These pass from the lymphatic circulation via the thoracic duct into the blood on an ongoing basis. The number circulating in the peripheral blood is about 1500–3000/mm^3, or 25–33% of the differential count. After entering the blood, lymphocytes will recirculate by passing into the tissue and eventually into the lymphatic circulation again. The life span of a lymphocyte is measured in months to years, depending on the tasks it is required to do. Lymphocytes are numerous in the lymph nodes, as well as other lymphoid tissues such as spleen, tonsils, submucosal areas of the gastrointestinal tract, and bone marrow.

There are two major populations of lymphocytes: T and B lymphocytes. The B lymphocytes, processed initially in the bone marrow, frequently become plasma cells. Plasma cells are the primary antibody-producing cells and can produce immunoglobulins at an extremely rapid rate—about 2000 molecules/sec for each plasma cell. Plasma cells occasionally circulate in the peripheral blood, usually in small numbers. The T lymphocytes, on the other hand, are processed initially in the thymus gland. Responsible for cell-mediated immunity, they are further subdivided into helper T cells, which aid in activation of B lymphocytes, and suppressor T cells.

Lymphocytopenia (lymphopenia) may be chronic in some congenital immunodeficiency syndromes. Other causes include lymphoid malignancies, impaired intestinal lymph drainage, kidney failure, severe right heart failure, malnutrition, aplastic anemia, and stress. Lymphocytosis may occur in lymphoid malignancy, "whooping cough," mononucleosis, tuberculosis, hepatitis, and toxoplasmosis. These conditions may cause a lymphocytosis significant enough to qualify as a lymphocytic leukemoid reaction. Abnormally large lymphocytes with reactive folded cytoplasmic borders may be present; these atypical lymphocytes are highly suggestive of certain viral infections. Relative lymphocytosis occurs with neutropenia or more generalized failure to produce the myelocytic leukocytes.

3. Platelet Measurements

Megakaryocytes are huge, multicellular bone marrow cells that fragment in the bone marrow into tiny cells called platelets. About a third of the platelets that form are immediately sequestered in the spleen, and the others circulate in the peripheral blood for 7–10 days. The normal blood platelet count is 150,000–450,000/mm^3. The function of platelets is primarily to promote blood clotting, especially at mucosal surfaces. Platelets release substances that cause nearby platelets to aggregate and form a clot. Platelet abnormalities can affect the clotting ability of the blood. Deviations from the normal include thrombocytopenia, thrombocytosis, and platelet function abnormalities.

Thrombocytopenia, an abnormally low platelet count, is caused by decreased production or increased destruction of platelets. Causes of decreased production include bone marrow failure or infiltration by malignant cells that crowd out the platelet precursors. Cytotoxic drugs that suppress most of the blood cell counts will also reduce platelets in a dose-dependent fashion. In these conditions, the bone marrow usually shows decreased megakaryocytes and it may also show abnormal cells or fibrosis. On the other hand, if thrombocytopenia results from platelet destruction, the bone marrow is usually full of megakaryocytes trying to keep pace with the ongoing platelet destruction. A number of conditions will result in reduced platelet life span. An enlarged spleen may sequester and destroy platelets and leukocytes; this is called hypersplenism. Artificial heart valves or conditions that cause diffuse intravascular clotting can result in mechanical injury and destruction of platelets. Antiplatelet antibodies induced by infections, drugs, or idiopathic causes can result in platelet destruction because antibody-coated platelets are quickly removed in the spleen or other tissues by phagocytes. Although medications can cause severe thrombocytopenia, the platelet count usually rises promptly once the offending agent is discontinued. More prolonged thrombocytopenia may occur with medications such as gold or phenytoin, probably because these drugs take longer to eliminate from the body.

Thrombocytosis, more than 500,000 platelets/mm^3, is most commonly seen with either iron deficiency or with inflammation because platelets act as acute phase reactants (i.e., counts rise with inflammation, stress, and infection). Thrombocytosis may also be seen with malignancy, especially if the malignancy is advanced, disseminated, or leukemic. Recent splenectomy usually results in a transient thrombocytosis.

Abnormalities of platelet function may occur regardless of the platelet count. Platelet defects may be inherited or acquired. One class of drugs that classically affects platelets, the nonsteroidal anti-inflammatory drugs (NSAIDs), inhibits the platelet enzyme that catalyzes production of a prostaglandin that is needed for normal platelet function. Aspirin irreversibly acetylates this platelet cyclo-oxygenase enzyme so that a single dose impairs hemostasis for 5–7 days, but the other NSAIDs cause reversible inhibition. As a result, NSAIDs may cause easy bruising and bleeding in the skin or even postsurgical or mucous membrane bleeding through their effects on platelets.

4.   Multiple Blood Cell Abnormalities

It is probably clear from the preceding paragraphs that an abnormality may involve only one type or multiple types of blood cells. Therefore, the cells involved in the abnormality should always be determined. In general, cytopenias are due to either decreased production or increased destruction of the cell involved. A bone marrow examination will often make this determination be-cause it will be lacking in precursors if there is a production problem and it will be packed with precursors if there is a destruction problem. Classic examples of factors that reduce all blood cell counts through reduced bone marrow production are radiation injury to the bone marrow, cytotoxic drugs, and aplastic anemia.

Aplastic anemia deserves special mention. The term should be applied to patients with pancytopenia, i.e., cytopenias of all the major blood cell lines (anemia, neutropenia, and thrombocytopenia). Aplastic anemia may result from damage to a common bone marrow stem cell. About half the cases in the United States are idiopathic, although there are congenital causes, physical causes (X-ray exposure), and chemical causes (benzene). Aplastic anemia may follow infectious hepatitis, usually non-A, non-B hepatitis, suggesting an etiological relationship with certain viral infections. Medications have been incriminated as well. Cytotoxic drugs that suppress the bone marrow in a dose-related fashion occasionally can cause irreversible aplasia, but aplastic anemia is usually an idiosyncratic adverse drug event. Chloramphenicol is the single most commonly incriminated drug in cases of aplastic anemia, though aplastic anemia only occurs in 1 of 50,000 patients taking the drug. Many other medications are classified as having definite or possible toxic potential.

The onset of aplastic anemia is usually insidious, with initial symptoms of mild weakness and fatigue from anemia, or mucosal hemorrhage from thrombocytopenia. The bone marrow is markedly hypoplastic, with very few blood cell precursors present. Complete or partial recovery may occur with time, or the condition may progress. Long-term survivors may maintain mild abnormalities of cellular number or size, and are at increased risk of subsequently developing leukemia and other related syndromes.

Leukemia and related diseases must also be considered with the onset of abnormalities in more than one blood cell type. Leukemia is the uncontrolled production of leukocytes arrested at some stage of development, and may involve either myelocytic or lymphocytic cells. In myelocytic leukemia, the malignant cells may be partly differentiated into a neutrophilic, eosinophilic, or monocytic leukemia. Usually, however, the malignant cells are bizarre, undifferentiated, and immature. The undifferentiated leukemias tend to be acute, and the differentiated leukemias tend to be chronic. Leukemic cells, especially the very undifferentiated cells, are usually nonfunctional. The effects of leukemia include infections, severe anemia, and a bleeding tendency because cytopenias are common as a result of displacement of the normal bone marrow by the nonfunctional leukemic cells. An important effect on the body is the excessive use of metabolic substrates by the growing cancerous cells, resulting in metabolic starvation from depletion of the patient's energy and protein tissues.

B. Erythrocyte Sedimentation Rate

The erythrocyte sedimentation rate (ESR) measures how far erythrocytes sediment toward the bottom of a capillary tube over the course of an hour. Of the two methods in common use, the Westergren method gives the most linear and reliable results in patients with significant elevations of the sedimentation rate. Increased plasma proteins cause an elevated sedimentation rate because proteins cause cells to clump together, and clumped cells sediment more quickly than single cells. The sedimentation rate is most sensitive to increases in fibrinogen, but it will increase with elevated γ-globulins and other plasma proteins as well. Elevated sedimentation rates are common in inflammatory conditions because some plasma proteins, including fibrinogen and γ-globulins, are significantly elevated by inflammatory states. The resulting increase of these so-called acute phase reactants results in an increase in the sedimentation rate. Examples of inflammatory conditions that are associated with increased sedimentation rates include infection, rheumatic diseases, and acute myocardial infarction. Overproduction of γ-globulins occurs in a malignancy called multiple myeloma, which therefore also causes increases in the sedimentation rate.

The amount of blood cells present also affects the sedimentation rate. The decreased erythrocytes present in anemia tend to sediment more rapidly, and the increased erythrocytes present in polycythemia tend to sediment to the bottom more slowly. Because males have slightly higher hemoglobin values than females, the normal sedimentation rate in males is lower. The sedimentation rate may be artifactitiously high if the test is carried out on a surface that is subject to frequent vibration, even from a source such as a radio.

There has been much written about the value of the sedimentation rate as a screening test, and the meaning of abnormalities in patients who otherwise appear to be healthy. In general, significant elevations of the sedimentation rate should probably be investigated with at least some measurements of plasma proteins and a good medical history and physical.

C.   Serum Electrolytes and Other Constituents

Electrolytes are substances that ionize in solution. An ion with a positive charge is called a cation and an ion with a negative charge is called an anion. The sum of the cations is always in balance with the sum of the anions. In the serum, the most numerous cationic electrolytes include potassium, sodium, calcium, and magnesium. The most numerous anionic substances include chloride, bicarbonate, phosphates, and proteins.

1.   Potassium

Potassium, a metallic element of the alkali group, is the chief intracellular cation (positively charged ion). Its concentration is maintained by active transport and is about 40 times higher in the cells than in the extracellular fluid. Because its concentration in cells is so high, it is the principal determinant of cell volume. It is also important in many metabolic processes, especially membrane potential in muscle tissues. The normal potassium concentration is about 4.5 mEq/L (3.5–5.0 mEq/L), which varies in an individual only by about ±0.3 mEq under normal conditions. The daily intake is about 100 mEq. The kidneys filter out about 800 mEq/day and then reabsorb the majority of it. If there is insufficient dietary intake of potassium, hypokalemia may occur because the kidneys take up to 2 weeks to fully conserve potassium.

Hyperkalemia, or increased serum potassium, is usually due to failure to excrete potassium by the kidneys. Some medications can cause hyperkalemia, including the "potassium-sparing" diuretics and antihypertensives, usually by reducing the kidney's potassium excretion. Interactions between these drugs can cause additive effects on serum potassium. Severe dehydration can cause hyperkalemia through a drop in renal blood flow, and acidosis shifts potassium out of the cells into the extracellular fluids. Hyperkalemia may also occur if enough potassium is released from tissues after severe injury, hemolysis, or prolonged seizures. Artifactitious elevation of potassium is commonly caused by hemolysis of erythrocytes during venipuncture or incomplete separation of the serum and clot; thrombocytosis may also result in a falsely elevated serum potassium.

Hypokalemia, or decreased serum potassium, is among the most common electrolyte disturbances seen in clinical practice, partly because of the extensive use of diuretics and corticosteroids, which cause potassium loss in the urine. Diuretics may also cause mild alkalosis, which shifts potassium from the extracellular space into the cells. Another common cause of hypokalemia is the loss of potassium-rich fluids from the body through the gastrointestinal tract as a result of vomiting or nasogastric suction, villous adenoma or cancer of the colon, laxative abuse, or chronic diarrhea. Renal sodium wasting can occur in some renal diseases, and it can also lead to significant hypokalemia if potassium is lost along with sodium.

Monitoring serum potassium in clinical trials is important because very slight changes in the extracellular fluid potassium can alter nervous and cardiac function seriously. The most serious clinical effect of hyperkalemia is cardiac arrhythmias, including asystole. Hypokalemia causes neuromuscular symptoms, including muscle weakness, but the most severe problem is cardiac irritability, which can lead to atrial or ventricular arrhythmias. Cardiac effects of hypokalemia are more likely to occur in patients with cardiac disease or patients using digitalis preparations. In fact, these patients are often recommended to maintain their serum potassium no lower than 4.0 mEq/L.

2. Sodium

Sodium, a metallic element of the alkali group, is the chief extracellular cation. The two major extracellular fluids are the blood plasma and the interstitial fluid, which have essentially equal compositions of electrolytes. Sodium salts account for more than 90% of the total osmolality of the extracellular fluid. Conversely, all but 2–5% of the sodium in the body is in the extracellular fluids, not considering the sodium that is in bone and is essentially static. A normal range for serum sodium is 136–145 mEq/L.

The development of abnormalities of serum sodium must always be combined with a clinical assessment of the patient's fluid status because of the close relationship between sodium and extracellular fluids. If fluid and sodium are lost together, the patient may be volume-depleted without any abnormality of the sodium value. Hyponatremia, or low serum sodium, may be caused by (a) volume depletion if more sodium than fluid is lost through the gastrointestinal tract, lung, skin, or kidney (depletional hyponatremia), (b) volume excess where pure water is retained (dilutional hyponatremia), or (c) inappropriate isolated loss of sodium. This third condition is often due to the syndrome of inappropriate secretion of antidiuretic hormone (SIADH), which causes pure water retention. SIADH is a fascinating syndrome that may occur with certain illnesses or medications, or as a postsurgical complication. Artifactitious hyponatremia results from significant elevations of blood lipids or blood glucose.

Development of significant hyponatremia during a clinical trial always warrants evaluation. First, the patient's fluid status must be assessed. Then, sources of fluid and sodium loss must be sought, such as gastrointestinal sources (diarrhea), renal sources (diuretic use), intra-abdominal sequestration, or skin sources (sweating). Other abnormalities of laboratory tests may be present, such as an elevated blood urea nitrogen (BUN) or decreased potassium. Hypernatremia, or elevated serum sodium, is caused by a water deficit relative to body sodium. In normal people, thirst is the primary mechanism for preventing hypernatremia. Comatose or immobile patients, or patients with an abnormal thirst mechanism, may become hypernatremic.

Hyponatremia usually does not cause clinical symptoms unless the sodium falls under 125 mEq/L, though a rapid fall can cause symptoms even at higher levels. Neurological dysfunction is the principal clinical symptom due to osmotic effects on the brain cells. In severe cases, convulsions may occur. Bizarre behavior and even overt psychosis have been attributed to occult hyponatremia. On the other hand, the symptoms of hypernatremia often relate to any associated volume depletion rather than to the hypernatremia itself, though central nervous symptoms such as seizures and coma may occur. As is true for hyponatremia, the symptoms of hypernatremia are more severe if the condition develops acutely.

3.   Bicarbonate and Chloride

Bicarbonate anion in equilibrium with dissolved carbon dioxide is the most important buffer system in the body. Normal serum levels of bicarbonate range from 23 to 29 mEq/L, and there is approximately a 20:1 ratio of bicarbonate ion to dissolved carbon dioxide. Although this buffer system is present in fairly low concentrations and has weak buffering capacity at the pH of plasma, the significance of the system depends on the body's ability to separately regulate concentrations of the two elements. The rate of bicarbonate excretion and regeneration is controlled by the kidney, and carbon dioxide, continually formed in the body by the different intracellular metabolic processes, is excreted through the lungs into expired air. To some extent, the respiratory rate can be varied to control the concentration (partial pressure) of carbon dioxide in the blood.

Understanding bicarbonate and chloride abnormalities involves understanding the acid–base status of the body and common acid–base abnormalities that may develop. If an abnormal acid–base status results from primary changes in the bicarbonate levels, it is usually referred to as "metabolic" acidosis or alkalosis. If an abnormal acid–base status results from primary changes in the carbon dioxide levels, it is usually referred to as "respiratory" acidosis or alkalosis. Primary abnormalities in either bicarbonate or carbon dioxide always result in secondary compensatory changes in the other component. Sometimes compensation may be complete, especially for primary respiratory alkalosis, but it is often incomplete. Complicated mixed conditions can also occur.

When metabolic acidosis occurs, it is further classified as "anion gap" or "nonanion gap" metabolic acidosis. The anion gap is calculated by comparing the numeric value of the primary serum anions—bicarbonate and chloride—to the numerical value of the cations—primarily sodium, though potassium may be included. The sum of the anions is roughly about 8–12 mEq less than the sum of the cations if potassium is included. This anion gap is actually not a gap, because the unseen negative charge is due to the serum proteins. When anion gap metabolic acidosis occurs, the anion gap increases because there are "unseen" anions of the organic acid causing the metabolic acidosis. The organic acid is most frequently lactic acid, a ketoacid, or an acidic compound like salicylic acid. When nonanion gap metabolic acidosis occurs, the anion gap remains normal because the acid involved is hydrochloric acid, whose anion is chloride. As a result, the bicarbonate falls and the chloride increases, but the anion gap does not change because both bicarbonate and chloride are included in the calculation.

Nonanion gap metabolic acidosis is caused by a primary decrease in serum bicarbonate, which is most commonly caused by losses of bicarbonate-rich fluids from the gastrointestinal tract (diarrhea) or through the kidney (diuretic use, renal failure, or renal tubular disease). Bicarbonate is secondarily decreased when the buffer system attempts to compensate for conditions that cause anion gap systemic acidosis, such as diabetic ketoacidosis, starvation, or salicylate poisoning. Metabolic alkalosis is caused by increased serum bicarbonate, which results from either exogenous administration of bicarbonate or loss of acid through protracted vomiting or nasogastric suction. Bicarbonate is secondarily increased when the buffer system attempts to compensate for respiratory acidosis from chronic obstructive lung disease.

Chloride is the most common extracellular anion, with serum concentrations ranging from 96 to 106 mEq/L. Abnormal chloride levels must always be correlated with bicarbonate levels because they are interdependent. Chloride anion is increased in dehydration or in any condition causing a decrease in bicarbonate. This includes nonanion gap metabolic acidosis and compensatory states resulting from primary respiratory alkalosis. Chloride anion is decreased in conditions causing pure water overload or in any condition causing an increase in bicarbonate. This includes primary metabolic alkalosis and compensatory states resulting from primary respiratory acidosis. The effect on chloride of an anion gap metabolic acidosis may be variable.

Changes in either bicarbonate or chloride anion during a clinical trial should always be evaluated carefully. Medications that stimulate or depress the central nervous system may affect the respiratory rate and result in secondary changes in bicarbonate and thus chloride levels. Medication effects on the kidney must be assessed. It may even become necessary to evaluate serum carbon dioxide (pCO_2) and pH values to determine if a significant acidosis or alkalosis is present. Mathematical equations and graphs are available in which to use a patient's bicarbonate, pH, and pCO_2 values to help determine what type of abnormality or combination of abnormalities is present.

4. Calcium

Calcium, a bivalent cation found in almost all tissues, is the most abundant mineral in the body. It is an essential element of bone and teeth, as well as a common extracellular and intracellular cation. Calcium plays many roles in blood coagulation and enzymatic processes. The concentration of calcium in the serum ranges from 9 to 11 mg/dl and is very narrowly regulated. The primary regulatory force is parathyroid hormone (PTH), a peptide hormone produced by the four tiny parathyroid glands nestled around the thyroid in the neck. Plasma calcium is present in three different forms. About 41% is complexed with plasma proteins and is therefore nondiffusible through the capillary membrane. About 9% is diffusible but is not ionized, being combined with other substances of the plasma and interstitial fluids such as citrate and phosphate. The remaining 50% is both diffusible through the capillary membrane and ionized. The normal concentration for ionized calcium is 4.25–5.25 mg/dl. Ionized calcium is important for the function of the heart and the nervous system.

About 0.4–1.0% (5–10 g) of total bone calcium, called exchangeable calcium, can be readily mobilized as a rapid buffering mechanism to keep the calcium ion concentration in the extracellular fluids from rising to excessive levels or falling too low under transient conditions of excess or hypoavailability of calcium. This buffering mechanism is so rapid that a single passage of blood through bone will remove almost all of the excess calcium. This buffer system is supplemented by the long-term control of PTH and vitamin D on calcium absorption from the gastrointestinal tract and calcium excretion in the urine.

Hypercalcemia is recognized much more commonly now than in the past because of routine surveillance and preventive medical care. The most common cause is hyperparathyroidism, or overproduction of PTH, which characteristically causes chronic hypercalcemia. The second most common cause of hypercalcemia is malignancy. Hypercalcemia of malignancy usually follows a rapid course, and may be due to direct tumor destruction of bone or to tumor-secreted cellular factors that can increase bone resorption systemically. Together hyperparathyroidism and malignancy account for 90% of all cases of hypercalcemia. Because vitamin D acts to increase calcium levels, hypercalcemia may also result from excessive vitamin D intake. In addition, hypercalcemia may result from conditions with high bone turnover such as hyperthyroidism, Paget's disease, and immobilization. Potentiating factors include medications that reduce calcium excretion, such as the commonly used thiazide diuretics. Paradoxically, hypocalcemia can result in hypercalcemia if it results in overcompensatory secondary hyperparathyroidism. This situation is commonly seen in chronic renal failure. Hypercalcemia that usually is not clinically significant can occur if the serum proteins that bind calcium are increased, especially albumin; an increase in the protein-bound calcium causes an increase in total serum calcium, but ionized calcium levels remain normal. False-positive elevations of calcium may occur from stasis during blood drawing.

Chronic hypocalcemia may occur from insufficient dietary intake or malabsorption of calcium, phosphorus, and vitamin D. Vitamin D deficiency can be induced by several anticonvulsants, which stimulate the hepatic microsomal mixed-oxidase enzymes and hence increase the rate of clearance of vitamin D and its metabolites. Liver disease can also lead to reduction in active vitamin D levels. Other causes of hypocalcemia include chronic renal failure, hereditary or acquired failure of PTH hormone function, and low serum magnesium. Transient but sometimes life-threatening hypocalcemia can occur quickly in patients with sepsis, burns, acute renal failure, acute pancreatitis, and extensive blood transfusions. Decreased serum albumin causes a decreased total calcium with a normal ionized calcium.

Calcium abnormalities can cause clinical symptoms that may be life threatening. Symptoms of hypercalcemia include fatigue, depression, mental confusion, anorexia, nausea, vomiting, constipation, and increased urination. There is a variable relationship between the severity of hypercalcemia and the presence of symptoms from one patient to the next. Symptoms are often present at calcium levels above 11.5–12.0 mg/dl, though some patients are asymptomatic at this level. Calcium levels over 13 mg/dl can result in renal failure, and deposition of calcium phosphate salts throughout body tissues may occur if blood phosphate levels are also elevated. Calcium levels of 15 mg/dl or above constitute a medical emergency because coma and cardiac arrest may occur. Hypercalcemia is commonly associated with hypercalciuria, which can result in calcium-containing kidney stones.

Symptoms of hypocalcemia primarily affect the nervous system and muscle, which become progressively more excitable as the hypocalcemia causes increased membrane permeability and decreased action potentials. As the calcium concentrations falls from 9.4 mg/dl to about 6 mg/dl, corresponding to a 35–50% reduction in ionized calcium, peripheral nerve fibers begin to discharge spontaneously, initiating tetanic skeletal muscle contractions. Tetany usually occurs in the hands and feet first, where it is called carpopedal spasm. Increased neuronal excitability may also result in convulsions. Hypocalcemia usually becomes lethal at about 4 mg/dl, frequently via cardiac arrhythmias from increased myocardial excitability. Laryngeal spasm, respiratory arrest, and increased intracranial pressure may occur.

The symptoms of chronic hypocalcemia may be more nonspecific, including irritability, depression, and psychosis. Gastrointestinal symptoms such as constipation, cramping, or chronic malabsorption may occur. Latent tetany may be demonstrable via certain diagnostic maneuvers. The electrocardiogram may demonstrate abnormalities, including signs of irritability such as premature ventricular contractions or other arrhythmias. Cardiac toxicity is increased in patients taking digitalis preparations. Chronic hypocalcemia, especially in association with hypophosphatemia, will also result in bony demineralization that may eventually become symptomatic with bone pain or fractures.

5. Phosphorus

Phosphorus, the most abundant intracellular anion, is present in all tissues. It is a major component of mineralized bone and is involved in almost all metabolic processes. Phosphorus is critical for membrane structure as well as for energy transport and storage. An average 700 g of phosphorus is present in the body, of which 85% is in the skeleton, 15% is in soft tissues, and 0.1% is in the extracellular fluid. Serum phosphorus levels range from 3.0 to 4.5 mg/dl in adults. A normal daily intake of phosphorus is about 1 g, which is almost completely absorbed. At a typical plasma pH of 7.4, inorganic phosphate in plasma exists in a 4:1 mixture of HPO_4^{2-} and $H_2PO_4^-$. As the pH becomes more acidic, there is a relative increase in the $H_2PO_4^-$ form and decrease in the HPO_4^{2-} form, whereas the opposite occurs when the fluid becomes more alkaline. This phosphate buffer system operates near its maximum buffering power at body pH, but its blood-buffering function is not very important because of its low concentration. However, the phosphate buffer is very important both inside cells and in the tubular fluid of the kidneys, where its function is to buffer hydrogen ions for excretion. The phosphorus in the extracellular fluid is freely diffusible into cells and into the urine.

Hyperphosphatemia results from excess vitamin D action, from reduced PTH hormonal effect (hypoparathyroidism), and from overcompensatory increase of PTH in hypocalcemic states such as chronic renal failure (secondary hyperparathyroidism). These states result in increased absorption and decreased excretion of phosphorus. Hyperphosphatemia can occur with extensive tissue damage or cellular destruction due to hypothermia, massive liver failure, muscle injury, intestinal obstruction, and leukemia. Some bone diseases may result in hyperphosphatemia, such as healing fractures, Paget's disease, or bone malignancy.

Of all these causes of hyperphosphatemia, the most common are renal failure and hypoparathyroidism.

Hypophosphatemia can result from nutritional causes in alcoholism or starvation, and serum phosphorus may decrease further during the "refeeding" period. Vitamin D deficiency causes hypophosphatemia and, because insulin transfers phosphate to cells, the treatment of diabetes may precipitate hypophosphatemia. Respiratory alkalosis is a common cause of hypophosphatemia, especially in such acute conditions as sepsis or alcohol withdrawal. Other causes of hypophosphatemia include hyperparathyroidism, renal tubular leaks of phosphate, low serum potassium or magnesium, diuretic treatment, and use of antacids that can bind phosphate in the gastrointestinal tract. Some rapidly growing malignancies take up enough phosphate to cause hypophosphatemia as well. Severe hypophosphatemia, defined as levels of 1.0 mg/dl or less, is most common when there is more than one contributing cause. Mild hyperphosphatemia does not usually cause symptoms. In fact, changing the extracellular fluid phosphate concentration from far below normal to four times normal does not affect the body significantly. However, if significant hyperphosphatemia is associated with hypercalcemia, widespread disposition of calcium phosphate salts, or calciphylaxis, may occur.

The primary consequences of hypophosphatemia include dysfunction of leukocytes and platelets, as well as reduced tissue oxygenation through an increase in erythrocyte oxygen affinity. Muscle effects include skeletal muscle weakness and breakdown (rhabdomyolysis), cardiac muscle dysfunction (cardiomyopathy), and respiratory insufficiency from weakness of the diaphragm. Liver dysfunction may occur, and nervous system dysfunction is one of the most distinctive and predictable abnormalities if the phosphate deficiency is severe. Early neurological effects include irritability, apprehension, and hyperventilation. This may progress to confusion, obtundation, convulsions, coma, and death. Effects on the muscles of the eyes and throat may mimic symptoms of botulism. Chronic hypophosphatemia also leads to skeletal demineralization.

6. Magnesium

Magnesium, the fourth most abundant cation in human tissues, is important in the activity of many enzymes. A typical serum magnesium concentration ranges from 1.5 to 2.5 mEq/L (about 1.8–3.0 mg/dl), and the total body magnesium content is about 25 mEq/kg. About 67% of magnesium is incorporated in bone, 31% in body cells, and only 1% in extracellular fluid. The ideal intake for an adult is 30–40 mEq/day, and both the gastrointestinal tract and the kidney are involved in regulation of magnesium levels. The kidney can retain all but 1–2 mEq/day through reabsorption in the renal tubule. Magnesium is measured less frequently in clinical trials than other electrolytes because most abnormalities occur in patients who are clinically ill and often hospitalized. It is rare to see clinically significant isolated abnormalities of serum magnesium levels.

Hypermagnesemia usually occurs when the kidney's ability to excrete magnesium is impaired by renal failure, especially when magnesium-containing antacids are administered. The use of magnesium sulfate to treat toxemia of pregnancy can also result in hypermagnesemia. Mild hypermagnesemia may be seen in diabetes and hypothyroidism.

Hypomagnesemia may occur in patients with hereditary defects in intestinal absorption or renal reabsorption of magnesium. Inadequate intake may occur in intestinal malabsorption syndromes, chronic alcoholism with poor nutritional intake, and parenteral nutrition that lacks magnesium. Excessive magnesium loss may occur with renal diseases or medications that reduce the kidney's ability to reabsorb magnesium in the renal tubules. This may be associated with urinary loss of potassium and calcium as well. Other causes of hypomagnesemia include insulin treatment of diabetic coma, hyperthyroidism, parathyroid disorders, bone tumors, acute pancreatitis, hypophosphatemia, and hypokalemia. In healthy individuals, slight hypomagnesemia may occur with cardiovascular conditioning and with hypermetabolic states such as cold acclimatization. Severely ill individuals often have drops in magnesium as well as calcium.

Hypermagnesemia results in depression of both neuromuscular transmission and central nervous system function. Symptoms usually correspond to serum levels. Between 4 and 5 mEq/L, nausea appears. From 4 to 7 mEq/L, patients may experience sedation and muscle weakness. Between 5 and 10 mEq/L, hypotension, bradycardia, and vasodilatation appear. Between 10 and 15 mEq/L, coma and respiratory paralysis may occur. Because calcium ion directly opposes magnesium ion at the site of action, the effects of hypermagnesemia can be emergently treated with intravenous infusion of calcium salts.

Symptoms of hypomagnesemia include poor appetite (anorexia), nausea, vomiting, lethargy, and weakness, which develop within weeks in chronic deficiency. Additional symptoms that may require months of deficiency to develop include paresthesias, muscle cramps, irritability, decreased attention span, and mental confusion. When the serum magnesium falls below 1.0 mEq/L, secondary hypocalcemia usually occurs, and all the symptoms of hypocalcemia may compound the clinical picture. The secondary hypocalcemia may be severe and is refractory to treatment with calcium replacement. About half the patients with hypomagnesemia also develop hypokalemia.

7. Glucose

Glucose, or dextrose, is the body's chief source of oxidative energy. The blood glucose concentration is very narrowly controlled, usually between 80 and 90 mg/dl in the fasting person before breakfast. Glucose increases to 120–140 mg/dl about an hour after a meal but returns to normal within about 2 hr after the last absorption of carbohydrates. The liver acts as a blood glucose buffer by either making needed glucose or by storing glucose as glycogen after a meal and then releasing glucose into the blood again during the succeeding hours after the meal. Insulin and glucagon are peptide hormones that are important to glucose balance. Insulin secretion results in a decrease in blood glucose, and glucagon secretion results in an increase in blood glucose. Hypoglycemia also directly affects the hypothalamus, which then stimulates epinephrine release, which cascades on to cause glucose formation (gluconeogenesis) by the liver. Most glucose formed by gluconeogenesis is used for metabolism in the brain.

Hyperglycemia most commonly results from diabetes mellitus, which is caused by undersecretion of insulin, resistance of body cells to insulin action, or a combination of both factors. Hyperglycemia can also be caused by excess cortisone, ACTH (adrenocorticotropic hormone, which releases cortisone), or HGH (human growth hormone). Because adrenalin causes gluconeogenesis, hyperglycemia may occur in conditions associated with increased adrenalin levels, such as stress or adrenalin-producing tumors (pheochromocytoma). Pancreatitis and central nervous system lesions may be associated with hyperglycemia.

Hypoglycemia may occur from insulin oversecretion by pancreatic tumors, from pancreatitis, from autonomic nervous system disease, and from excess use of insulin or medications that lower blood glucose. "Factitious hypoglycemia" is usually caused by surreptitious administration of insulin. Hypoglycemia may be precipitated by inadequate hepatic glycogen reserves in malnutrition, in certain hereditary liver enzyme disorders, and in severe diffuse liver disease. Recurrent hypoglycemia is one of the "dumping syndromes" that can develop after gastrectomy; these patients no longer have the normal delay in carbohydrate absorption provided by the stomach and the sudden "dumping" of carbohydrate into the small intestine causes oversecretion of insulin. Some tumors can release systemic factors that cause hypoglycemia, such as fibrosarcomas.

Hypoglycemia can be characterized into two patterns—fasting (food-deprived) or reactive (food-stimulated or functional) hypoglycemia. Fasting hypoglycemia usually occurs after many hours of fasting and is more likely to indicate an insulin-secreting tumor or other pathology. Reactive hypoglycemia tends to occur an hour or two after a meal and results from excessive insulin release. Reactive hypoglycemia is usually not clinically significant although it has been blamed for more symptoms than it probably deserves.

Symptoms of hyperglycemia include the immediate effects of the elevated serum glucose such as cellular dehydration and osmotic diuresis. The osmotic diuresis occurs when the renal glucose threshold is surpassed, usually at about 200 mg/dl blood glucose, and is driven by the glucose loss in the urine. The diuresis results in excessive thirst (polydipsia), excessive urination (polyuria), nocturnal urination (nocturia), and symptoms from depletion of other electrolytes such as potassium and magnesium. Hyperglycemia may lead to obesity if excess glucose is converted to fat and stored in adipose tissue, or to weight loss if insulin lack is so severe that the glucose is lost in the urine rather than incorporated into cells. In a sense, this latter situation results in cell starvation in the midst of plenty. Other symptoms of diabetes include weakness, fatigue, dizziness, and blurred vision. Insulin lack hyperglycemia can lead to nausea, vomiting, keto-acidosis, and coma. Diabetes also results in a number of less explainable though serious effects such as peripheral neuropathy, accelerated atherosclerotic disease, neovascularization of the retina with the potential for bleeding and blindness, decreased resistance to infections, and chronic renal failure.

Symptoms of hypoglycemia usually occur when the blood glucose falls to 40 mg/dl or less. Rapid falls in glucose where values remain in the normal range probably do not consistently elicit symptoms. Symptoms of central nervous system impairment can occur, such as confusion, bizarre behavior, convulsions, and coma. These symptoms are most characteristic of the food-deprived, or fasting, hypoglycemias. Prolonged or recurrent severe hypoglycemia can lead to neuronal death and reduced intellectual capacity. Less significant though uncomfortable symptoms include those from secondary adrenalin release, such as weakness, tremors, anxiety, sweating, and palpitations. These symptoms are characteristic of the food-stimulated, or reactive, hypoglycemias.

8.   Uric Acid

Uric acid is the end product of purine breakdown in primates. Uric acid in solution does not appear to have any toxicity, but problems arise when the solubility is exceeded and the uric acid forms crystals. Uric acid can form stable supersaturated solutions, but these solutions are prone to crystal formation if any precipitating event occurs. The normal solubility of uric acid in plasma is 6.4–6.8 mg/dl. The normal range for uric acid based on population studies ranges from about 1.5 to 8.0 mg/dl, with males falling into the higher end of this range.

The most frequent cause of hyperuricemia is decreased renal tubular clearance of uric acid because renal tubular secretion is the primary mechanism of uric acid excretion. Diuretic therapy, hypertension-induced renal disease, and chronic renal failure commonly reduce uric acid excretion. Excessive dietary intake of purines probably does not cause hyperuricemia although it may aggravate symptoms of hyperuricemia in an affected individual. Excessive alcohol intake may also increase serum uric acid levels because alcohol reduces uric acid excretion. A small subpopulation of individuals are overproducers of uric acid, and specific enzyme defects may be demonstrable. Overproduction of uric acid may also result from disseminated cancers or leukemias, tissue breakdown from cancer chemotherapy (tumor lysis syndrome), hemolysis, and psoriasis. In many cases of chronic hyperuricemia, a combination of overproduction and underexcretion may be present. Hypouricemia occurs from reduced dietary intake of uric acid, enzyme deficiencies, or increased renal tubular excretion of uric acid. Increased tubular excretion of uric acid may result as an isolated defect or as a generalized effect on the renal tubule, such as in Fanconi's syndrome.

Symptoms of hyperuricemia occur when uric acid crystals form in body tissues. One of the most familiar disorders is gouty arthritis, an inflammatory arthritis involving one or more joints with uric acid crystals demonstrable in the synovial fluid. Uric acid stones may result from chronic hyperuricemia, and renal failure may occur from either chronic or acute hyperuricemia. Hypo-uricemia itself does not cause any clinical symptoms.

9. Albumin

The total protein content of serum is about 6.0–8.0 g/dl, of which the two primary proteins are albumin and globulins. Plasma also contains the third primary protein, fibrinogen. Almost all the albumin and fibrinogen, as well as 50–80% of the globulins, are formed in the liver. Albumin is quantitatively the most important protein made by the liver, and a normal serum albumin ranges from 3.5–5.5 g/dl. The principal function of albumin is to provide colloid osmotic pressure in the plasma, which prevents plasma loss from the capillaries into other body tissues. Albumin and other proteins also form the most plentiful buffer in the body because they are present in blood and in large amounts in the cells, although the slow movement of hydrogen and bicarbonate ions through cell membranes often delays maximum protein buffering for several hours.

The liver can make plasma proteins at a maximum rate of 15–50 g/day. When plasma protein depletion occurs, the liver cells will divide rapidly to keep up with the protein demand; this can actually result in growth of the liver to a larger size. The liver has other functions important in protein metabolism, including the removal of nitrogen from amino acids, formation of urea for removal of ammo-nia, and interconversions among the different amino acids and other compounds important to the metabolic processes of the body.

Hypoalbuminemia can result from liver failure if albumin synthesis does not keep pace with degradation. More commonly, hypoalbuminemia is caused by loss of albumin, although both factors must be considered because the serum albumin results from the balance of albumin loss and the liver's ability to form new albumin in replacement. Albumin loss may occur rapidly with severe burns, renal disease, or denuding skin disorders; or the loss may be more chronic through the kidney or gastrointestinal tract. Fluid overload can dilute albumin as well as other plasma constituents; this occurs most commonly in congestive heart failure, chronic renal failure, and ascites. Elevated serum albumin is rarely significant.

Hypoalbuminemia causes symptoms via the lowering of serum oncotic pressure. Fluid leakage from the capillaries results in edema, which can be massive if the serum albumin is extremely low. Other proteins may be affected by the same factors that have depleted albumin, and associated symptoms may occur related to the loss of those other proteins or to the etiological condition.

D. Creatinine/BUN

The kidney is vital for the balance of fluids, acids and bases, and many other body constituents. The kidney is especially vulnerable to insults because of its high blood flow—almost a quarter of the total blood flow—and high use of oxygen. Many medications are included among the substances or conditions that can affect renal function through their effects on renal blood flow and thus oxygen delivery, or through their effects on the rate that the kidney filters fluid and substances from the blood (glomerular filtration rate). Creatinine and BUN are important measurements for determining renal function. Both creatinine and urea are produced at a reasonably constant rate, urea by the liver and creatinine by the muscles. Because production and excretion are in equilibrium and excretion is primarily accomplished by the kidney, determination of serum values gives an estimate of renal efficiency in excreting these substances. Because medications can affect renal function through many mechanisms, monitoring of creatinine and BUN is an essential part of safety follow-up in clinical trials. Significant changes in either parameter do not occur in isolation; therefore, comparisons of the values for both tests gives more information than either test alone.

1. Creatinine

Creatinine is the anhydride form of creatine, which is involved in storage of energy in muscle and brain tissue. The amount of creatinine formed daily is proportional to muscle mass and is normally constant as long as muscle mass remains constant. Daily formation and urinary excretion of creatinine result in an equilibrium serum level that normally ranges from 0.6 to 1.2 mg/dl.

   Elevated creatinine values should be compared with the associated degree of BUN elevation. A normal ratio of BUN to creatinine is 10:1. If the BUN/ creatinine ratio is less than 10:1, it suggests a dilutional effect, low protein intake, protein loss (repeated dialysis, severe diarrhea or vomiting), or hepatic inability to make sufficient protein. If renal failure is associated, both BUN and creatinine will also be elevated. If the BUN/creatinine ratio is about 10:1 with elevation of both creatinine and BUN, primary renal failure is the most likely cause. If the BUN/creatinine ratio is greater than 10:1 with elevations of BUN and, to a lesser extent, creatinine, it suggests contraction of the effective blood volume from dehydration, shock, congestive heart failure, or liver disease. An elevated BUN/creatinine ratio with a normal or only slightly elevated creatinine suggests tetracycline or corticosteroid use, excess protein intake, breakdown of blood in the gastrointestinal tract, or other causes of increased tissue breakdown and turnover (cachexia, burns, high fever). Urinary tract obstruction with renal failure also tends to be associated with an elevated BUN/creatinine ratio.

Symptoms of an elevated serum creatinine are described in the next section. In addition, there will be associated symptoms of the etiological disorder and associated electrolyte abnormalities. A low serum creatinine is asymptomatic and not clinically significant; the cause is usually a low muscle mass.

2. BUN

BUN (blood urea nitrogen) is a measure of the urea content of blood. Urea is the principal end product of protein catabolism and constitutes about one half of the total urinary solids. The body removes nitrogen from amino acids and incorporates it into ammonia. The ammonia is converted to urea by combining two molecules of ammonia with one molecule of carbon dioxide, and the urea is then excreted in the urine in direct relationship to the glomerular filtration rate. The body forms an average of 25–30 g of urea each day, depending on the amount of protein in the diet, resulting in a normal BUN ranging from 15 to 35 mg/dl.

Increased BUN is called azotemia and is usually associated with an increased creatinine. When blood volume contraction occurs with elevations of BUN, creatinine, and the BUN/creatinine ratio, the condition is called prerenal azotemia. In prerenal azotemia, there is a proportionally greater increase in BUN than in creatinine. Causes of prerenal azotemia were described in the preceding section. Any cause of azotemia can result in BUN values up to about 50 mg/dl, but values of 50–150 mg/dl imply serious renal impairment and values ranging greater than 150 mg/dl are almost conclusive evidence of severe renal insufficiency.

A low BUN may occur from failure of protein synthesis from severe liver damage (liver failure) and during periods of increased protein utilization such as late pregnancy or infancy. A low BUN may also be due to inadequate protein intake from malnutrition, low-protein and high-carbohydrate diets, and intravenous feedings. Protein loss through the kidney or the gastrointestinal tract can cause a low BUN. Last, overhydration causes a dilutional effect that frequently decreases the BUN below 10 mg/dl.

Symptoms of prerenal azotemia would be those of the contracted blood volume and of the underlying etiological disorder. If azotemia is due to renal failure, symptoms depend on the severity of the renal insufficiency. Because the kidney has a large reserve, an elevation of the creatinine to about twice the patient's normal value implies almost 90% loss of renal function, and symptoms usually appear when about 80–90% of renal function is lost. Symptoms of severe renal azotemia, or uremia, include loss of appetite, nausea, vomiting, weight loss, polyuria, nocturia, itching, and edema. Other associated problems may include hypertension, heart failure with pulmonary congestion, pericardial fluid formation, hypertriglyceridemia and accelerated atherosclerosis, multiple abnormalities of serum electrolytes, abnormal serum pH balance, anemia, leukocyte and platelet dysfunction, secondary hyperparathyroidism, and neuropathy. Some of the abnormalities that occur are not well understood but may be related to other substances not cleared properly by the failing kidney.

E.   Liver Function Tests

Liver injury may follow the use of a number of medications and chemical agents. Dose–response injury occurs most commonly with agents that are systemic poisons, like carbon tetrachloride, or with agents that are converted to toxic metabolites that cause liver damage, such as overdosage of acetaminophen. Idiosyncratic liver injury is more common, although it is now known that some adverse drug events characterized as idiosyncratic are actually due to idiosyncratic metabolism that results in toxic metabolites. Examples include liver toxicity from halothane and isoniazid.

Drug-induced hepatotoxicity may be asymptomatic or it may be accompanied by systemic symptoms and signs such as fever, rash, arthralgias, anorexia, fatigue, nausea, itching, leukocytosis, and eosinophilia. The liver may become tender or enlarged. The most serious consequences of drug-induced liver injury are either death from massive liver injury or the initiation of chronic liver injury that could ultimately lead to hepatic scarring (cirrhosis) and/or death. Many drugs have been incriminated in acute liver injury, making serial determinations of liver function tests of paramount importance in clinical trials. Some drugs have been incriminated in chronic hepatitis, cirrhosis, or syndromes of intrahepatic biliary stasis resembling primary biliary cirrhosis.

Liver function tests are measurements of serum enzymes whose abnormalities may indicate liver disease. In clinical trials, there are some basic guidelines regarding liver function test abnormalities [3]. First, it is wise to exclude patients from clinical trials for more than very mild elevations of liver function tests because of the possibility of preexisting liver disease. Once a patient has begun double-blind therapy, subsequent liver function values should be compared to the upper limit of normal or to baseline values if they were slightly elevated. Repeat testing within a week should be considered for SGPT or SGOT elevations between two and three times the upper limit of normal, for alkaline phosphatase elevations between about 1.5 and 2 times the upper limit of normal, or for bilirubin elevations between about 1.2 and 1.5 times the upper limit of normal. It is wise to cease study drug therapy and repeat testing as soon as possible for marked elevations such as SGPT or SGOT more than 3 times the upper limit of normal, alkaline phosphatase more than 2 times the upper limit of normal, or bilirubin more than 1.5 times the upper limit of normal. If the marked elevation is confirmed, the patient should be discontinued from the study.

Milder liver function abnormalities that occur during a clinical trial should be followed weekly for up to 4 weeks. If the abnormalities disappear or stabilize, routine follow-up may be resumed. If there is a progressive increase in the abnormal value(s) over that month or additional liver function tests become abnormal, discontinuation of study drug is generally advisable. When liver function test elevations are severe or persistent, hepatitis screening tests should be performed and liver biopsy considered.

1. Transaminases

The tests used most often to monitor for liver cell injury are the transaminases, enzymes involved in nitrogen transfer reactions from amino acids to other substrates for eventual disposal in the urea cycle. Serum glutamic-oxaloacetic transaminase (SGOT), also known as aspartate aminotransferase (AST), is an enzyme that is present in the cytoplasm and mitochondria of most cells. Because SGOT is found in many tissues, abnormalities are not specific for liver injury. SGOT is elevated in conditions as disparate as liver cell injury, acute myocardial infarction, muscle trauma or intramuscular injection, acute pancreatitis, intestinal injury, radiation injury, pulmonary infarction, cerebral infarction, or renal infarction. Levels may be falsely elevated by administration of medications such as polycillin, opiates, or erythromycin. Levels may be falsely decreased during diabetic ketoacidosis, beriberi (thiamine deficiency), severe liver disease, and chronic renal failure.

Serum glutamate pyruvate transaminase (SGPT), also known as alanine aminotransferase (ALT), is an enzyme found in many cells but most abundant in the liver. Though it may increase in a number of conditions, elevations of SGPT are most specific for liver cell injury, including hepatic necrosis and acute hepatitis. It is important to remember that actual levels of SGPT or SGOT do not necessarily correlate with the degree of liver cell injury and thus do not have prognostic value in themselves.

2. Alkaline Phosphatase

This hydrolase enzyme is present in a variety of tissues, including bone, liver, intestine, and placenta. Elevations are most commonly of bone or liver etiology. The bone fraction of alkaline phosphatase may be increased in hyperparathyroidism, Paget's disease, healing fractures, bone tumors, osteomalacia, rickets, or late pregnancy. The liver fraction of alkaline phosphatase is predominantly elevated by biliary system obstruction, whether in the liver itself (intrahepatic) or in the ducts beyond the liver (extrahepatic). Hepatitis and certain drug reactions can cause intrahepatic biliary obstruction, usually of the tiny bile canaliculi. The most striking increases of alkaline phosphatase are found with biliary obstruction. Some miscellaneous conditions that cause elevations of the serum alkaline phosphatase include severe hyperthyroidism, myocardial infarction, and pulmonary infarction. A number of conditions cause decreases in alkaline phosphatase although the decrease itself is not clinically important. Blood collection in an EDTA tube can falsely lower alkaline phosphatase levels.

3. GGT

γ-Glutamyl transpeptidase/transferase (GGT) is an enzyme that is present in the plasma membrane of all cells and is involved in transmembrane transfer of amino acids. Elevations of GGT are very sensitive for liver disease, especially biliary obstruction, and the degree of GGT elevation in liver disease tends to correlate with alkaline phosphatase levels. Liver diseases associated with marked GGT elevations include primary biliary cirrhosis, fatty liver, obstructive jaundice, and liver cancer. After acute hepatitis, GGT is usually the last enzyme to recover, and it may be the only enzyme elevated in the dormant stage of chronic hepatitis or cirrhosis. Elevated GGT is not specific for liver disease, however, as it may be increased in acute pancreatitis, kidney disease, and myocardial infarction. Because bone disease does not cause elevations of serum GGT, concurrent elevation of alkaline phosphatase and GGT is very suggestive of a liver etiology for both enzymes. GGT may be elevated by agents that induce microsomal enzymes, such as alcohol, making elevations of GGT a sensitive but not specific indicator of heavy alcohol use.

4. Bilirubin

Bilirubin is the major end product of the breakdown of hemoglobin and related compounds. In its unconjugated (free) form, it normally circulates in plasma as a complex with albumin. Within hours, unconjugated bilirubin is taken up by the liver, absorbed through the hepatic cell membrane, and conjugated to a water-soluble form called direct bilirubin (80% is the diglucuronide conjugate). The newly formed conjugated (direct) bilirubin is excreted via active transport into the bile canaliculi and then moves through the common bile duct into the small intestine. Once in the intestine, about half is converted by bacterial action into urobilinogen. Some of the urobilinogen is reabsorbed into the portal circulation and then excreted by the liver back into the gastrointestinal tract, although about 5% of reabsorbed urobilinogen is excreted by the kidneys into the urine.

The test for serum bilirubin detects both the conjugated and unconjugated forms. The normal bilirubin concentration ranges from 0.3 to 1.1 mg/dl; the majority of this—from 0.2 to 0.7 mg/dl—is in the unconjugated form. Total bilirubin can rise as high as 40 mg/dl and much of it can become of the conjugated type. When the level is about three times normal, or about 1.5 mg/dl, the skin usually begins to appear jaundiced. Unconjugated hyperbilirubinemia is most common in diseases associated with excessive breakdown of hemoglobin, such as hemolysis. These conditions cause unconjugated bilirubin to overload the liver's ability to conjugate bilirubin quickly enough to keep serum bilirubin levels normal. Despite the increased serum bilirubin in these conditions, unconjugated bilirubin is not excreted in the urine because it is not water-soluble. However, the increased excretion of conjugated bilirubin into the intestine results in increased intestinal reabsorption and urinary excretion of urobilinogen.

Conjugated hyperbilirubinemia is usually due to biliary obstruction. Bilirubin continues to be conjugated despite the liver disease unless liver cell injury is extremely severe, but the bilirubin cannot pass into the intestine if there is total biliary obstruction. Therefore, no urobilinogen is formed and the stools become clay-colored for lack of stercobilin and other bile pigments. Some conjugated bilirubin enters the blood, probably from rupture of congested bile canaliculi and direct emptying of the bile into the lymph exiting the liver. Because the kidney can excrete conjugated bilirubin, the urine becomes foamy and intensely yellow or yellow-brown.

There are several congenital disorders associated with hyperbilirubinemia. These are usually recognized at a fairly early age, though mild forms may become evident during a clinical trial. In some of these syndromes, the bilirubin level may increase with fasting, fever, infection, surgery, exertion, or alcohol ingestion. Elevated bilirubin levels are usually not harmful in themselves in adults, though chronic overproduction can lead to gallstones.

F. Lipids (Fats) and Lipoproteins

Abnormalities of blood lipoproteins have been increasingly connected to atherosclerosis (arteriosclerosis). Atherosclerosis involves the deposition of lipids into "plaques" lining the blood vessels, often with associated narrowing, sclerosis (hardening), and thickening of the vessels. The abnormality can involve blood vessels of major organs such as brain, heart, and kidney. Atherosclerosis is a leading cause of morbidity (illness) and mortality (death) in the United States. Physician and public awareness of the importance of lipids in the etiology of atherosclerosis has increased in the past few years. In clinical trials, it is more important than ever to be aware of any effects of new medications on lipoproteins. This is especially true for medications used to treat diseases in patients already at higher risk for atherosclerosis, including patients who smoke and patients with hypertension. Although the clinical significance of elevated plasma lipoproteins is primarily due to their effects on atherosclerosis, another potentially life-threatening disease known to be caused by elevated lipoproteins is pancreatitis.

1. Lipids

The most commonly measured lipids are triglycerides and cholesterol, though phospholipids and other lipid compounds also play important roles in the body. Triglycerides are neutral fats with a backbone of glycerol, to which three molecules of fatty acid have been esterified. Fatty acids, long-chain hydrocarbon organic acids, are the basic lipid portion of triglycerides. In addition to dietary intake of triglycerides, excess dietary carbohydrate increases triglyceride stores because the liver uses it to synthesize triglyceride for storage in adipose (fat) tissue. When fat stored in adipose tissue needs to be used to provide energy, fatty acids exit the adipose cells and enter the circulation. In the circulation, they are transported as a complex of free fatty acids with albumin. Triglycerides share almost equally with carbohydrates in providing energy for metabolic processes. There is a wide population range in triglyceride values, though values ranging from 40 to 150 mg/dl are considered to be normal, and older patients have higher ranges.

Cholesterol is a steroid alcohol that shares many of the physical and chemical properties of other lipid substances. Like triglycerides, cholesterol is obtained both from the diet (exogenous cholesterol) and from endogenous production. More than half of cholesterol is endogenous. Cholesterol and other lipids are used throughout the body in cell membranes; cholesterol is also the precursor to the steroid hormones. Because cholesterol is highly fat-soluble but only slightly soluble in water, it tends to form esters with fatty acids. In fact, about 70% of the cholesterol in plasma lipoproteins is in the form of cholesterol esters. Cholesterol levels are highly variable, although levels of 150–200 mg/dl are usually considered normal, and levels of 200–240 mg/dl are considered borderline or slightly elevated. The value given for cholesterol represents the total cholesterol, which includes both the cholesterol esters (cholesteryl esters) in plasma lipoproteins and the unesterified cholesterol circulating freely in plasma.

2.   Apolipoproteins (Apoproteins)

Apolipoproteins are the proteins that associate with blood lipids to form particles called lipoproteins. These proteins are grouped by their function in classes A, B, C, and E. The A apolipoproteins (subgroups I, II, III, IV) occur primarily in high-density lipoproteins (HDLs) and in lesser amounts in chylomicrons. The A-1 apolipoprotein is important because it activates lecithin-cholesterol acyltransferase (LCAT), the enzyme in HDL particles that catalyzes the esterification of cholesterol. The B apolipoproteins are primarily found in very-low-density lipoproteins (VLDLs), low-density lipoproteins (LDLs), and intermediate-density lipoproteins (IDLs). The B apolipoproteins are recognized by cell surface receptors that mediate endocytosis and cellular intake of lipoprotein particles. The C apolipoproteins (subgroups I, II, III) occur in chylomicrons and in VLDL and HDL. Apolipoprotein C-II is important because it activates lipoprotein lipase, the enzyme that hydrolyzes triglycerides to allow their transfer from the lipoprotein particles to body tissues. Apolipoprotein E is found in all lipoprotein classes and may be involved in the conversion of VLDL to IDL, and the clearance of IDL from the circulation.

3.   Lipoproteins

Blood fats are often transported in lipoproteins, complexes of lipids and apolipoproteins. Lipoproteins are globular particles of high molecular weight that transport nonpolar lipids, primarily triglycerides and cholesterol esters, through the plasma. Each lipoprotein particle contains a nonpolar core where the water-insoluble lipids are packed in an oil droplet. The lipids account for most of the mass of the particle, and the proportion of triglycerides and cholesterol esters varies. The outer surface coat of the lipoprotein consists of polar phospholipids that stabilize the particle in solution in the plasma. The apolipoproteins are exposed at the surface for binding to specific enzymes or transport proteins on cell membranes.

There are five major groups of lipoproteins based on size, density, electrophoretic mobility, and composition. Chylomicrons have very little protein content, while the protein content of the other lipoproteins varies from about 25% to 35%. A description of the lipoproteins in order of descending size follows:

1. *Chylomicrons* are the largest lipoproteins, ranging in size from 0.08 to 0.5 μm. Chylomicrons contain primarily triglycerides, but they also contain about 9% phospholipids, 3% cholesterol, and 1% apolipoprotein B. Chylomicrons are qualitatively similar in composition to other lipoproteins although their size and triglyceride content are so much greater that they are sometimes considered to be in a class in themselves.

2. *VLDLs*, or very-low-density lipoproteins, are the second largest lipoproteins and contain the largest amount of triglyceride after the chylomicrons. VLDL particles are synthesized by the liver and, to a small degree, by the gastrointestinal tract. They have a lipid core that consists primarily of triglycerides with a moderate amount of cholesterol esters and phospholipids. VLDL particles contain apolipoproteins B-100 and E. VLDL particles carry lipids to the body. As they circulate, triglycerides are removed, resulting in an increase in density until the VLDL particle becomes an IDL particle.

3. *IDLs*, or intermediate-density lipoproteins, are intermediate in density between VLDLs and LDLs. IDLs are formed from VLDLs from which a large share of the triglyceride has been removed. As a result, compared to VLDL particles, IDL particles have a higher concentration of cholesterol and phospholipids, and a lower concentration of triglycerides. About half these particles eventually become LDL particles.

4. *LDLs*, or low-density lipoproteins, result from the continued removal of triglyceride from IDL. With much of the triglyceride removed, LDLs primarily carry esterified cholesterol. In fact, LDLs carry about three fourths of the total cholesterol in normal human plasma. The cholesterol esters are in the heart of the particle, and the surface contains phospholipids, some unesterified cholesterol, and apolipoprotein B-100. The LDL particles will eventually supply cholesterol to many extrahepatic cells, which have LDL receptors on their surfaces.

5. *HDLs*, or high-density lipoproteins, have the highest density and smallest size of all the lipoproteins. HDL is sometimes called α-lipoprotein. Most HDL is made in the liver, but small quantities are also synthesized in the

intestinal epithelium during the absorption of dietary fatty acids. HDL is synthesized as a discoidal particle that becomes spheroidal as it acquires more protein. HDL eventually consists of about 50% protein with smaller amounts of phospholipids and a cholesterol ester core. Associated with HDL are apolipoproteins A-I and A-II, which lie on the outer surface of the particle. HDL may be responsible for the transport of cholesterol from the tissues to the liver for excretion.

4. Lipoprotein ''Pathways'' and Functions

1. The exogenous pathway involves the moving of dietary fat into the body by the chylomicrons. During digestion, most of the dietary triglycerides are split into their constituent monoglycerides and fatty acids. While passing through the intestinal epithelial cells, they are reassembled and aggregate into chylomicrons. A small amount of apolipoprotein B adsorbs to the surface to prevent adherence to lymphatic vessel walls. Most of the cholesterol and phospholipids absorbed from the gastrointestinal tract also enter the chylomicrons. The chylomicrons pass into the lymph and thus into the general circulation via the thoracic duct. An hour or so after a fatty meal, the plasma volume may consist of up to 1–2% chylomicrons, resulting in a turbid and occasionally yellow appearance. Because the half-life of chylomicrons is less than 1 hr, the plasma becomes clear again within a few hours. The chylomicrons bind to capillary walls in fat and muscle, lipoprotein lipase is activated by apolipoprotein C-II, and free fatty acids and monoglycerides are released from the chylomicrons. The fatty acids and monoglycerides immediately diffuse into the cells and are resynthesized into new triglycerides there. The chylomicron remnant particles are taken up by the liver.

2. The endogenous pathway transports triglycerides synthesized in the liver to other tissues, primarily adipose tissues. This pathway is also responsible for the transport of phospholipid and cholesterol between the liver and peripheral tissues. The endogenous pathway involves VLDL, IDL, and LDL. Of these three lipoproteins, only the VLDL is synthesized by the liver. As VLDL particles move through the circulation, the low-density triglycerides are gradually unloaded to form IDL particles. About half of these IDL particles are then removed from circulation by the liver, while the other half continue to lose triglycerides progressively until their density increases to the point where they become LDL particles. The associated apolipoprotein B-100 is recognized by cellular LDL receptors, causing the LDL particle to attach to the cell. The cholesterol is liberated by lysosomal cholesteryl esterase and the entire LDL particle is transported into the cell and digested internally. Cellular receptors remove 70–80% of the LDL from circulation each day and the remainder is degraded by phagocytic cells. Cholesterol

from degraded LDL particles is eventually released into the plasma again, where it is usually picked up by HDL.

3. HDL appears to function as a cholesterol scavenger. When HDL encounters the free cholesterol released by degradation of LDL particles and cell membranes, the associated apolipoprotein A-I activates LCAT to esterify the cholesterol. These cholesterol esters are formed on the surface of the HDL particle and then transferred to VLDL and eventually to LDL. Some of the cholesterol is transported by HDL to the liver, where it is incorporated into bile salts. Overall, much less is known about the function of HDL than about other lipoproteins.

5. Lipoprotein Abnormalities

Abnormalities of lipoproteins correlate with abnormalities of cholesterol and/or triglycerides in a sensible way. An isolated elevation of triglycerides indicates an elevation of chylomicrons and/or VLDL because those lipoproteins are the primary carriers of triglycerides. An isolated elevation of plasma cholesterol nearly always indicates an increase in LDL because that is the primary carrier of cholesterol. Often both triglycerides and cholesterol are elevated. In this situation, a triglyceride/cholesterol ratio greater than 5:1 indicates an increase in chylomicrons and/or VLDL, and a triglyceride/cholesterol ratio less than 5:1 indicates an increase in LDL as well as in chylomicrons and/or VLDL. In some conditions, abnormal lipoproteins are formed in association with elevations of triglycerides and/or cholesterol.

There has been disagreement in the past regarding where the upper level of normal should be set for plasma cholesterol and triglycerides, although it is agreed that measurement should be preceded by at least a 12-hr fast. The National Institutes of Health made a consensus statement that there is a high risk of atherosclerosis if the cholesterol is over the 90th percentile, and a moderate risk if cholesterol is in the 75th to 90th percentile [4,5]. The absolute values associated with these percentiles change somewhat with age and vary somewhat with gender. Cholesterol levels for the 75th percentile range from about 200 mg/dl for ages 0–19 and about 240 mg/dl for ages over 40, while cholesterol levels for the 90th percentile range from about 220 mg/dl for ages 0–19 and about 260 mg/dl for ages over 40. Clinically, the definition of borderline elevation of cholesterol is values from 200–239 mg/dl, and definite elevation of cholesterol is values of 240 mg/dl and above. If the cholesterol is normal, the risk of atherosclerosis may be increased if the fasting triglyceride level is over 250 mg/dl. Fasting triglyceride levels of 250–500 mg/dl and greater than 500 mg/dl are defined as borderline and definite hypertriglyceridemia, respectively.

If the total cholesterol is over 240 mg/dl, measurement of HDL is recommended to help assess the risk of coronary artery disease because many studies have suggested an inverse relationship between HDL levels and coronary artery disease. Whereas an average HDL level is 50 mg/dl, levels under 25 mg/dl are associated with a twofold to threefold increase in the risk of coronary artery disease, and levels over 75 mg/dl are associated with a 50% decrease in the risk of coronary artery disease. It may be that HDL can actually scavenge cholesterol crystals that are beginning to deposit as atherosclerotic plaques in arterial walls. In Tangier disease, a familial disease with HDL levels below the 10th percentile, premature coronary artery disease is common.

Genetic factors play a major role in many of the hyperlipoproteinemias. About 15% of inherited hyperlipoproteinemias can be traced to single-gene abnormalities, whereas about 85% are polygenic. Genetic factors can also predispose an individual to acquired hyperlipoproteinemia. For example, alcoholism often produces mild elevations in plasma triglycerides due to an elevation of VLDL. However, the genetics of a subgroup of patients with alcoholism results in clinically significant hyperlipidemia with elevations in both VLDL and chylomicrons.

Other causes of hypercholesterolemia and hypertriglyceridemia include diabetes, hypothyroidism, liver disease, kidney disease (nephrotic syndrome), pregnancy, acute myocardial infarction, and pancreatic disease. Medications that may cause hyperlipidemia include estrogen-containing oral contraceptives, corticosteroids, thiazide diuretics, and some antihypertensives. Hypertriglyceridemia may also occur in gout, obesity, excess carbohydrate intake, and chronic renal failure. Elevations of HDL may occur as a familial autosomal dominant trait, or may result from alcoholism, exposure to chlorinated hydrocarbon pesticides, and estrogen administration. Women tend to have higher HDL levels than men, probably because of endogenous estrogen.

Hypolipidemia may occur as a genetic trait or may be due to malnutrition or malabsorption. Hypocholesterolemia may occur in hyperthyroidism, severe liver injury, chronic anemia, corticosteroid therapy, infection, acute myocardial infarction, or acute trauma. Marked decreases in HDL levels and apolipoproteins A-I and A-II occur in the hereditary condition called Tangier disease, or hypoalphaproteinemia.

To close this section on plasma lipoproteins, it is interesting to note some aspects of lipid regulation. Endogenous cholesterol regulation occurs at the cellular and hepatic levels. Each cell controls its own internal concentration of cholesterol by regulating its production of LDL receptors. When the cellular cholesterol concentration is high, the receptor number drops. Then the rising concentration of cholesterol inhibits the most essential hepatic enzyme for endogenous synthesis of cholesterol, 3-hydroxy-3-methylglutaryl CoA reductase. The result is reduced synthesis of cholesterol by the liver. Exogenous regulation of cholesterol levels is better achieved by reducing dietary saturated fat than by reducing dietary cholesterol. It makes sense that reducing dietary cholesterol would reduce plasma cholesterol, and indeed up to an average 15% reduction in plasma cholesterol can be achieved this way. However, if the diet is also high in saturated fats, the resulting deposition of fat in the liver may cause increased liver synthesis of cholesterol that could increase the cholesterol concentration as much as 15–25%. Dietary reduction of saturated fat can result in greater reductions in cholesterol levels than dietary reduction of cholesterol alone, although the mechanism is not clear.

G. Urinalysis

The urinalysis (UA) has been called "the poor man's kidney biopsy," and indeed it gives a significant amount of information regarding fluid and electrolyte balance, pH regulation, and overall kidney function. Though it is one of the most fruitful laboratory screening tests, it is the most poorly performed test in laboratory medicine. It suffers from improper collection techniques, failure to perform while the sample is fresh, and incomplete examination of the sediment. Improper collection leading to specimen contamination is more common in females, and is almost inevitable in the obese, the elderly, and those in late pregnancy. Catheterization may be utilized to obtain a specimen if prevention of contamination is essential, though this may result in increased urinary erythrocytes. Once obtained, the sample should be stored at 4°C unless it is viewed within 2 hr to avoid cell breakdown and organism growth in the sample. Use of preservative tablets may help reduce these effects, especially in samples that are shipped to a central laboratory.

Following is a brief discussion of some of the standard parameters involved in a urinalysis.

1. Color/Appearance

The color and appearance of the sample are generally nonspecific. Endogenous substances as well as some foods and medications can color the urine; these effects may be pH-dependent. Endogenous pigments include porphyrins, melanin, and urates. Exogenous pigments include drugs such as pyridium (orange), phenytoin, robaxin, methyldopa, adriamycin (pink), phenolphthalein, some sulfonamides, and phenothiazines; organisms such as *Serratia marcescens*; and substances present in beets (pink), rhubarb (red), blackberries (red), paprika (orange), and vegetable dyes. Pink discoloration can give the appearance of pseudohematuria. Dark urine has been reported with a number of medications. The appearance of a urine sample is usually described as either clear or some descriptor such as cloudy, turbid, or hazy. Lack of clarity can be caused by cellular elements, casts, and crystals. Samples that are not examined immediately tend to become hazy due to formation of urate crystals.

2. Specific Gravity

The specific gravity, a measure of urinary solutes, gives an indication of the kidney's concentrating ability. The specific gravity of urine may vary from 1.001 to 1.035, though a normally hydrated patient usually has values in the range of 1.016–1.022. Loss of the ability to concentrate urine is a common and sometimes early sign of renal disease. Because these patients cannot concentrate their urine, they have isosthenuria, which is a urinary specific gravity slightly less than or equal to that of a typical serum specific gravity of 1.010. Specific gravity values greater than 1.040 usually occur only after an exogenous dye load.

3. pH

Urinary pH is a measure of urine acidity, which normally ranges from 4.5 to 7.5. The pH of water is 7, and values less than 7 reflect an acidity greater than that of water. Plasma has a pH of about 7.4 and is thus slightly more alkaline than water. An abnormally high urinary pH should suggest the possibility of urinary tract infection with an organism that can split urinary urea into ammonia. Otherwise, random urinary pH results do not usually have diagnostic value by themselves. Comparison of urinary and systemic pH may be useful. For example, urine that is not maximally acidic in a patient with systemic acidosis should suggest renal tubular dysfunction because most bicarbonate regulation occurs in the tubules.

4. Dipstick Parameters

Protein The most commonly used qualitative urine protein test is included on the Ames Multistix reagent strip. This test utilizes the indicators methyl red and bromophenol blue with buffering salts. Because protein lowers the pH at which the indicators change color, the test square becomes progressively more green in response to increasing protein concentrations. This test is particularly sensitive to albumin but not to some other proteins that can be present in the urine (light chains of immunoglobulins). The test is also subject to reader variability, as are many of the dipstick tests in which a color change must be qualitatively interpreted. Results correlate roughly with quantitative urinary protein: trace-positive is about 10 mg/dl protein, 1 + is about 30 mg/dl protein, 2 + is about 100 mg/dl protein, 3 + is about 300 mg/dl protein, and 4 + is at least 1000 mg/dl protein. Trace and even 1 + results can occur if a patient is dehydrated and the urine is maximally concentrated. It is also not unusual to see trace and 1 + results in patients with fever or congestive heart failure. Orthostatic and exercise-induced proteinuria have been described, and patients with proteinuria from any cause may have an orthostatic component with lower protein excretion at night while they are recumbent.

False-positive results for urinary protein may occur with extremely alkaline urine, with observer error, and with medications such as the skin cleanser chlorhexidine. Protein detection tests other than the Ames procedures may result in false-positive or negative results from other medications characteristic for the specific test. Once a false positive has been rule out as the cause of a positive dipstick test for proteinuria, the amount of urinary protein should be determined quantitatively from a 24-hr urine collection.

Twenty-four-hour urinary collections show that normal adults may excrete up to 150 mg of urinary protein per day. Only about 10–15 mg is albumin; the rest consists of over 30 different plasma proteins and renal glycoproteins. The most common renally derived protein is Tamm–Horsfall mucoprotein, which is produced in the renal tubule; about 25 mg/day is excreted. If a 24-hr urine collection demonstrates proteinuria, further workup is usually indicated. Proteinuria is usually due to renal glomerular disease or to renal tubular disease. Glomerular proteinuria consists primarily of albumin and can be very heavy, even up to 10 g or more per day. Tubular proteinuria consists of the range of serum proteins and usually does not exceed 1–2 g/day. Both types of proteinuria are often associated with hyaline or granular casts.

Blood   The qualitative test for urinary blood in the Ames Multistix panel is very sensitive to the presence of heme pigments, including hemoglobin and myoglobin. Hematuria usually is associated with enough erythrocyte lysis to show a uniformly positive test for blood, which corresponds to a uniformly green color change in the test square. Individual erythrocytes may produce green spotting on the test square also. The test square generally shows a positive result when about three erythrocytes per high-power field are present. The association of a positive test for urine blood with pigmented urine may suggest hemoglobinuria or myoglobinuria, especially if no erythrocytes are seen on microscopy. Proteinuria or highly concentrated urine may result in a false-negative result, and false positives may occur with hypochlorite, ascorbic acid (vitamin C), or bacteria that can produce peroxidase.

Glucose   The test square for urine glucose contains glucose oxidase, which is specific for dextrose (glucose). Positive tests are most likely to occur with diabetes, heavy proteinuria, during pregnancy, and in patients with renal tubular disorders such as Fanconi's syndrome or renal glycosuria. The presence of ascorbic acid (vitamin C) decreases test sensitivity.

Nitrate   A positive test for urinary nitrate occurs when gram-negative organisms in the urine reduce the nitrate on the test square to nitrite. The nitrite then produces a uniformly reddish pink color in the test square. This is a relatively insensitive test for the presence of urinary tract infection, and bacterial overgrowth may result in a positive test if a sample is left standing at room temperature.

Leukocyte esterase   The leukocyte esterase dipstick test becomes positive when leukocytes present in the urine produce esterases, which react with the test square. Usually urinary microscopy will also reveal the presence of urinary leukocytes.

Bilirubin   The urinary test for bilirubin generally detects conjugated (direct) bilirubin, which can be excreted in the urine. The test is not very sensitive to small amounts of bilirubin, and the presence of ascorbic acid can cause false-negative results.

Ketones   The urinary test for ketones detects only one of the ketone bodies, acetoacetic acid; it does not detect acetone or β-hydroxybutyric acid. Borderline positive tests may result from fasting, exercise, pregnancy, highly pigmented urine specimens, or levodopa metabolites. Sulfhydryl-containing compounds may cause positive or atypical results.

Urobilinogen   Urobilinogen is a product of bacterial metabolism of bilirubin in the gastrointestinal tract. Once formed, it is reabsorbed from the bowel and a small portion is eventually excreted in the urine. The urobilinogen reagent square may also react with substances such as *p*-aminosalicylic acid and sulfonamide antibiotics. Formalin may cause false-negative results. Absence of urobilinogen cannot be confirmed with this test because it is not very sensitive, but a negative test result in a jaundiced patient does suggest complete biliary obstruction.

5.   Microscopy

The key to accurate urinary microscopy is a fresh sample. If the sample must be transported to a central laboratory, a preservative should be used so that the microscopy can be delayed for several hours if necessary. A trace of formalin will preserve cells and casts, and boric acid 0.5 g/30 ml of urine will inhibit bacterial growth. The urine should be centrifuged before examination to concentrate cellular elements and casts, and the slide should be properly stained. Low-illumination light microscopy highlights the urinary elements, phase contrast microscopy may help identify morphological features of cells, and polarized light may aid in identification of crystals.

Bacteria   The presence of bacteria on a stained slide of uncentrifuged, well-mixed urine examined under high power generally correlates with a culture colony count of greater than 100,000/ml and is diagnostic of infection unless the sample has been contaminated or improperly handled in such a way that bacterial overgrowth could occur.

White blood cells   On high-power examination of uncentrifuged urine, more than 10 leukocytes per high-power field is abnormal. Contamination from the vagina in women and the prostate in men may falsely increase the urinary leukocytes. The amount of vaginal contamination tends to correlate with the number of squamous epithelial cells present. Increased urinary leukocytes, called pyuria, suggest urinary tract infection, but pyuria may occur without bacteriuria in conditions such as urinary tuberculosis, renal stones, analgesic nephropathy, chemical cystitis, acute glomerulonephritis, chlamydial urethral infections, or antiseptic contamination of the sample. If more than 5% of the leukocytes are eosinophils, this suggests acute interstitial nephritis. Unfortunately, the presence of urinary eosinophils is neither sensitive nor specific for this syndrome.

Red blood cells There should not be enough erythrocytes in the urine for them to be observed in uncentrifuged urine with high-power light microscopy. After centrifugation, there should be three or fewer erythrocytes per high-power field. Observer error may occur when erythrocytes are confused with small oxalate crystals, yeast, or air bubbles. This is less likely to occur if careful high-power examination is done. If erythrocytes are crenated, or wrinkled, it is more likely that they originated in the upper urinary tract. Menstruation is a very common cause of urinary contamination with erythrocytes. After observer error and contamination are accounted for, about 3–4% of the adult population is found microscopically to have increased urinary erythrocytes, or microhematuria. There are multiple causes of microhematuria, and a cause cannot be found in 8–15% of these patients. The identifiable causes include hematological conditions (hemoglobinopathies, coagulopathies, anticoagulant therapy), renal glomerular disease, renal interstitial disease, renal vascular disease, urinary tract malignancy, renal stones, urinary tract instrumentation, and urinary tract infection. The most common causes of hematuria are inflammation of the bladder or urethra (25%) from infection or other cause, renal stones (20%), and urinary tract neoplasms (15%). Unexplained persistent or recurrent microhematuria warrants a diagnostic workup, especially in a high-risk patient population, because of the possibility of malignancy. This is true even in patients on appropriate anticoagulant therapy.

Epithelial cells Epithelial cells are frequently present in urine. They derive most commonly from vulvar epithelium and therefore are seen most frequently in urine from women patients. Transitional epithelial cells are smaller and have a more uniform oval shape. Normal urine may contain a few transitional epithelial cells, especially in female patients, where the cells usually originate from the urethra or bladder neck. Transitional epithelial cells may be increased if a urinary tract infection is present.

Other cells Foreign cellular elements that are frequently seen include yeast and *Trichomonas*, usually as contaminants from vaginal infections. Yeast overgrowth in the bladder may occur in patients on broad-spectrum antibacterial therapy. The presence of sperm in the urine indicates retrograde ejaculation, which occurs most commonly in men who have had urinary tract surgery or instrumentation. Special staining techniques may be used to examine the morphology of other cells found in the urine. A Pap or methylene blue stain is generally used for this cytology examination, which is more likely to be diagnostic for malignancy if the malignancy originates in the lower urinary tract rather than in the kidney.

Urinary casts These cylindrical bodies form in the lumen of the distal tubules of the kidney, especially the collecting tubule where flow and pH are low and osmolality is high. The matrix of urinary casts is formed from Tamm–Horsfall mucoprotein, a viscous glycoprotein with a molecular weight of about 85,000. This Tamm–Horsfall protein gel is secreted by cells lining part of the renal tubule. Whole cells, cellular debris, and other proteins in the tubular lumen may be aggregated and caught up in the protein gel to form the different varieties of casts. Centrifuged urine is examined for casts, with low-power light microscopy.

Hyaline casts consist entirely of Tamm–Horsfall protein, and are clear and colorless. Hyaline casts may be seen in normal urine after exercise or in concentrated urine. Showers of hyaline casts may occur during febrile illness or after administration of a loop diuretic such as furosemide. Granular casts are pale but show a granular appearance from disintegrated cells or aggregated serum proteins. Immunofluorescence has identified albumin, lipoproteins, and immunoglobulins in the granules. Finely granular casts usually have the same significance as hyaline casts, but densely granular casts are always pathological. Densely granular casts are most common in conditions with heavy proteinuria.

Fatty casts contain highly refractile fat globules that may be mistaken for erythrocytes. In addition to these free fat globules, fatty casts also may contain oval fat bodies, which are epithelial cells filled with fat granules. Fatty casts are seen in patients with moderate to heavy proteinuria. Polarized light microscopy will reveal the classic Maltese cross pattern that has been attributed to the presence of cholesterol esters.

Cellular casts are much less common. The presence of even one red blood cell cast is pathognomonic for glomerular bleeding and is thus diagnostic for renal disease. A red blood cell cast may contain many densely packed erythrocytes or the erythrocytes may be few in number. The erythrocytes may be degenerated, resulting in a rust-colored granular cast called a hemoglobin cast. Leukocyte casts indicate pyelonephritis and are relatively rare. Epithelial cell casts are found in acute tubular necrosis or acute glomerulonephritis. Hyaline or finely granular casts that contain relatively few epithelial cells are less specific. Casts or cellular clumps containing transitional epithelial cells may indicate a bladder tumor.

Urinary crystals The presence of urinary crystals is very common and usually nondiagnostic because oxalate crystals and amorphous urate crystals commonly form in urine samples that are left standing before examination. This is usually because these substances crystallize as the urine sample cools. When urine is kept at body temperature and then examined on a warm-stage microscope, the presence of oxalate crystals suggests a tendency to form oxalate stones. The acid–base status of the urine also affects the formation of crystals. Calcium oxalate and amorphous or crystalline uric acid crystals tend to form in acidic urine. Conversely, amorphous phosphates, triple phosphate, and calcium phosphate crystals tend to form in more alkaline urine.

III. SUMMARY

The laboratory is an invaluable tool to help assess the risks and benefits of established or new medical therapies. The assessment of patient safety through laboratory measurements, however, is only a part of the larger issue of medication safety and must be considered in the context of each patient's clinical picture. The physician must consider all known factors contributing to the total benefit–risk equation before the optimal therapeutic decision can be made.

REFERENCES

1. Guyton AC, ed. *Textbook of Medical Physiology*. 8th ed. Philadelphia: WB Saunders; 1991.
2. Wilson JD, Braunwald E, Isselbacher KJ, Petersdorf RG, Martin JB, Fauci AS, et al. *Harrison's Principles of Internal Medicine*. 12th ed. New York: McGraw-Hill; 1991.
3. Davidson CS, Leevy CM, Chamberlayne EC, eds. Guidelines for Detection of Hepatotoxicity Due to Drugs and Chemicals. National Institutes of Health (NIH Publication No. 79-313), 1979.
4. Consensus development conference on lowering blood cholesterol to prevent heart disease. *JAMA*. 1985;253:2080–2086.
5. Report of the National Cholesterol Education Program Expert Panel on Detection, Evaluation, and Treatment of High Blood Cholesterol in Adults. *Arch Intern Med*. 1988;148:36–69.

4

Drug Research in the Elderly

Piet M. Hooymans and Robert Janknegt

Maasland Hospital
Sittard, The Netherlands

I. INTRODUCTION

A major part of total drug consumption is attributable to elderly patients. This is due on the one hand to the increasing number of elderly people in most countries and on the other hand to multipathology and polymedication in these patients. However, drug research has for the most part been performed in young, healthy volunteers. The information obtained from these pharmacokinetic and clinical studies gives us indications concerning the pharmacokinetics and pharmacodynamics of these drugs in the elderly, but these data are insufficient for an optimal use of drugs in older patients. Significant advances have been made in understanding the age-related changes in organ functions and their effects on the pharmacokinetic behavior of drugs in the elderly. This knowledge emphasizes the need for more research on pharmacokinetics and pharmacodynamics in old age. In most countries pharmacokinetic studies in elderly patients have to be performed for the registration files. Many drugs already marketed should be examined, especially those with a narrow therapeutic range.

Much less is known on the pharmacodynamics of drugs in elderly patients. It is widely recognized that a drug must be studied in patients for whom it is intended. Drugs to be investigated are first of all the ones most frequently used in the elderly. These might be different from those used in young patients because of the difference in the intention to treat. The goals of treatment are different in young and in elderly patients. In the elderly improvement in the quality of life is a more important criterion than extension of life. Also, clinical studies in the elderly are complicated by multipathology and polymedication in these patients, resulting in an increased risk of drug interactions.

Several practical and ethical problems are encountered in the performance of clinical studies in the elderly, but it is now widely accepted that drugs should be tested in clinical studies involving those patients who are most likely to be treated with these drugs, e.g., elderly patients. The increased awareness of the specific problems of drug use in the elderly recently resulted in the first review journal devoted to this topic entitled *Drugs and Aging*.

II. ALTERATIONS IN PHARMACOKINETICS IN THE ELDERLY

Several pharmacokinetic parameters, such as absorption, distribution, metabolism, and elimination, may be significantly altered in elderly patients. These are summarized in Table 1.

A. Absorption

Gastric acidity is usually reduced in elderly people because of atrophic changes in the gastric mucosa. This may be a problem with drugs requiring sufficient gastric acidity for a reliable absorption, such as the antimycotic drug ketoconazole [2]. The effects of decreased gastrointestinal motility on the absorption of drugs is less clear. Elevation of pH may increase gastric emptying rate. Most studies have failed to show evidence of a significantly reduced enteric absorption

Table 1   Alterations in Pharmacokinetics in the Elderly

Function	Alteration
Absorption	Reduced gastric acidity
	Reduced gastric emptying rate
	Reduced small bowel motility
	Reduced splanchic blood flow
Distribution	Lower albumin levels
	Reduced lean body mass
	Increased fat tissue mass
	Dehydration
Metabolism	Reduced liver size
	Reduced liver blood flow
Elimination	Decreased glomerular filtration rate
	Reduced renal blood flow
	Decreased tubular secretion

in the elderly. A relatively slow absorption after intramuscular injection may be observed in elderly patients. This has been shown in the case of the antimicrobial agents cefuroxime and depot penicillin G [2].

B. Distribution

Many drugs are bound to serum proteins. This binding is usually reversible. The most important binding proteins are albumin and α_1-acid glycoprotein. This protein binds basic drugs such as lidocaine, disopyramide, and erythromycin. The binding of drugs to albumin or α_1-acid glycoprotein is highly variable and ranges from 0% for hydrophilic drugs such as aminoglycosides to >99% for most nonsteroidal anti-inflammatory drugs. Only the unbound fraction is considered to be pharmacologically active although there is no consensus on the clinical relevance of protein binding.

Age has a significant influence on serum albumin levels. The serum levels of this important drug-binding protein are approximately 20% lower at age 80 years than when compared to 20 years, with a resulting effect on the free fraction of highly protein-bound drugs. The serum levels of α_1-acid glycoprotein are highly variable in elderly patients but the mean level is not significantly different from that of younger people [3].

In general the effects of lower circulating levels of albumin do not have significant effects on the protein binding of drugs in elderly people, but it may contribute to the wide variation in pharmacokinetics observed in this group. The free fraction is changed by greater than 50% in the elderly for only a limited number of drugs, such as acetazolamide, diflunisal, etomidate, naproxen, salicylate and valproate [3].

The volume of distribution relates the amount of drug in the body to the serum concentration. This volume does not necessarily refer to a given physiological volume but merely to the fluid volume that would be required to account for all the drug in the body. Generally hydrophilic drugs have a lower volume of distribution than more lipophilic drugs because the latter drugs may penetrate into cells to a higher degree. Most (hydrophilic) β-lactam antibiotics have a volume of distribution of about 0.25–0.4 L/kg which corresponds to the extracellular fluid volume. Highly lipophilic drugs such as flecainide, verapamil, and neuroleptics have a large volume of distribution of >5 L/kg. Theoretically an increased volume of distribution might be expected in the elderly for lipid-soluble drugs due to the increased fat tissue mass, and the reverse would be expected for water-soluble drugs due to a reduced lean body mass and extracellular and intracellular dehydration. Lean body mass (as a percentage of body weight) in men is 64% at the age of 70 years and 81% at 25 years. In women the values were 68% and 51%, respectively [4]. In practice, however, the differences in volumes of distribution observed in young and elderly people are usually small and do not correlate well with the above expectations. In individual patients the volume of distribution may be quite different from that observed in young patients. A smaller volume of distribution has been shown in the case of the water-soluble drugs digoxin and cimetidine but there are several notable exceptions, e.g., tobramycin, which has an increased volume of distribution in the elderly. The lipid-soluble drugs diazepam and nitrazepam have a larger volume of distribution in older patients. However, lorazepam has a reduced distribution [1].

C. Metabolism

The liver is by far the most important metabolizing organ. However, no reliable tests for the metabolizing capacity of the liver are available. With advancing age, the size of the liver decreases both in absolute terms and in relation to body weight. Regional blood flow to the liver is also markedly lower in elderly patients. A fall of over 35% is observed in apparent blow flow to the liver and liver perfusion falls by 10–15% [5]. These reductions in blood flow to the liver, as a result of the decreased cardiac output (1% per year during adult life), result in a decreased clearance of drugs having a high hepatic extraction ratio, such as propranolol and labetalol. The clearance of these drugs depends on liver blood flow and is reduced by 30–40% in elderly patients. The clearance of drugs with a low extraction ratio depends primarily on the hepatocellular function. Oxidation, reduction, and hydrolysis are mostly reduced in the elderly, but glucuronidation, acetylation, and sulfation are generally unaffected. Chlordiazepoxide, diazepam, clorazepate, and prazepam all undergo oxidative metabolism and have prolonged elimination in the elderly. Oxazepam, lorazepam, and temazepam are only conjugated in the liver and their elimination rate is therefore not changed in old age [1]. These alterations of liver function may be partly responsible for the high incidence of type A (dose-related) adverse drug reactions observed in elderly patients. The activity of drug-metabolizing enzymes is more or less preserved in healthy elderly subjects but may be significantly reduced in frail elderly patients [5].

D. Elimination

An important factor of impaired drug clearance in the elderly is the reduction in glomerular filtration rate (GFR). It is estimated that the GFR decreases 0.4 ml/min/year between the ages 20–50 years and by 1 ml/min/year thereafter. However, serum creatinine levels are not markedly higher in elderly patients. Therefore, serum creatinine levels are not a reliable parameter of renal function in the elderly. If the GFR is estimated from the serum creatinine level, it is important that this level is corrected for age.

Dosages of drugs that are excreted predominantly by the kidney, in particular those with a narrow therapeutic range such as gentamicin, lithium, and digoxin, have to be corrected for the diminished renal function in elderly patients [5].

III. PHARMACODYNAMICS

A. Drug Action

Only limited information is available concerning the action of drugs on their specific receptors in the elderly. The number of β receptors in the sympathetic nervous system declines with advancing age, but the affinity of β receptors does not change. The clinical relevance of these findings requires further investigation. Elderly persons appear to be more sensitive to the effects of benzodiazepines. Elderly patients are sedated at lower drug concentrations than those required by young adults [1]. In considering the action of antibacterial drugs in elderly patients, it is important to realize the fact that several changes in host defense occur in these patients. Both cell-mediated immunity and humoral immunity are less effective in elderly patients in comparison with young or middle-aged people. Both colonization and infections are more frequent in elderly patients [6].

B. Side Effects

Elderly patients are known to suffer from adverse effects of drugs more frequently than other age groups. The Medicine Adverse Reactions Committee of New Zealand has studied the number of adverse drug reactions (ADR) per 10,000 population in different age groups. This number was at its lowest value at age 10–19 years, with only five ADR per 10,000. The number of ADR increases with age to reach 31 at the age range 50–59 years and to 54 in patients above 80 years [7].

This increase in ADR is caused by both a higher incidence of side effects of drugs in elderly patients and a marked increase in drug use in this age group. Important changes in homeostatic responses occur in elderly subjects, e.g., tachycardia as a response to exercise and posture, baroreceptor function, glucose tolerance, body temperature regulation, bowel and bladder function, and body stability. These changes make old patients more vulnerable to adverse effects of drugs regarding these homeostatic responses [8]. In particular, benzodiazepines, cardiovascular drugs, drugs for respiratory diseases, antiparkinson drugs, and antimicrobial agents are used by many elderly patients.

Adverse reactions leading to hospitalization have received considerable attention, and it has been estimated that 3–8% of hospital admissions are a consequence of adverse drug reactions [9]. Drugs that are frequently involved in hospitalization due to side effects are hypnotics, tranquillizers, sedatives, antiepileptic drugs, antidepressants, cardiac glycosides, and antiparkinson drugs.

Psychoactive drugs often cause serious side effects in elderly patients. The risk of falling (with the possibility of hip fracture) increases significantly in elderly patients using benzodiazepines [10]. The indication for these drugs in (normal!) sleep disturbances in the elderly is often questionable.

Elderly patients are highly susceptible to the anticholinergic and hypotensive effects of tricyclic antidepressants, resulting in tachycardia, accommodation disturbances, raised intraocular pressure, urinary retention, and obstipation (leading to laxative usage). These effects are most marked in the case of amitryptiline, and as a result this drug should not be prescribed to elderly patients. During the first few years of experience with newly approved medications the physician must use them with great caution and with a high index of suspicion for toxocity in the elderly [11]. Postmarketing surveillance is especially of interest in old patients.

The relative high incidence of side effects in elderly patients stresses the need for the performance of clinical studies in the elderly in order to optimize drug efficacy in this age group.

IV. SPECIFIC PROBLEMS IN PERFORMING CLINICAL STUDIES IN THE ELDERLY

The interest in geriatric pharmacology has increased considerably in recent years. In the past old people were systematically excluded from drug studies. Most drug regulatory authorities now require the testing of new drugs in an elderly population. Morley and coworkers studied the number of published clinical studies that included at least one subject over 65 years of age. Only about 14% of all these studies published in general journals, such as *New England Journal of Medicine*, *Journal of the American Medical Association*, *Lancet*, and the *British Medical Journal*, included at least one elderly patient. This percentage did not change markedly in the period 1966–1988 [12]. However, the number of journals that deal specifically with elderly patients has increased steadily over the last 10 years [7].

The need to study drugs in the population for which they are intended will be clear, but many specific problems are encountered in the performance of clinical studies in the elderly. These are summarized in Table 2. Because of the great variability in drug disposition and response in the elderly it is advisable to perform clinical studies in different groups of old patients. Four groups are of special interest:

Subjects aged 65 or above, who are drug-free and show no evidence of systemic disease on clinical examination, electrocardiography, and routine tests of hematological, liver, and renal function
Patients with stable diseases that might affect the pharmacokinetics of the investigated drug, such as hepatic or renal impairment and heart failure
Patients taking drugs chronically that are frequently prescribed for the elderly and involved in drug interactions, such as nonsteroidal anti-inflammatory drugs, digoxin, and diuretics
Patients suffering from the condition for which the drug is indicated [9].

Table 2 Problems in Clinical Studies in Elderly Patients

Aspect	Problem
Multipathology	Identification of drug action
	Causal relationship of ADR
Polypharmacy	Causal relationship of ADR
	Drug interactions
Practical aspects	Administration problems
	Drug sampling
	Identification of drug action
	Identification of side effects
	Patient compliance
	Selection of patients
Ethical aspects	Informed consent
	Disruption of daily routine
	Mentally incompetent patients

A. Multipathology and Polypharmacy

An important problem in interpreting the results of clinical studies in elderly patients is the fact that many elderly patients use more than one drug and suffer from different diseases. Therefore, it is difficult to select patients suffering only from the disease for which the drug to be studied is indicated. Usually patients with different diseases participate in clinical drug research. As a result of the multipathology several drugs are used that can interfere with the drug to be investigated. The interpretation of the results can therefore be complicated by unexpected drug interactions. In the Netherlands, the percentage of people using at least one drug increases from 15–25% (men and women, respectively) at 20 years to 67–80% in people over 80 years of age [13]. Elderly residents of nursing homes in particular take impressive amounts of drugs. Forty percent of these patients use five or more drugs at the same time and 20% take eight or more drugs simultaneously [13] !

It will be clear that the risk of drug interactions is very high in this patient population. Although only a limited number of studies have investigated this problem, it is evident that potentially dangerous interactions include hypo-kalemia due to diuretics, interactions with oral anticoagulants, and interactions between psychoactive drugs. These potential drug interactions may affect the clinical efficacy and tolerance of any new, investigational drug added to the medication of the patients.

Quite often, the use of certain (groups of) drugs is excluded before entry into the study, which causes a bias in the selection of patients to be treated with the study drug. Frail elderly patients, taking many other drugs for a variety of illnesses, are often excluded from these studies, although they are the population most likely to receive the drug after registration.

B. Practical Aspects

Many practical problems are encountered in clinical and pharmacokinetic studies in elderly patients.

Selection of patients is difficult because the ill elderly can cause diagnostic difficulties due to problems in obtaining an accurate history, altered symptoms, and nonspecific presentation of disease. Pharmacokinetic studies in frail elderly patients are difficult to perform due to problems with administration of the study drug, such as difficulties in swallowing, difficulties in ingesting the required volume of water with the drug after oral administration, and intolerance of intravenous infusions. Sampling of relevant serum or urine samples may also pose significant problems due to inability to maintain vascular access and urinary and fecal incontinence [14]. It is also very difficult to collect information concerning clinical efficacy and side effects of drugs in this patient population, especially those showing varying degrees of confusion.

Most clinical studies are performed on nursing home patients to guarantee a high degree of patient compliance. This compliance may be very low in elderly patients living at home, especially those who must take several drugs at the same time.

C. Ethical Aspects

In all clinical studies and even more so in elderly patients it is necessary to obtain informed consent from the patient, before he or she is included in the trial. The patient should be free to refuse participating in the study at any time, for any reason. Elderly patients, especially those in a nursing home, do not always feel free and are in a dependent position to the physician. The disruption of every day routine in the nursing home may be very troublesome to most patients. Quite often they regret their participation in the study, without asking their doctor to stop the study. Informed consent is of special significance if research, rather than or in addition to rational therapy, is the reason for drug use [15].

Mentally incompetent patients should not be included in trials unrelated to their problems but with the consent of close family may serve as subjects for trials of drugs intended for these patients, such as drugs for the treatment of Alzheimer's disease. At all times they require special protection against abuse as research subjects [15].

V. CONCLUSIONS

It is now widely accepted that drugs should be tested in the patient groups in whom they are most likely to be used. Elderly patients use significantly more drugs than younger patients. Due to alterations in pharmacokinetics and pharmacodynamics, it is necessary to test drugs in the elderly.

The high incidence of side effects in elderly patients is caused by both polymedication and improper dosage. Studies to investigate the proper usage of drugs in elderly people are often troublesome but are nevertheless necessary to improve the quality of pharmacotherapy in this population. Many clinical studies involving elderly patients (e.g., treatment of hypertension) still have important shortcomings [16]. Therefore clinicians must be able to evaluate these reports critically.

REFERENCES

1. Montamat SC, Cusack BJ, Vestal RE. Management of drug therapy in the elderly. *N Engl J Med*. 1989;321:303–309.
2. Ljungberg B, Nilsson-Ehle I. Pharmacokinetics of antimicrobial agents in the elderly. *Rev Infect Dis*. 1987;9:250–262.
3. Wallace SM, Verbeeck RK. Plasma protein binding of drugs in the elderly. *Clin Pharmacokinet*. 1987;12:41–72.
4. Norrby SR. Antibiotic therapy in aging patients. *Bull NY Acad Med*. 1987;63:519–532.
5. Woodhouse KW, Wynne HA. Age-related changes in liver size and hepatic blood flow. *Clin Pharmacokinet*. 1988;15:287–294.
6. Hirsch BE, Weksler ME. Normal changes in host defence. In: Abrams WE, Berkow R, eds. *The Merck Manual of Geriatrics*. Rahway, NJ: MSD Research Laboratories; 1990;876–883.
7. Ohose K. The need for a review journal of drug use and the elderly. *Drugs and Aging*. 1991;1:2–5.
8. Turner P. Medicine in the elderly. Clinical trials in elderly. *Postgrad Med J*. 1989;65:218–220.
9. Nolan L, O'Malley K. Prescribing for the elderly: part I. Sensitivity of the elderly to adverse drug reactions. *J Am Geriatr Soc*. 1988;36:142–149.
10. Sorock GS, Shimkin EE. Benzodiazepine sedatives and the risk of falling in a community-dwelling elderly cohort. *Arch Intern Med*. 1988;148:2441–2444.
11. Beers MH, Ouslander JG. Risk factors in geriatric drug prescribing. A practical guide to avoiding problems. *Drugs*. 1989;37:105–112.
12. Morley JE, Vogel K, Solomon DH. Prevalence of geriatric articles in general medical journals. *J Am Geriatr Soc*. 1990;38:173–176.
13. Van Bezooijen CFA. Side effects and hospitalization due to drug use in elderly patients (in Dutch). *Ger Inf*. 1989; section E3035:1–19.
14. Janknegt R, Boogaard-van den Born J. Hameleers BA, et al. Pharmacokinetics of amoxicillin in elderly in-patients. *Pharm Weekbl Sci*. 1992;14:27–29.
15. Goldstein MK. Ethical considerations in pharmacotherapy of the aged. *Drugs and Aging*. 1991;1:91–97.
16. Kitler ME. Clinical trials and clinical practice in the elderly: a focus on hypertension. *Drugs and Aging*. 1962;2:85–94.

5

Drug Assessment in Critical Illness

M. I. Bowden and J. F. Bion

Queen Elizabeth Hospital, The University of Birmingham
Edgbaston, Birmingham, England

I. INTRODUCTION

In 1982 the medical staff working in the intensive care unit (ICU) of the Western Infirmary, Glasgow, noticed an unexpected increase in mortality among their multiple-trauma patients who were undergoing mechanical ventilation. Clinical suspicions were confirmed by a retrospective survey [1] of this diagnostic group, which showed that whereas from 1969 to 1980 the mortality rate had remained relatively constant at 19–29%, it had indeed risen during 1981–1982, to 47%. The most likely reason for this was that the patients were more seriously injured, but this hypothesis was discounted by calculating the mean injury severity scores (ISS) for each year: there had been no increase in ISS during 1981–1982, and so an alternative explanation had to be found. The only change in clinical practice which had occurred in the unit was the introduction of the anesthetic hypnotic agent etomidate, which was being used by continuous infusion for days or weeks to sedate critically ill patients who were receiving mechanical respiratory support. Etomidate was licensed only for induction and short-term maintenance of anesthesia by infusion in patients in the operating theater; but its cardiovascular stability, short half-life, and absence of accumulation were perceived as giving it a significant advantage over other currently available agents for sedation in intensive care.

What was not known at the time, however, was that etomidate is also the most potent inhibitor of adrenocortical function yet discovered, exceeding metyrapone by several orders of magnitude [2,3]. In retrospect it seems remarkable that this side effect should have been undetected at a time when stress response inhibition during surgery was being studied so closely. While no direct causal relationship has been established, during 1979–1982 the mortality among those patients sedated with morphine with or without a benzodiazepine was 28% but in those sedated with morphine and etomidate was 77% [1]. Moreover, the withdrawal of etomidate for infusion sedation of critically ill patients was associated with a reduction in mortality rates to 25% the following year.

Three morals can be drawn from this episode. The first is that the absence of clinically apparent side effects does not mean that a drug is necessarily safe. The second is that drugs licensed for use in one patient population must not be applied to a different population without revalidation. The third is that measures of severity of illness should form an integral part of drug assessment in intensive care. We will return to these principles when we examine specific issues relating to drug assessment in critically ill patients in this chapter, but before doing so we need to define the term *critical illness*.

A. What Is Critical Illness?

Critical illness means the unstable failure of one or more of the body's organ systems, limiting the capacity for independent survival and requiring specialized organ system support. Definitions of organ system failures (OSFs) have been proposed by Dr. Knaus and his colleagues [4]. Organ system support in its widest sense encompasses all therapeutic activities, but in intensive care it is generally used to mean major interventions such as mechanical ventilation, renal dialysis, use of vasoactive drugs to support blood pressure or oxygen delivery, total parenteral nutrition, or frequent infusions of blood and blood products. All these activities either directly or indirectly involve the use of drugs.

Three factors determine survival from critical illness: the severity of disease, the extent of physiological reserve, and the specificity and timing of treatment. In mechanical terms these may be likened to the size of the applied load, engine capacity, and the skill of the operator. There are now several scoring systems that assess severity of illness (for a recent review, see Ref. 5). The ISS [6] mentioned above is based on the anatomical extent of injury, but of more general application is the physiologically based Acute Physiology and Chronic Health Evaluation (APACHE) system [7,8], which has now been extensively validated for severity stratification in research and for prediction of outcome of groups of patients. The relationship between severity of illness and therapy is complex, but two aspects are of particular importance in the context of this chapter and are illustrated by Figures 1 and 2.

Figure 1 demonstrates the relationship between severity of illness and mortality for three disease processes: sepsis, congestive heart failure, and diabetic ketoacidotic coma. It is evident that for any given degree of physiological

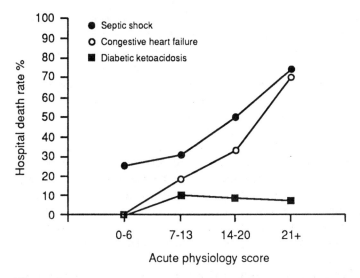

Figure 1   Hospital death rate plotted against APACHE score for three different diagnostic categories. (From Ref. 9.)

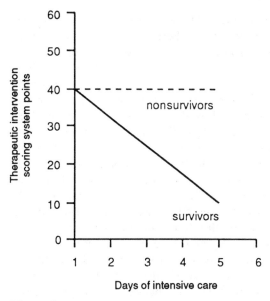

Figure 2   TISS score plotted against duration of stay on intensive care for survivors and nonsurvivors. (From Ref. 10.)

disturbance diabetics have better survival rates than patients with heart failure, who in turn do better than patients with sepsis. This difference is explicable in part on the basis of *therapeutic specificity*, which is high for diabetes (insulin), intermediate for heart failure (vasoactive drugs and mechanical devices), and low for sepsis (antibiotics and supportive therapy only). It is also possible that chronic disease and limitation of physiological reserve are more common features in patients with sepsis or heart failure than in those with insulin-dependent diabetes, who are therefore better able to respond to treatment.

Figure 2 presents similar information in a different way by using a measure of therapeutic workload, the Therapeutic Intervention Scoring System (TISS) [10], to show that patients who survive critical illness require less therapy as time passes, whereas those who subsequently die require continuing high levels of support. The machinery of the nonsurvivors has been irretrievably wrecked, and organ system support under these circumstances is like towing a car without an engine. Organ system support is only useful if the underlying disease process is reversible.

These three illustrations serve as reminders that the detection of both adverse and beneficial drug effects is made easier by severity stratification. Conversely, both adverse and beneficial effects of drugs can be masked by the severity of the underlying disease.

B. Implications of Critical Illness for Drug Assessment

The pathology of critical illness and the therapeutic maneuvers of organ system support make patients in ICUs very different from those in ordinary hospital wards or operating theaters. ICU patients are a heterogeneous population in terms of both diagnosis and severity of illness, ranging from patients admitted electively for invasive monitoring following surgery to those who are admitted as emergencies with unstable failure of several organ systems. This diversity complicates analysis and has encouraged the development of physiological indices of severity of illness typified by the APACHE system. Physiological disturbance of varying degrees, either actual or potential, is a property shared by all ICU patients, and this has two important implications for drug assessment and safety. The first and most obvious is that physiological disturbance affects drug pharmacokinetics and pharmacodynamics. Second, variations in pathophysiology can mask, expose, or mimic both beneficial and adverse drug affects. Stratification for severity of illness is therefore important for increasing the signal-to-noise ratio [11]. Reliance solely on diagnostic groups is unwise even when the groups are large because of variations in severity of illness between patients. Small numbers of patients within specific diagnostic groups (the main problem for intensive care research) increase the likelihood of a type 2 error (failure to detect a difference), and confidence intervals should from an integral part of the analysis. Similarly, the chance of detecting an adverse drug effect is substantially reduced if the population is small. A simple rule of thumb for calculating the 95% confidence interval is to use $300/n$ where n is the number of patients receiving the drug [12]; thus if 50 patients are studied without apparent adverse effects, there is still the risk that 6% (300/50) of a different or larger population may not be so fortunate.

In addition to these general principles, there are several practical problems that complicate drug assessment in this population. Because of the nature of critical illness, supportive treatment often has to precede diagnosis and specific therapy of the underlying disease. There is considerable potential for drug interactions because many ICU patients have significant comorbidities for which they are already receiving treatment, and during their ICU stay they will receive many more; indeed it is common for 10–15 different medications to be prescribed concurrently. Supportive therapy such as inotropic drugs or mechanical ventilation may affect drug handling by altering regional blood flow to organs with biotransforming or excretory functions such as liver, gut, kidneys, and lungs. Finally, pharmacological monitoring is limited by the absence of clinically useful bedside drug assays, by uncertainty about the relationship between blood and tissue levels of a drug and its clinical effect, and by alterations in drug receptor populations. These points will be considered in more detail below.

II. DRUG FACTORS

Critically ill patients receive drugs for three main reasons: for definitive therapy of the underlying disease, for the prevention or management of complications, and to facilitate organ system support. The range and number of compounds prescribed are considerable. Superimposed on drug therapy are many other nonpharmacological forms of treatment that may have an impact on pharmacokinetics (Table 1).

The majority of drugs prescribed in intensive care are given intravenously, usually via a central vein. This allows more rapid onset of action, facilitates control, and circumvents the problems with absorption that occur with other sites, such as gastrointestinal stasis, hepatic first-pass effects, or altered skin or muscle blood flow. Enteral administration is reserved for nutrition if the gut is intact, and for specifically enteral therapies such as sucralfate for stress ulcer prophylaxis, vancomycin for pseudomembranous colitis, and selective antibiotic decontamination of the gut. The lungs can be used for giving emergency drugs during cardiopulmonary resuscitation, and β_2 agonists, anticholinergics, and certain antibiotics can all be nebulized; the lung is also a logical route for the administration of volatile sedative agents in patients undergoing mechanical ventilation [13].

Problems with drug interactions start before the drug reaches the biophase. The concurrent administration of a number of drugs via a limited number of

Table 1 Examples of Forms of Therapy in Intensive Care

Specific	*Organ system support*
Antibiotics	Oxygen, intravenous fluids
Antidysrhythmics	Vasoactive drugs, inotropes
Hormones	Analgesics, sedatives
Immunomodulators	Muscle relaxants
Anticonvulsants	Parenteral nutrition
	Blood and blood products
Prophylactic	*Nonpharmacological*
H-2 blockers	Mechanical ventilation
Selective antibiotic decontamination (SDD)	Dialysis
Anticoagulants	Surgery
	Extracorporeal oxygenation

intravenous cannulae can lead to interactions within the drug delivery system itself. In one study [14] investigating 45 two-drug combinations commonly encountered in the ICU, 19 produced obvious visible evidence of incompatibility, such as nicardipine forming a precipitate with a number of antibiotics [15]. However, the absence of obvious precipitation is no guarantee of physical compatibility; some drugs lose their potency when mixed with others or with their diluents (e.g., verapamil with aminophylline in 5% glucose [16]), and other drugs can precipitate out as microcrystals causing damage to various vascular beds. Drug trials must be preceded by an investigation of physical incompatibilities with commonly used intensive care drugs before clinical testing and, if given intravenously, should be infused through a single dedicated cannula.

Once in the biophase, polypharmacy complicates the assessment of competition for protein-binding sites, target organ receptors, and for the enzyme systems responsible for biotransformation and elimination. It is difficult to ascertain the contribution of each of these processes. There are only a small number of drugs whose concentrations can be measured, and because of variation in protein binding, free fraction, and tissue uptake in critically ill patients, the relationships between plasma levels, tissue concentrations, and clinical effects are complex [17].

The analysis of body fluids requires considerable care with the way samples are taken, processed, and stored prior to analysis, and lapses in technique may invalidate results. For example, the muscle relaxant atracurium undergoes rapid spontaneous degradation at body temperature and pH by a process of Hoffman elimination and ester hydrolysis [18]. Consequently, a known volume of plasma has to be separated, acidified, and frozen within 3 min [19] if a meaningful result is to be obtained. This is relatively easy to achieve in the laboratory but is a considerable challenge in the context of a busy ICU. Once processed, assay specificity for some drugs may be impaired by the presence of others—highly likely to occur in the context of polypharmacy [20].

A. Problems of Drug Delivery

Drug prescription or preparation errors are common in medical practice, though they are usually identified before any harm occurs. Even in the controlled circumstances of a laboratory study, when 20 nurses or pharmacists were asked to add potassium to a bag of intravenous fluid there were variations in the resulting potassium concentration of over 1000-fold [21]. Given the multiplicity of therapies and the need for rapid interventions in intensive care, it is perhaps surprising that prescribing and dispensing errors are not more frequent. This is in part because of high staffing ratios, close supervision, good standards of care, and protocol-guided therapy. In a clinical environment, particular care must be taken to ensure that research drugs reach the patient in the concentration that was initially prescribed, and assays of the solution infused into the patient may need to form part of drug assessment.

Once the drug has been correctly prescribed and dispensed there are two further problems that can occur before the drug reaches the patient. First, drugs can be adsorbed onto the surface of the delivery system. Several drugs used in intensive care have this property. Insulin [22] and nitroglycerin [23] are notable examples, and may result in a reduction in the received dose. Second, there are substantial variations in syringe driver performance. Most countries have published performance standards for pumps and syringe drivers, but the measurement of volume delivered over time does not guarantee linearly continuous infusion rates; many syringe drivers actually deliver small, intermittent boluses, though they may exceed the standards for averaged delivery rates. For many drugs this is not of clinical importance, but for those with a short onset and offset of action (such as vasoactive drugs), this will produce significant fluctuations in blood pressure (Figure 3) with potentially serious physiological consequences. Similar effects may arise if there is friction between the rubber flange of the syringe piston and the inner surface of the body of the syringe, and with kinking of the intravenous infusion cannula or delivery tubing.

B. Monitoring Drug Effects

Studies of drug efficacy and safety require clear definitions of therapeutic end points and objective systems of measurement. Some drugs have effects that are relatively easy to detect and to quantify, such as neuromuscular blocking agents [24], but even these may present difficulties in critically ill patients who may have significant muscle wasting or polyneuropathies. Antibiotics are relatively easy to test in the laboratory but more difficult to assess in the context of clinical efficacy. Analgesic and sedative drugs are particularly difficult to assess in crit-

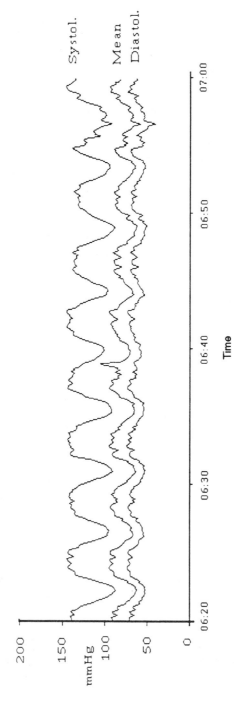

Figure 3 Cyclical variations in arterial pressure plotted against time. This was discovered to be due to the nonlinear delivery of an infusion of noradrenaline (norepinephrine) by a faulty syringe driver. (Unpublished data courtesy of Dr. T. H. Clutton-Brock.)

ically ill patients because they are generally prescribed for intubated patients receiving mechanical ventilation, and the combination of the tracheal tube, septic encephalopathy, and sedation will all impede communication; assessments must be made by observers using scoring systems such as rating scales [25] or linear analog scales [26]. Similarly, postdischarge interviews are limited by the amnesia engendered by drugs and by the impaired cerebral function of critical illness, and one can in any case only interview the survivors.

The high mortality of critical illness makes improvements in survival rates a natural aim of many drug studies but, as the earlier discussion has shown, stratification for severity of illness is essential when mortality is used as an end point. This becomes even more important when there are difficulties in identifying which patient population is likely to benefit from the drug being tested and when the pharmaceutical industry pays investigators for each patient recruited. Monoclonal immunotherapy for sepsis is a good example, whereby the benefits of drug therapy are either modest or unproven, the criteria for patient selection ill defined, and the costs of the drugs (both development and purchase) high. Under these circumstances there may be pressure on investigators to relax the criteria for study entry, thereby biasing results. Conversely, the absence of severity stratification may mean that a genuinely beneficial effect of therapy on survival is obscured. The way to deal with this is to stratify patients on study entry by severity of illness as part of the randomization procedure and then to calculate observed expected mortality ratios for each treatment group.

If demonstrating drug effectiveness is complex, proving its safety is even more so, as the etomidate story shows. The problem is that the end point of interest is the *absence* of demonstrable undesirable effects, and this presupposes a knowledge of what effects may occur, a method for detecting them, and some idea of their incidence so that the investigator can select a sufficient sample size. Physiologically unstable, immunodepressed, critically ill patients receiving large numbers of drugs are not a secure testing ground to determine the absence of side effects of a drug. A high index of suspicion is required of the clinician. The most commonly perceived problems are drug-related hypotension resulting from vasodilatation or a reduction in myocardial contractility, and cutaneous reactions. Skin rashes may be caused by the disease process itself or by many drugs, particularly antibiotics.

III. PATHOPHYSIOLOGY

Multiple organ failure (MOF) typifies intensive care practice but was only described as a clinical entity as recently as 1975 [27]. MOF complicates between 7% and 22% of all emergency operations and up to 50% of all operations for intra-abdominal sepsis. The mortality of the condition varies from 30% to 100%, with a close relationship between the number and duration of organ system failures, and mortality [28]. The pathophysiology of MOF is slowly being unraveled; in outline, a comparatively small number of forms of physiological injury (sepsis, trauma, inflammatory and infective lesions) stimulate a very wide variety of complex intermediary processes, the end results of which are expressed in a limited number of ways as organ system failures. Part of the pathophysiological process involves alterations in regional blood flow and in cellular oxygen delivery as well as changes in cellular function, and this has important implications for drug handling.

A. Hepatic Failure

Liver dysfunction is common in multiple organ failure, manifested as a progressive cholestatic jaundice with modest hepatomegaly that may be a consequence of prolonged sepsis or result from the absence of enteral stimuli for bile drainage. The extent to which liver involvement in MOF contributes to the development of the syndrome is uncertain. In contrast, primary acute hepatic failure, such as following paracetamol poisoning or viral hepatitis, is the direct and inevitable cause of failure of all other organ systems, and without liver transplantation is rapidly fatal in the majority of cases. Acute (fulminant) hepatic failure is a useful model for pharmacokinetic analysis because of the extreme nature of the pathological process, and (in centers that can offer transplantation) it offers the opportunity to explore both the anhepatic period and the effect of a new liver on drug handling.

Drug clearance by the liver depends on the lipid solubility of the drug, hepatic blood flow, and hepatocellular function. Clearance of lipid-soluble drugs is affected primarily by liver blood flow ("flow-limited"). Other substances are dependent more on liver enzymes for their metabolism ("rate-limited") [29]. Liver blood flow has been shown to decrease during anesthesia and surgery [30], sepsis [31], and during mechanical ventilation [32]. The changes in liver blood flow brought about by positive pressure ventilation are sufficiently marked for this to have been proposed as a model of disease states [33]. Hepatocellular function also changes in critical illness. Hypoxia and hepatocellular damage can cause rate-limited drugs to accumulate. Other drugs can depress enzyme activity, such as H-2 blocking agents [34] that are routinely prescribed for the prophylaxis of stress ulceration.

Changes in liver blood flow and hepatocellular function are likely to affect the pharmacokinetics of most drugs [35] and therefore these variables should be measured in pharmacological research in intensive care. The problem is that the methodology is poorly developed. Hepatocellular function is commonly assessed by measuring the serum concentration of enzymes such as alanine transaminase and alkaline phosphatase, and serum bilirubin levels, but the relationship between these tests and the extent of liver damage is weak [36]. The synthetic function of the liver can be estimated by monitoring serum albumin and the prothrombin time, but again these variables are poor predictors of impaired drug clearance [37]. Antipyrine clearance has been used as a measure of hepatocellular function, but this drug actually induces microsomal enzymes and the test is of doubtful value when employed repetitively. The duration of sampling required for the test (up to 48 hr) makes it too cumbersome in critical care practice [38]. Hepatic blood flow can be estimated at the bedside using a modification of the Fick principle applied to indocyanine green (ICG) clearance [39] detected with a dichromatic earpiece densitometer, and this technique has been shown to be a reliable and repeatable noninvasive estimate of liver blood flow [40]. However, marked impairment of hepatocellular function is likely to interfere with ICG clearance, which should therefore be interpreted with caution. Measurements of liver blood flow should be related to the cardiac output estimated at the same time as there is a near-linear relationship between the two [41]. The double blood supply of the liver (hepatic arterial and portal venous) complicates accurate noninvasive measurement of hepatic blood flow and oxygen delivery, though hepatic venous oxygen saturation monitoring has been used as an indirect estimate [42]. Recently, an indirect measure of gut mucosal perfusion has been developed using tonometry [43], and this might have some relevance for hepatic blood flow measurement as part of the assessment of splanchnic perfusion.

B. Renal Failure

In health the kidneys receive 20% of the cardiac output and have the highest blood flow per gram of tissue of any organ in the body. They are therefore at risk from any humoral mediator of MOF, and renal impairment is indeed one of the most common manifestations of this syndrome, giving rise to the associated problem of impaired clearance of certain water-soluble drugs or their metabolites. As with hepatic function, routine tests of renal function, such as creatinine clearance, may be unreliable [44], and this limits the validity of dosage nomograms published by manufacturers. Serum creatinine is used routinely by most clinicians in intensive care as a marker of renal function, but its relation to muscle mass and its nonlinear relationship to creatinine clearance limit its usefulness as an early warning sign of renal impairment. Urinary sodium excretion can help to distinguish the oliguria of normal renal function from that of renal tubular failure only if the patient has not received natriuretic agents; but the majority of critically ill oliguric patients will have been given dopamine or frusemide.

In contrast to liver failure, there are a variety of therapies available to replace the function of failing kidneys. Peritoneal dialysis and intermittent hemodialysis are useful in patients who are physiologically stable or those with limited vascular access; but the former cannot be applied to patients following abdominal surgery, and the latter provides only a few hours of dialysis, may cause undesirable shifts in fluids and circulating volume, and requires the permanent presence of a dialysis nurse. Neither method may be able to cope with the hypercatabolic state of sepsis, and both have tended to be replaced by forms of continous dialysis such as continuous arteriovenous hemodiafiltration (CAVHD) and its many modifications. These techniques have been extensively reviewed elsewhere [45]; in essence the devices consist of hollow-fiber or plate membranes acting as glomeruli, with dialyzate fluid passing against the direction of blood flow. The amount of serum removed is dependent on modifying hydrostatic pressures in the extracorporeal circuit. There is limited information as to how such devices clear drugs [46]. They are most efficient at clearing low molecular weight water-soluble molecules with a small volume of distribution [47]. Solute removal by CAVHD depends on convective clearance by mass transfer across the semipermeable membrane and by diffusion resulting from the osmotic gradient produced by the dialysis fluid. The membrane allows passage of molecules up to a molecular weight of 15,000. Clearance therefore depends on the molecular size, protein binding, electrical charge, plasma flow through the filter, and dialyzate flow across the membrane. Drug clearance is expressed as an extraction ratio that can be calculated from the mean arterial concentration of the drug and the mean filtrate concentration, together with the total filtrate volume from which the sample was taken.

Combined hepatic and renal impairment presents particular challenges for drug assessment. Morphine is metabolized by the liver to morphine-3- and 6-glucuronide, and even the markedly cirrhotic liver retains this capacity; however, the glucuronides are dependent on renal clearance and will accumulate in renal failure. As morphine-6-glucuronide is considerably more potent than morphine [48], significant cerebral and respiratory depression may result from the use of morphine in patients with renal impairment. The phosphodiesterase inhibitor enoximone is metabolized to an active sulfoxide metabolite; hepatic failure will prolong the life of the parent compound, renal failure the life of the metabolite [49], and prolonged vasodilatation may result that is difficult to override.

C. The Lung

The contribution of the lung to drug sequestration and metabolism [50] is largely ignored in clinical practice. It is, however, a significant site for the metabolism of hormones such as noradrenaline (norepinephrine) and the activation of angiotensin, and avidly takes up basic, lipophilic drugs such as fentanyl which it may later release [51,52]. The clinical significance and the effects of pulmonary insufficiency are simply not known. This is surprising as it is relatively easy to measure pulmonary blood flow and to sample blood entering and leaving the pulmonary circuit. Respiratory failure is usually associated with changes in pulmonary blood flow, but there are few studies of the effects on pulmonary drug uptake; lignocaine has been examined, and does not appear to be affected by mechanical ventilation [53], which therapeutic modality may itself affect lung blood flow.

D. Other Organ Systems

Although the liver and kidneys are primarily responsible for drug metabolism and clearance, studies in anhepatic animals [54,55] and humans during the anhepatic phase of liver transplantation [56,57] have demonstrated the existence of extrahepatic sites of metabolism. The enzyme systems important for the biotransformation of drugs have been found in the gut, lung, kidneys, brain, and other tissues [58]. The contribution of these organs to drug metabolism in critically ill patients is largely unknown. One of the main problems preventing the advancement of knowledge in this field is that in the human it is difficult to justify selectively cannulating various organs to measure effluent drug concentrations and regional blood flow; animal models remain an important source of information [59].

IV. PHARMACOKINETICS AND PHARMACODYNAMICS

A. Pharmacokinetics

In affluent countries, critically ill patients tend to be an elderly population [60]. They therefore have reduced volumes of distribution and altered protein binding [61] before being subjected to MOF and organ system support. Furthermore alterations in the volume of distribution in renal, cardiac, and hepatic disease have been documented for some drugs [62,63].

Plasma protein binding influences the volume of distribution and the elimination of many drugs. Hypoalbuminemia is common in critical illness, and as albumin is an important carrier protein and binds many acidic drugs, a reduction in serum albumin may result in an increase in the free fraction of such drugs. It also implies that more of the drug is presented to the liver for extraction and more to the kidney for excretion. Albumin can also alter the way in which it binds drugs in certain pathological processes [64,65], and this may minimize the pharmacodynamic impact of reduced binding. The serum albumin concentration should be recorded during drug research and when possible assays should measure the free (and therefore active) fraction of drug. The acute phase protein α_1-glycoprotein can bind many basic drugs. Concentrations of this protein rise as a response to stress, trauma, and surgery. The clinical consequences of this process for drug kinetics in intensive care have not been determined.

The physiological instability of critical illness has two particular implications for practical pharmacokinetic analysis. First, steady-state conditions may be difficult to attain, either because the drug being studied is a necessary part of therapy and the dose is frequently being adjusted, or because abrupt changes in systemic or regional blood flow alter drug distribution and elimination. Second, patients may die during the study period, and the terminal half-life of the drug cannot be measured. Model-independent calculations should be used to determine clearance and volumes of distribution [66]. Further discussion of this subject can be found in two recent reviews [67,68].

B. Pharmacodynamics

Physiological interactions between drugs are almost inevitable given the extent of necessary polypharmacy and organ system support in intensive care. As an example of the many levels at which pharmacodynamic effects may operate, consider the patient with acute respiratory failure secondary to a pneumonia, and preexisting stable ischemic heart disease, who needs mechanical ventilation. Mechanical ventilation causes a reduction in cardiac output and blood pressure, for which a catecholamine infusion is required. Sedative or analgesic agents prescribed for the patient's comfort aggravate this effect. β-Receptor downregulation develops as a result of myocardial impairment [69] and chronic exposure to the drug [70]. Renal blood flow deteriorates and the sedative drugs accumulate, making assessment of cerebral function difficult by contributing to the encephalopathy of MOF [71]. An H-2 blocking drug is prescribed to minimize the risk of gastric stress ulceration, and the alkaline conditions permit gastric colonization with gram-negative bacteria, which then proceed to colonize the oropharynx and lungs, contributing to the problem of pulmonary sepsis. This is treated with an aminoglycoside antibiotic, which together with sepsis contributes to further renal damage. Renal support with CAVHD is eventually needed, which improves drug clearance. The extracorporeal circuit is prevented from clotting using the platelet-inhibiting effect of a prostacyline infusion, but the associated vasodilatation caused by this drug necessitates the prescription of noradrenaline (norepinephrine) to maintain an adequate systemic pressure. This not uncommon sequence of events demonstrates the difficulty of identifying cause and effect, and may explain why so few drugs have been examined and validated specifically for use in intensive care.

V. CONCLUSION

Throughout the chapter we have tried to describe the "scientific" difficulties that may be encountered when conducting drug research in the ICU. There are many other difficulties of a practical, social, and even emotional nature. It has been suggested that if a drug has a narrow therapeutic range, a clinical effect that is difficult to measure, and no reliable assay, then its use should be avoided in this environment [68]. It is difficult to obtain informed consent from the relatives of a moribund patient and it can be difficult dealing with those relatives throughout the study whatever the clinical outcome. These difficulties must all be addressed as many publications describing drug research in critically ill patients have in fact been conducted in patients with stable single-organ failures or patients who merely require overnight respiratory support following surgery. Such patients bear little relation to those with MOF. The challenge for drug research in intensive care is to develop models and methods that permit more detailed knowledge of both regional and cellular drug handling in critical illness.

REFERENCES

1. Watt I, Ledingham IMcA. Mortality amongst multiple trauma patients admitted to an intensive therapy unit. *Anaesthesia.* 1984;39:973–981.
2. Lambert A, Mitchell R, Frost J, Ratcliffe JG, Robertson WR. Direct in vitro inhibition of adrenal steroidogenesis by etomidate. *Lancet.* 1983;2:1085–1086.
3. Wagner RL, White PF, Kan PB, Rosenthal HH, Feldman D. Inhibition of adrenal steroidogenesis by the anaesthetic etomidate. *N Engl J Med.* 1984;310:1415–1421.
4. Knaus WA, Draper EA, Wagner DP. Prognosis in acute organ system failure. *Ann Surg.* 1985;202:685–693.
5. Bion JF. Severity scoring: principles, methods, and applications. In: Atkinson RS, Adams AP, Eds. *Recent Advances in Anaesthesia and Analgesia.* Vol 17. Edinburgh, UK: Churchill Livingstone; 1992:173–196.
6. Baker SP. O'Neil B, Haddon W. The injury severity score: a method for describing patients with multiple injuries and evaluating emergency care. *Trauma.* 1974; 14:187–196.
7. Knaus WA, Wagner DP, Draper EA, Zimmerman JE. APACHE II: a severity of disease classification. *Crit Care Med.* 1985;13:818–829.
8. Wagner DR, Draper EA, Knaus WA. Development of APACHE III. *Crit Care Med.* 1989;17:s199–s203.
9. Wagner DP, Knaus WA, Draper EA. Physiologic abnormalities and outcome from acute disease. Evidence of a predictable relationship. *Arch Intern Med.* 1986; 146:1389–1396.
10. Cullen DJ. Results and costs of intensive care. *Anesthesiology.* 1977;47:203–216.
11. Knaus WA, Wagner DP, Draper EA. The value of measuring severity of disease in clinical research on critically ill patients. *J Chron Dis.* 1984;37:455–463.
12. Hanley JA, Lippman-Hand A. If nothing goes wrong, is everything all right? Interpreting zero numerators. *JAMA.* 1983;249:1743–1745.
13. Kong KL, Willatts SM, Prys-Roberts C. Isoflurane compared to midazolam for sedation of ventilated patients in the intensive therapy unit. *Br Med J.* 1989;298:1277–1280.
14. Dasta JF, Hale KN, Stauffer GL, Tschampel MM. Comparison of visible and turbidimetric methods for determining short-term compatability of intravenous critical care drugs. *Am J Hosp Pharm.* 1988;45:2361–2368.
15. Halpern NA, Colucci RD, Alicea M, Greenstein R. The compatability of nicardipine hydrochloride with various ICU medications during simulated Y-site injection. *Int J Clin Pharmacol Ther Toxicol.* 1989;27:250–254.
16. Johnson CE, Lloyd CW, Mesaros JL, Rubley GJ. Compatability of aminophylline and verapamil in intravenous admixtures. *Am J Hosp Pharm.* 1989;46:97–100.

17. Perucca E, Grimaldi R, Crema A. Interpreation of drug levels in acute and chronic disease states. *Clin Pharmacokinet*. 1985;10:498–513.
18. Hughes R, Chapple DJ. The pharmacology of atracurium: a new competitive neuromuscular blocking agent. *Br J Anaesth*. 1981;53:31–44.
19. Simmonds R. Determination of atracurium, laudonasine and related compounds. *J Chromatogr*. 1985;343:431–436.
20. McDowall RD. Sample preparation for biomedical analysis. *J Chromatogr*. 1989; 492:3–58.
21. Thompson WL, Feer TD. Incomplete mixing of drugs in intravenous infusions. *Crit Care Med*. 1980;8:603–607.
22. Petty G, Cunningham NL. Insulin adsorption by glass infusion bottles, polyvinyl chloride infusion containers, and intravenous tubing. *Anesthesiology*. 1974;40: 400–404.
23. Cote DD, Torchia MG. Nitroglycerin adsorption to polyvinyl chloride seriously interferes with its clinical use. *Anesth Analg*. 1982;61:541–543.
24. Viby-Mogensen J. Neuromuscular monitoring. In: Miller RD, ed. *Anesthesia*. 3rd ed. New York: Churchill Livingstone; 1990:1209–1226.
25. Ramsay MAE, Savege TH, Simpson BRG, Goodwin R. Controlled sedation with alphaxalone and alphadalone. *Br Med J*. 1974;2:656–659.
26. Bion JF, Chow BFM, Bowden MI. Aims and methods of assessment of sedation in intensive care. *J Drug Dev*. 1991;4(Suppl 3):19–25.
27. Baue A. Multiple, progressive, or sequential systems failure: a syndrome of the 1970s. *Arch Surg*. 1975;110:779–781.
28. Carrico CJ, Meakins JL, Marshall JC, Fry D, Maier RV. Multiple organ failure syndrome. *Arch Surg*. 1986;121:196–208.
29. Wilkinson GHR, Shand DG. A physiological approach to hepatic drug clearance. *Clin Pharmacol Ther*. 1975;18:377–390.
30. Gelman SI. Disturbances in hepatic blood flow during anaesthesia and surgery. *Arch Surg*. 1976;111:881–883.
31. Banks JG, Fowlis AK, Ledingham IMcA, MacSween RNM. Liver function in septic shock. *J Clin Path*. 1982;35:1249–1262.
32. Bonnet F, Richard C, Glaser P, Lafay M, Guesde R. Changes in hepatic blood flow induced by continuous positive pressure ventilation in critically ill patients. *Crit Care Med*. 1982;10:703–705.
33. Perkins MW, Dasta JF, De Haven B, Halpern P, Downs JB. A model to decrease hepatic blood flow and cardiac output with positive pressure breathing. *Clin Pharmacol Ther*. 1989;45:548–552.
34. Dunk AA, Jenkins AK, Burroughs AK, Walt RP, Osuafor TOK, Sherlock S, et al. The effect on the plasma clearance and hepatic extraction of indocyanine green in patients with chronic liver disease. *Br Clin Pharmacol*. 1983;16:117–120.
35. MacNab MSP, Macrae OJ, Guy E, Grant IS, Feely J. Profound reduction in morphine clearance and liver blood flow in shock. *Intensive Care Med*. 1986; 12:366–369.
36. Corless JK, Middleton HM. Normal liver function a basis for understanding hepatic disease. *Arch Intern Med*. 1983;143:2291–2294.

37. Krann J, Jonkman JHE, Koeter GH, Gips CH, De Jong PE, Van Der Mark THW, et al. The pharmacokinetics of theophylline and endprofylline in patients with liver cirrhosis and patients with chronic renal failure. *Eur J Clin Pharmacol.* 1988; 35:357–362.

38. Mirvis L, Buchanan N, Eyberg C. Antipyrine elimination in critically ill patients. *Intensive Care Med.* 1979;5:69–71.

39. Leevy CM, Stein SW, Cherivck GR. Indocyanine green clearance as a test for hepatic function. *JAMA.* 1967;200:148–152.

40. Anderson MN, Kuchiba K. Measurement of acute changes in liver function and blood flow. *Arch Surg.* 1970;100:541–545.

41. Bulkley GB, Oshima A, Bailey RW. Pathophysiology of hepatic ischaemia in cardiogenic shock. *Am J Surg.* 1986;151:87–97.

42. Dahn MS, Lange MP, Jacobs LA. Central mixed and splanchnic venous oxygen saturation monitoring. *Intensive Care Med.* 1988;373–378.

43. Landow L, Phillips DA, Heard SO, Prevost D, Vandersalm TJ, Fink MP. Gastric tonometry and venous oximetry in cardiac surgery patients. *Crit Care Med* 1991;19:1226–1233.

44. Gabriel R. Time to scrap creatinine clearance. *Br Med J.* 1986;293:1119–1120.

45. Sweny P. Haemofiltration and haemodiafiltration: theoretical and practical aspects. *Curr Anaesth Crit Care.* 1991;2:37–43.

46. Maher JF. Pharmacokinetic alterations with renal failure and dialysis. In: Chernow B, ed. *The Pharmacologic Approach to the Critically Ill Patient.* Baltimore: Williams & Wilkins;1988:47–68.

47. Gibson TP, Nelson HA. Drug kinetics and artificial kidneys. *Clin Pharmacokine.* 1977;2:403–426.

48. Shimomura K, Kamata O, Ueki S, Ida S, Oguri K, Yoshimura H, et al. Analgesic effects of morphine glucuronides. *Tohoku Exp Med.* 1971;105:45–52.

49. Okerholm RA, Chan KY, Lang JF, et al. Biotransformation and pharmacokinetic overview of enoximone and its sulphoxide metabolite. *Am J Pharmacol.* 1987;60:21C–26C.

50. Hook GER. The metabolic potential of the lungs. In: George, Shands, eds. *Presystemic Drug Elimination.* London: Butterworths Scientific;1982:117–146.

51. Roerig DL, Kortly KJ, Vucins EJ, Ahlf SB, Dawson CA. First pass uptake of fentanyl, meperidine and morphine in the human lung. *Anesthesiology.* 1987; 67:466–472.

52. Boer F, Bovill JG, Burm AGL, Mooren RAG. Uptake of sufentanil, alfentanil and morphine in the lungs of patients about to undergo coronary artery surgery. *Br J Anaesth.* 1992;68:370–375.

53. Jorfeldt L, Lewis DH, Lolfstrom B, Post C. Lung uptake of lidocaine in man as influenced by anaesthetics, mepivicaine infusion or lung insufficiency. *Acta Anaesth Scand.* 1983;27:5–9.

54. Hug CC Jr, Murphy MR, Sampson JF, Terblanche J, Aldrete JA. Biotransformation of morphine and fentanyl in anhepatic dogs. *Anesthesiology.* 1981;55:A261.

55. Gerkens JF, Desmond PV, Branch RA. Hepatic and anhepatic glucuronidation of lorazepam in the dog. *Hepatology.* 1981;1:329–335.

56. Park GR, Manara AR, Dawling S. Extrahepatic metabolism of midazolam. *Br J Clin Pharmacol.* 1989;27:634–637.
57. Bodenham A, Quinn K, Park GR. Extrahepatic morphine metabolism in man during the anhepatic phase of orthotopic liver transplantations. *Br J Anaesth.* 1989;63: 380–384.
58. Rawlins MD. Extrahepatic drug metabolism. In: Wilkinson GR, Rawlins MD, eds. *Drug Metabolism and Distribution: Considerations in Clinical Pharmacology.* Lancaster, UK: MPT Press;1985:21–33.
59. Runciman WBH, Ilsley AH, Mather LE, Carapetis RJ, Mao MM. A sheep preparation for studying the interactions between blood flow and drug disposition: I. Physiological profile. *Br J Anaesth.* 1984;57:1239–1245.
60. Knaus WA. Too sick and too old for intensive care. *Br J Hosp Med.* 1987;37:381.
61. Richey DP, Bender AD. Pharmacokinetic consequences of ageing. *Ann Rev Pharmacol Toxicol.* 1979;17:49–54.
62. Thomson PD, Melmon KL, Richardson JA, Cohn K, Steinbrunn W, Cudihee R, et al. Lidocaine pharmacokinetics in advanced heart failure, liver disease, and renal failure in humans. *Ann Intern Med.* 1973;78:499–508.
63. Klotz U. Pathophysiologic and disease-induced changes in drug distribution volume: pharmacokinetic implications. *Clin Pharmacokinet.* 1976;1:204–218.
64. Koch-Weser J, Sellers EM. Binding of drugs to serum albumin. *N Engl J Med.* 1976;294:311–316, 526–531.
65. Piafsky KM. Disease-induced changes in plasma binding of basic drugs. *Clin Pharmacokinet.* 1980;5:246–262.
66. Benet LZ, Galeazzi RL. Non-compartmental determination of the steady-state volume of distribution. *J Pharm Sci.* 1979;68:1071–1074.
67. Bodenham A, Shelly MP, Park GR. The altered pharmacokinetics and pharmacodynamics of drugs commonly used in critically ill patients. *Clin Pharmacokinet.* 1988;14:347–373.
68. Runciman WB, Myburgh JA, Upton RN. Pharmacokinetics and pharmacodynamics in the critically ill. In: Dobb GJ, ed. *Intensive Care: Developments and Controversies.* Ballieres Clinical Anaesthesiology International Practice and Research. Vol 4. 1990:271–304.
69. Ruffolo RR. Cardiovascular adrenoreceptors; physiology and critical care implications. In: Chernow B, ed. *The Pharmacological Approach to the Critically Ill Patient.* Baltimore: Williams & Wilkins; 1988:166–183.
70. Unverferth DV, Blandford M, Kates RE. Tolerance to dobutamine after 72 hours infusion. *Am J Med.* 1982;69:262–266.
71. Bion JF, Logan BK, Newman PM, Brodie MJ. Sedation in intensive care: morphine and renal function. *Intensive Care Med.* 1986;12:359–365.

6

Laboratory Data in Multicenter Trials: Monitoring, Adjustment, and Summarization

Lawrence K. Oliver and Christy Chuang-Stein

The Upjohn Company
Kalamazoo, Michigan

I. INTRODUCTION

Lab specimens are routinely collected and assayed in clinical trials to ensure that patients are not experiencing untoward toxicities. Lab results are by far the best indicators of systemic toxicities and provide vital information regarding a patient's safety. The importance of such data is demonstrated by their conspicuous role in all clinical trials. Clinical interpretation of lab results is commonly done by utilization of a reference range (once called the normal range, a term that fortunately has fallen into disfavor because of its misleading connotations). The interpretation is typically conducted with the clinical understanding that a reference range defines a region of lab results within which the likelihood of there being a biochemical abnormality in the patient is relatively small. This concept arose from the need to identify *diagnostically* useful labs. The evaluation of lab abnormalities with the use of reference ranges is illustrated and exemplified in Ref. 1 and discussed by Sogliero-Gilbert, Zubkoff-Schulz, and Ting in Chapter 7 of this book.

Multicenter clinical trials are typically used in the phase III development of an investigational drug, even though the heavy emphasis on expediting the drug development process has also led to an increase in the use of multiple centers for late phase II dose–response studies in recent years. There are many reasons to use multiple centers in a trial to confirm or refute a conjecture. First, the required sample size for a randomized phase III or late phase II trial is usually high, making it impossible for a single center to recruit the necessary number of patients in a timely fashion. In addition to the time factor, a multicenter trial generally produces results that are applicable to a wider patient population because the results are less likely to be confounded with the characteristics unique to a particular center [2]. These are some of the advantages of conducting a trial at multiple sites. The disadvantages of multicenter trials include a more complex study design and a more elaborate analysis strategy. In addition, there are issues such as protocol compliance, comparable patient care, and uniform data collection that need to be addressed. The concern with the uniformity of data collection is the greatest with lab data generated at the various study sites. Despite the recent attempt to utilize a centralized laboratory for multicenter trials, using a centralized laboratory is not always possible, especially when a trial is conducted under the auspices of a cooperative group. Individual investigators in a cooperative group are generally allowed to use or choose their own laboratories. Because laboratories frequently use different equipment and assay procedures, they rely on their own reference ranges for interpretation and there is the belief that as long as the clinical interpretation of lab results is done using the lab-specific references ranges, the interpretation is sound. We will argue later in this chapter that there are at least two basic problems with this concept. First, most of the laboratories participating in a clinical trial use assays intended for diagnostic evaluations of a disease state, and not for the continued assurance of a preexisting status of a patient's biochemistry. Second, there is no universal definition for the reference population and the method to determine the reference range. Although there has been some recent effort to revisit the issue of constructing reference ranges (e.g., see Ref. 3), the consensus does not exist and no one single method has been accepted universally. Besides the mathematical algorithms involved, it is not unusual to find that the reference population chosen by a laboratory depends on the lab site's typical demographic makeup. The heterogeneity in the selection of the reference population and the method to construct a reference range alluded to in Section II casts some doubt on the usefulness of the reference ranges as they are currently being provided.

In addition to evaluating lab abnormality in a clinical trial, we routinely look at the changes in the lab values from their respective baselines and frequently construct statistics for inferential purposes. This inevitably leads to the pooling of data from different laboratories. The validity of the inference based on the data pooled from different laboratories can be in jeopardy when different laboratories produce very different results due to either procedural or methodological differences. Chuang-Stein [4] proposed a method to pool data from different sites. Her procedure basically calls for first standardizing lab values with respect to their reference ranges, computing inferential statistics using the standardized values, and restoring the units at the end. The procedure is based on the premise that reference ranges are sound markers and that data are fundamentally poolable.

One should ask the question of just how reasonable this premise is considering our earlier comments on the reference ranges in general.

In this chapter, we will discuss issues and mysteries concerning reference ranges. We will propose a way to conduct interlab comparisons that does not use reference ranges. We will also propose a method to adjust lab results from different laboratories for statistical summarization. Furthermore, we will comment on how the adjusted lab values can be used to construct protocol-specific reference ranges that take into consideration the underlying disease presentation. As a result, the study-specific reference ranges are more relevant to the target patient population insofar as clinical trials are concerned.

II. REFERENCE RANGES

A. Analytical Variables in the Definition of a Reference Range

All properly validated lab assays meet numerous criteria. The ones that are of importance to our discussion are as follows:

They give results that are linear over a specified range of values (dilutions of the specimen give results that are in proportion to the dilution).

They can be controlled such that results on the same sample have a known variability over time (precision).

They have a defined analytical sensitivity (limits of detection).

Although analytical accuracy is preferred for obvious reasons, it is an ill-defined target even for such common analytes as cholesterol for which no universally accepted set of reference standards exist. (For a more complete description of acceptable performance of clinical lab procedures, the reader is referred to the documents produced by the National Committee for Clinical Laboratory Standards.) When setting up an assay, a laboratory must take into account the clinical intentions of its users, optimize the analytical procedure, and select the operating characteristics appropriately. The key factor in the selection of operating characteristics is the clinical decision points. A laboratory will balance the reagents in such a way that the resulting biochemistry is the most precise (has the least imprecision) at or near the points where clinical decisions are to be made. The latter are usually the upper and lower ends of the reference population range. In other words, precision obtained in an assay outside the reference range is of less importance when the assay is used primarily for the diagnostic purpose. The prime consideration is to confidently identify a result as clinically abnormal. On the other hand, a clinical trial laboratory has to follow a different set of criteria because it is rarely in the diagnostic business. Clinical trial laboratories must optimize precision in the ranges appropriate for making decisions that are relevant to the objectives of the clinical trials. For example, the optimum monitoring of the activity of a drug or its efficacy in a patient population requires that precision of the results outside the reference range be as or more important than that at the upper and lower ends of the range. A common example is insulin and C-peptide levels that are used for assessing the performance of antidiabetic medications.

Ideally, a clinical trial laboratory should develop its assays according to the criteria pertinent to the clinical trials. However, the laboratory is often limited to usage of existing reagents and kits, for which the operating characteristics are set by the manufacturer. In contrast, multicenter trials are often conducted at sites where a clinical specialty is practiced and an in-house method developed for that specialty may be in place. Therefore, one should allow for such differences in analytical validation when conducting interlab comparisons.

B. Clinical Considerations in the Definition of a Reference Range

Using a lab test diagnostically requires that the clinician have a high degree of confidence that his or her interpretation of the results vis-à-vis the quoted reference range could identify the actions needed to complete the diagnosis or initiate a treatment. Unfortunately, the analyte level for many disease entities is very close to, or even overlaps, the range of values observed in a normal healthy population. In other words, a level that is consistent with a nondisease state for one person may be indicative of existing disease in another. The evaluation of thyroid function is a good example of this phenomenon. A histogram of results for T4 from a healthy population will extend up to 12–14 mcg/dl, whereas a similar histogram from a population of patients known to be suffering from hyperthyroidism can have results as low as 9–10 mcg/dl.

The definition of the upper limit of a reference range is thus determined by the clinical sensitivity and specificity one wishes to obtain. The cutoff point selected is a matter of probability: *what degree of confidence does one want that a result outside the reference range is indeed abnormal* (sensitivity)? If one's goal is to identify the maximum number of hyperthyroid patients, the upper limit is placed low. However, a low upper limit will result in the inclusion of a number of false-positive cases, i.e., people who are outside the range but do not have the disease. The other end of the diagnostic spectrum is to set the upper limit high so that one can have a high degree of confidence that a result outside the range does indeed identify a diseased patient. In the first case, a clinical sensitivity is high while clinical specificity is low, and in the second case the opposite is true. Which approach to select is a function of a laboratory's clientele since a general practitioner's patient population is considerably different from that coming to a tertiary care hospital. The reference range limits will therefore be different, even if the analytical procedures are identical.

C. Mathematical Differences in the Definition of a Reference Range

The usual definition of a reference range is the 95% limits obtained by excluding 2.5% of the nondiseased population at each end of the range. The choice of the 95% limits is not universal, however, and neither is the method to determine the cutoff points. It is beyond the scope of this chapter to detail the different approaches and their pros and cons, but we will illustrate a variety of current practices to caution the readers against making unwarranted assumptions about the meaning of the 95% limits.

A long-used and common approach is the simplistic one of analyzing 40 laboratory or hospital employees who are self-diagnosed as healthy, excluding the highest and the lowest result and calling the remainder the 95% limits on the range. (Note that the top and the bottom constitute 5% of the 40 lab results.) Variations of this method include assaying 40 individuals of each sex, grouping individuals into different age intervals, or assaying a large number of subjects. When the number of subjects gets higher, the construction of the 95% limits is usually based on the method to construct a 95% confidence interval using the normal approximation if the data look "reasonably" normally distributed. In other words, one would first compute the sample mean and the sample standard deviation. One would then set the 95% limits as 2 SD below and above the mean. On the other hand, if the data look "skewed," one would chop off 2.5% at each end of the data ordered from the smallest to the highest.

One can increase the utility of the 95% limits by including a more complete assessment of a subject's health such as a questionnaire on the medical history of the subject and/or a physical exam. Unfortunately, the cost of a reference range determined this way increases quite rapidly and becomes prohibitive in terms of time and money for many laboratories even though the approach seems logical. When a commercially available kit is used, it is a common practice to adopt the manufacturer's range without regard to the population that the manufacturer used to determine the range.

Other methods of determining the 95% limits include the use of the Battacharya plot [5], a technique that is more common in Europe. This plot is often applied when there is tailing at one end or the other.

The application of more sophisticated techniques begins with the recognition that the population of results associated with an assay rarely follows a normal distribution and the use of the normal approximation in constructing 95% limits is only applicable after the data are properly transformed. Among the possible choices, logarithmic transformation is the most commonly used. Unfortunately, a laboratory often does not have the access or the time to consult someone on the proper transformation necessary to employ the normal approximation.

It should be apparent by now that different clinical and mathematical considerations can lead to different sets of 95% limits even if one starts with the same set of lab results. The point that we want to drive home is that *all the above approaches are in use and there is no accepted set of guidelines for defining a reference population or mathematically deriving the reference range from a set of obtained results.*

III. INTERLAB COMPARISONS

A. Adjustment or Normalization of Lab Data

The conversion of U.S. laboratories to the use of SI (Systéme Internationale) units has created a widespread belief that many or all of the interlab comparisons will be made simpler. Many people even think that the problem of interlab differences can be solved by use of a common system of units. To a certain extent, there is some truth in that belief if one confines the discussion to small molecules of a clearly defined and stable structure, and restricts the comparisons to methodologies utilizing similar chemistry. In other words, if various laboratories measure the same biological component (exactly) using procedures with comparable analytical sensitivity and specificity, then the application of a common set of units may be all that is needed to make clinically relevant comparisons across laboratories. These assumptions must be verified for other common but more complex analytes such as enzymes where even the reaction temperature is not standardized. The assumptions break down completely for protein hormones such as prolactin or angiotensin II when analyte recognition is based on immunological recognition.

Given that the first step in making interlab comparisons is to convert all data to a common set of units and that this has been accomplished, one is still left with the task of combining data from disparate laboratories in order to conduct statistical analysis for inferential purposes. A number of approaches have been proposed in the literature to accomplish this task. The most commonly used ones are those based on reference ranges. As we discussed before, approaches based on reference ranges suffer from the weaknesses that reference ranges are not consistently determined and that methodological differences do exist and can be significant at times. The bottom line is that the assumptions underlying those approaches based on reference ranges are frequently not true. As a result, using reference ranges as a basis for interlab comparisons and data standardization can be misleading and an alternative approach ought to be sought.

B. Interlab Comparisons Through Proficiency Surveys

Interlab comparisons of results require a common set of specimens to be analyzed by all laboratories under comparison. Proficiency testing programs mandated by the Clinical Laboratory Improvement Act of 1988 (CLIA 88) [6] provides the opportunity for exactly such a comparison.

Proficiency surveys are intended to serve as a means to identify aberrant lab performance by having all enrolled laboratories analyze a common set of specimens. The specimens are prepared under conditions that maximize the chance that the specimens will be identical from laboratory to laboratory. While some differences exist between survey sponsors, a typical approach is to have all laboratories send their results on the specimens to one coordinating center. The results are collated and sorted by methodology for an "apples-to-apples" comparison. Mean and standard deviation within each group defined by the assay methodology are calculated for each specimen. A lab's performance is determined by taking the difference between their result and the group mean and dividing it by the corresponding group standard deviation on the same specimen. This ratio is called the standard deviation index (SDI). Within a group, outliers are determined by the usual statistical methods with an acceptable performance defined as within 2 SD of the group mean. The test samples are sent to individual laboratories several times a year with multiple samples each time, so that numerous data points on each assay can be gathered each year. The testing programs cover virtually all lab procedures that have a proven diagnostic utility. The laboratories are, under CLIA 88, required to run the test samples in the same manner as they analyze patient specimens to ensure that the proficiency testing gives a true picture of the performance expected of the laboratories when they run samples for clinical interpretations.

While individual lab results are sent only to the participating laboratories as well as the state and federal agencies that regulate them, all results at the group level are made available to each participating laboratory. As mentioned earlier, these results are classified by methodology and separate means and standard deviations are given for each sample specimen. Thus, one can compare methodologies and determine the expected difference between any two methodologies based on the corresponding two sets of group statistics.

The use of the group results from proficiency surveys provides an objective way to compare the relative accuracy of the methods used by different laboratories. Bias and linearity can be determined from the results collected over time. Interlab differences in precision cannot be estimated from the group results and are only poorly estimated from an individual lab's results on the samples. A laboratory's internal quality control results (obtainable directly from the laboratory) must be used for that determination.

The preparation of samples that are presumably equivalent for all sites to run is of course a formidable task and the technology to accomplish that goal is difficult to control. While the agencies in charge of a proficiency testing program do a superb job of maintaining consistency, there are instances when a set of samples do not behave linearly for all procedures. However, this usually takes place when new analytical methodologies or new kits are entering the market. The latter situation is often corrected by the kit or reagent manufacturer within a relatively short period of time. Nevertheless, when evaluating interlab comparisons using proficiency testing results on newly introduced kits, one should check linearity by comparing the group means at different levels of analyte. If the ratio of the group means on the same sample (see Section IV.B.2 below) is not relatively constant from sample to sample, then the assay may not be linear.

An individual pharmaceutical company can apply the principles underlying a proficiency survey to perform a split-sample comparison itself. In doing so, care should be exerted to ensure homogeneity in specimens and in the shipping and handling conditions. Unfortunately, the complexities and time-consuming nature of specimen preparation, data collection, and summarization usually prohibit such an undertaking.

The advantage of using proficiency testing results from established surveys of interlab comparisons comes from the fact that comparisons are performed on the basis of comparable (or identical) methodologies applied to the same set of specimens. Use of proficiency testing results avoids the problems associated with no common definition for a reference population, no single method to calculate the ranges, and the absence of adequate assurance that the reference ranges provided are current. In addition, we will illustrate in the next section that proficiency testing results even provide a way to adjust lab results from different sites, which in turn facilitates statistical analysis.

Before proceeding to the next section, we want to emphasize one point. When complex analytes such as protein hormones or variably glycosylated species are being analyzed, the exact nature of the species being measured has a great deal of variability from one method to another. The specificity of the recognition system used (e.g., the antibody used in immunological assays) will determine the component being assayed. In addition, variations in seemingly similar reagents from various manufacturers will give widely disparate results. The differences are usually magnified in disease situations. In those cases, only an in-depth evaluation of the methods and reagents used can give an assessment of the comparability of the results obtained.

IV. A PROPOSAL TO ADJUST LAB DATA FROM DIFFERENT SITES

In this section we propose a method to adjust lab data from different sites using a two-stage procedure. The adjustment procedure is based on the proficiency testing results. The purpose of the adjustment is to make the data from different sites more "comparable" so that statistical summarization and analysis can be conducted by pooling data across sites.

A. Choice of a Reference Procedure

For a multicenter study, one needs to first choose a reference procedure for each analyte. This procedure can be the methodology employed at the principal site or a methodology in use at several sites to reduce the amount of adjustment necessary. One should also give consideration to selecting a methodology that is likely to be in use for an extended period of time to facilitate comparisons throughout the lifetime of the drug being studied.

B. Two-Stage Adjustment Procedure

Laboratories that intend to participate in a multicenter study will be asked to submit the following documents:

A copy of their standard operating procedure (SOP) for each procedure
Proficiency testing results for the most recent 1-year period
Internal quality control data for the immediately preceding 6 months

The first two documents define the methodology and confirm that the analyte being measured and the procedure employed can be properly referenced to the proficiency testing results. The third document is to verify the precision of a lab procedure. Once the above documents are obtained, we can adjust the lab results relative to the reference procedure using a two-stage procedure described below.

1. Within-Group Adjustment

The first stage consists of a within-group adjustment. To conduct the within-group adjustment, we require that the SDIs pertaining to the methodology for an analyte at a laboratory be available for the most recent 1-year period. Along with each SDI, we record the standard deviation calculated for the corresponding group. For example, suppose that the SDIs for bilirubin (total, mg/dl) for a laboratory from the most recent 1-year proficiency surveys are {0.5, −0.7, 0.6, 0.2, −0.5, 0.8, 0.3, −0.4, −0.5, 0.3, 1.0, −0.3} and that the standard deviations for the group for the same survey period are {0.11, 0.17, 0.10, 0.19, 0.11, 0.20, 0.13, 0.11, 0.13, 0.12, 0.10, 0.15 mg/dl}. The median SDI is 0.25 and the median group standard deviation is 0.125 mg/dl. We propose to adjust a bilirubin (total) value from this laboratory by the following formula:

New value = old value − (0.25 × 0.125)

In other words, we adjust the bilirubin (total) value relative to the group mean with an amount suggested by the pattern in the SDIs. If a laboratory tends to have positive SDI values (suggesting higher-than-group-mean values for most test specimens) for an assay, a lab value for the same assay from such a laboratory will be adjusted downward. On the other hand, if the laboratory tends to have negative SDI values (suggesting lower-than-group-mean values for most test specimens) for an analyte, a corresponding lab value will be adjusted upward. If the laboratory has a zero median SDI, this will result in no within-group adjustment because the laboratory does not demonstrate any consistent pattern of departure from the corresponding group mean.

The general formula to conduct the within-group adjustment is

New value = old value − median {SDI} × median {group standard deviation}

Thus, a bilirubin (total) of 0.9 mg/dl from the lab mentioned above will have an adjusted value of 0.9 − (0.25) × (0.125) = 0.87 after the within-group adjustment. The adjustment does not have much effect on the initial bilirubin (total) value in this case because the median SDI is 0.25, which does not suggest much deviation from the group's average performance.

2. Between-Group Adjustment

The second-stage adjustment concerns the between-group differences. In this stage, we will first compute the ratio of a group mean for each sample to the corresponding mean of the reference procedure (see Section IV.A) using results from the most recent 1-year period. Denote the group representing the reference procedure for an analyte by G_R and assume that we are to adjust lab values obtained using the procedure defining the group G. The means for group G_R and group G for each sample are available to all participating laboratories. We can compute the ratio (group mean of G)/(group mean of G_R) for each sample. Since the mean for each group is typically based on more than 20 laboratories, the ratio is relatively stable. Denote the median of these ratios from the most recent 1-year period by R. We propose to adjust the value obtained from the first stage by

Second-stage adjusted value = (first-stage adjusted value) × $\frac{1}{R}$

In other words, the value adjusted for within-group difference in the first stage is further adjusted by a multiplier of $1/R$. Thus, if one procedure produces values higher than the reference procedure because of the differences in the two procedures, lab values obtained under the former will be adjusted downward by a factor that reflects the relative size of the mean results pertaining to these two procedures.

For example, suppose that the median ratio between the group mean of a procedure and that of the reference procedure from the most recent 1-year period is 0.75 in our bilirubin (total) example, then a bilirubin (total) value of 0.9 mg/dl will be first adjusted according to the rule specified in Section IV.A.1 to 0.87 mg/dl and then adjusted for between-group difference to be 0.87(1/0.75) = 1.16 mg/dl.

One might question the choice of the 1-year data to carry out the adjustment. It is true that a better estimate for the median can be obtained with more data. Nevertheless, since we are dealing with medians that are generally calculated based on approximately 15 figures (4–5 samples per survey and about 4 surveys per year), we feel that 1-year data are adequate for the adjustment without undue burden to the laboratories.

V. SUMMARIZATION OF LAB DATA

Once lab values are adjusted according to the procedure specified in the previous section, one can proceed with the routine summarization using the adjusted values. For example, one can compute the mean, median, standard error of the mean, minimum, maximum, and range in the usual way. Furthermore, one can carry out hypothesis testing and conduct other statistical analyses.

In addition to the above summary statistics, individual patient results should be rechecked to identify outliers. This consists of reevaluating those flagged as abnormal by the ranges supplied by the participating laboratories and examining those which are at the extreme ends of the combined data for the pretreatment evaluations. A clinical determination needs to be made as to whether or not those identified in the above should be treated as clinically abnormal.

VI. COMMENTS

In this chapter, we stress the importance of comparing lab data from different laboratories in multicenter clinical trials. We dismiss the notion that one can simply rely on the reference ranges provided by the participating laboratories for toxicity evaluation and data analyses. Instead, we propose to monitor the performance of the laboratories using their results from proficiency surveys. Not only can the proficiency survey results provide us with a method to adjust the lab data, but the knowledge of such results can give us a higher degree of confidence (or no confidence) in the lab data, which in some instances are the primary end points such as in trials of cholesterol-reducing agents or regimens for diabetes. Since so much clinical interpretation relies on lab data, we feel it vitally important that results from the quality control programs at the national as well as the individual laboratory levels be utilized to help monitor the quality of the data generated by laboratories that participate in a research program like the development of a new drug or treatment entity.

The acquisition of proficiency survey results from laboratories that intend to participate in a trial might be a delicate issue. It is possible that some laboratories could regard such information as internal and be reluctant to supply such information to a research program. It is our conjecture that laboratories which have a good quality control record will be proud to share their survey results, which can only add to their credibility. On the other hand, laboratories that refuse to supply their survey results might have problems with their lab procedures and therefore are the ones that a research program should probably avoid anyway. In the latter case, a research program sponsor should arrange to have the specimens collected at the site in question shipped to a different laboratory for processing.

It is true that to monitor laboratories for their comparative performance requires some effort on the part of a research program sponsor. In our opinion, such effort will pay off in the long run because the sponsor will have control over what they will get from the laboratories. Considering the amount of effort needed to start a clinical trial and the amount of time spent on collecting the specimens for processing, one should ask only for *quality* data. In addition, once one has established the relative performance of a laboratory, the effort in the future studies that utilize the same laboratory will be minimum because one only needs to update the available information with respect to the most recent survey results. Since a research program tends to use the same investigators and therefore the same laboratories, the effort to monitor the laboratories can be much less than it appears to be.

If lab results are adjusted according to the proposed approach, concerns discussed in Section II in relation to the definition of a reference range largely disappear. In addition, the inclusion/exclusion criteria in the protocol for a multicenter study define a reference population. A set of study-specific reference ranges can be calculated based on the adjusted lab data obtained prior to treatment. For example, one can compute the 95% limits using the normal approximation if the combined adjusted lab data appear to follow a normal distribution, or one can simply chop off the top and bottom 2.5% of the adjusted data. The reference range thus constructed is only for the underlying study with a reference population defined by the inclusion/exclusion criteria specified in the protocol. The study-specific reference ranges can be used to evaluate the post-treatment lab results for treatment-related clinical toxicity. These reference ranges are more relevant in monitoring treatment-related lab toxicity because they take into account patients' disease presentation prior to the treatment.

Undoubtedly, there are other ways to adjust lab values using results from the proficiency surveys. In this chapter, we propose a simple method based on the median statistics. The advantage of the median statistics is that they are easy to compute and are relatively robust to outliers.

There are occasions whereby even with the adjustment proposed in this paper lab data are still considered not poolable due to the very nature of the assays and the methodology. The decision on whether lab data are fundamentally poolable or not is a scientific, and at times a difficult, one. The decision has to be made by individuals who are familiar with lab procedures and lab methodologies.

REFERENCES

1. Sogliero-Gilbert G, Mosher K, Zubkoff L. A procedure for the simplification and assessment of lab parameters in clinical trials. *Drug Inform J.* 1986;20:279–296.

2. Fleiss JL. Analysis of data from multiclinic trials. *Controlled Clin Trials*. 1986; 7:267–275.
3. Roystom P, Matthews JNS. Estimation of reference ranges from normal samples. *Stat Med*. 1991;10:691–695.
4. Chuang-Stein, C. Summarizing laboratory data with different reference ranges in multi-center clinical trials. *Drug Inform J*. 1992;26:77–84.
5. Hemel JB, Hindriks FR, van der Slik W. Critical discussion on a method for derivation of reference units in clinical chemistry from a patient population. *J Aut Chem*. 1985;7(1):20–30.
6. *Federal Register* 1992; 57(40):7002–7288.

7

The Genie Score:
A Multivariate Assessment of Laboratory Abnormalities

Gene Sogliero-Gilbert, Lonni Zubkoff-Schulz, and Naitee Ting

Pfizer Inc.
Groton, Connecticut

I. INTRODUCTION

One important aspect of statistical science is *data compression*. Statisticians perform data compression all the time. For example, a sample mean of *n* observations is a compression of *n* data points into a single statistic; a simple linear regression compresses many pairs of data down to a simple mathematical expression; other examples include multivariate techniques, meta-analysis, etc. We do not attempt to define the term data compression here. However, we want to illustrate the importance of this idea and apply it to the assessment of lab abnormality in clinical trials.

In this chapter we introduce the Genie Score as an application of data compression. The purpose of the Genie Score is to help identify and assess lab abnormalities in clinical trials. The procedure is to first compress each measurement together with the upper and lower reference ranges associated with this measurement into a percentage expression, then to compress several such percentages into a function group, and then further compress it into other forms.

Looking ahead, the need for data compression is increasing. T.A. Lewis [1] had a good discussion about this need in his article. Even though his article appeared in *Challenges for the '90s*, most of his arguments can be applied to fields other than just biometrics. We feel that as long as data collection persists (either data from controlled experiments, sample survey, market research, or other resources), the need for data compression will be tremendous.

A. Data Collection in Clinical Trials

During the course of a year, most of the large pharmaceutical companies have several drugs that are under development in clinical trials. Each trial is governed by a protocol that states the purpose of the study, the design in use, the indication under investigation, the drugs and dosing required, the duration of therapy, the type of patients that are appropriate, and many other topics that for the investigators explain how the study is to be run and for multicenter trials ensure a degree of uniformity that enables the results to be combined across centers.

Accompanying each protocol is a case report form (CRF) that has been specifically prepared for that protocol in order to capture the essential measurements and information that enables the clinical researchers to interpret and analyze the data.

At a minimum, a CRF will have information collected at baseline, during therapy, and at the end of therapy. Baseline information will usually include demographic and diagnostic information, previous medicines used, previous illnesses, factors predisposing the patient to the illness being studied, as well as a host of baseline tests that establish the start of efficacy and safety needed to perform subsequent analyses. As the trial progresses, these same tests will be performed as many times as specified in the protocol. At the end of therapy, a final assessment will be made by the investigator as to the safety and effectiveness of the drugs being studied.

When all the data contained in the CRF have been checked for errors, they are entered into the sponsor's database. The statistician then prepares and analyzes the data. The results are then reviewed by the clinical researchers and given medical interpretation. The investigators and sponsors then come to an agreement on the outcome of the study.

B. The Need for Data Compression in Clinical Trials

For single-dose studies, such as might occur in anti-infective drug trials, analgesic studies, and so forth, the number of pages in the CRF might be as few as 10, but such studies are not the rule. Most short-term studies (from 2 weeks to 6 months) would have 20–30 pages per CRF per patient, while long-term studies for chronic diseases could have CRFs of 300 pages or more for each patient.

Consider, for example, a large multicenter trial for the equivalence of two antiarthritic drugs. Such equivalence studies usually require several hundred patients to show adequate power. Each patient might be followed for 5 years for a total of 30 visits. At the end of the study, the case report form will contain 300 pages for each patient who completes therapy. So for this study alone, 120,000 pages of data must be entered into the database for analysis.

All of this background has been presented to prepare the reader for an appreciation of the enormous quantities of data that must be summarized, analyzed, and interpreted in order to determine if a test drug has a therapeutic effect on a patient and if the drug was successfully tolerated.

Safety data is the term used for the collection of adverse event data and the measurement of lab values. At every visit patients are queried about side effects they may have experienced since their last visit, and at every visit a new battery of lab tests is done on samples of blood and urine and sometimes other body fluids.

Tracking and noting the occurrences of unwanted side effects while receiving an experimental drug is a necessary and important component of drug safety assessment, but it is not the topic of this chapter. Here we will focus on lab parameters and their role in drug safety assessment.

In the example mentioned above (the antiarthritic study), at the end of the trial there would be more than 12,000 pages of lab data. Each page would have up to 120 lab test values recorded along with the reference ranges and the units, giving a total of 480 items of information per page. In a more typical situation, relevant to most other studies, measurements would be taken on 20–50 parameters per visit.

While it is true that extremely abnormal lab values are flagged by the lab doing the assays, over a year's time with such a large number of patients to monitor, it is obvious that only the most extreme problems would be noted. For the study as a whole, there is no objective way to quantify the abnormalities within the treatment group or to compare them between different treatment groups.

Until the development of the Genie Score, the lab parameters did not lend themselves *easily* to analysis or summarization. With the creation of the Genie Score, the monitoring of lab data over whole studies and the summarization and comparison of lab parameters between treatment groups became a reality. The subsequent sections in this chapter will explain how this can be done via the Genie Score.

II. THE GENIE SCORE CONCEPT

A. What Is the Genie Score?

Monitoring of lab parameters as part of all clinical trials for the safety assessment of a new drug is of paramount importance to the sponsor company and the U.S. Food and Drug Administration (FDA). This monitoring is data-intensive, since it requires knowledge of all lab abnormalities encountered by any patient during the course of therapy, and it is review-intensive in that these abnormalities must be judged as to whether they were due to the drug being administered or not. Complicating this process is the fact that there are many lab parameters being measured by many different laboratories, each with its own set of reference ranges and units of measurement.

The measured parameter alone conveys little information unless it is accompanied by the "reference range." Each laboratory establishes its own set of values called the "upper limit of reference range" (UL) and the "lower limit of reference range" (LL), for each lab test. These limits are intended to encompass about 95% of the values that would result from measuring a population of healthy people. What exactly is a "healthy" person? How do the labs establish their reference ranges?

Each of these questions could be answered in several ways and could require a chapter or more to discuss, but it is not our intention to do so here. We will accept as a given that each laboratory has developed a reasonable set of reference ranges for the parameters being assayed. All abnormal values are determined by noting whether the measured value is outside the reference range. A value two or three times higher than the UL is usually a clinically significant abnormality, whereas a value that is 10% lower than the LL will often be significant if the measured parameter is red blood cells (RBC), for example.

With all of these problems, is there anything that can be done to simplify, organize, and interpret the lab values for more than just one patient at a time or for just one patient *over* time? In order to make this complex problem more tractable, two concepts essential to the creation of a Genie Score [2] will be presented. These two concepts are as follows:

1. *Normalization* (or standardization) of lab parameters by a division of each value by its "upper limit of reference range" as established by the laboratory producing the measurement, and
2. A *multivariate scoring system* that assigns to each patient a number produced from a function of the normalized values over a functionally related group of parameters (e.g., hepatic function group, renal function group, etc.).

The main advantage of normalization is that all the transformed lab values become dimensionless—the units are not needed. This important property enables the parameters to be mathematically combined and, if desired, analyzed.

Another advantage of normalizing lab values is that the values can be directly interpreted. Since all normalized values have a 1 for their upper limit of the reference range, the condition of "abnormality or not" can be quickly determined and, if abnormal, the degree of abnormality can be obtained without reference to any other numbers.

By choosing the transformation for normalizing the measured values as division of each value by its upper limit of normal, several important properties are achieved:

1. All the transformed values are positive.
2. All the parameters have an upper limit for the reference range equal to 1.

3.   All the normalized values are dimensionless.
4.   Values outside the upper limit (>1) are easy to recognize and interpret.

B.   Definition of the Genie Score

The Genie Score is defined as follows:

A "Genie Score" is a summary statistic produced (for a functional group of parameters) from a weighted linear combination of *absolute normalized deviations from the reference range* for a single patient.

The Genie Score is defined for several functional groups and across functional groups. To illustrate, let X_i be the measurement of the ith lab parameter in a defined functional group, where $i = 1, \ldots, N$ and $N = $ the number of lab parameters in the function group; let UL_i and LL_i be the corresponding upper limit and lower limit of the reference range for the ith parameter; and let D_i, the normalized deviation from the reference range for the ith parameter, be defined as

$$
D_i = \begin{cases}
\left[\left(\dfrac{X_i}{UL_i}\right) - 1\right] \times 100, & \text{if } X_i \text{ is } > UL_i \\[2mm]
0 & \text{if } LL_i \leq X_i \leq UL_i \\[2mm]
\left[\left(\dfrac{X_i}{LL_i}\right) - 1\right] \times 100, & \text{if } X_i \text{ is } < LL_i
\end{cases}
\tag{1}
$$

Then the Genie Score (GS) is defined as

$$
GS = K \times \left(\frac{1}{N} \sum_{i=1}^{N} |D_i|\right)
\tag{2}
$$

where K assigns weight to the score according to the number of parameters outside the reference range and accounts for missing values (see Appendix 1 for details on K).

C.   Properties of the Genie Score

From this definition several important properties follow:

Any abnormality will produce a positive, nonzero Genie Score.
A Genie Score $= 0$ implies that all the parameters measured within the function group are within the reference range.
The higher the Genie Score the more (or more severe) the abnormalities a patient has. This can be expected generally to correlate with the severity of the disease (or drug toxicity).

A Genie Score is a measure of the degree of lab abnormalities a patient had at the time the lab tests were administered.

The advantage of the multivariate scoring system is that it yields a type of average assessment of abnormality for each patient within a prespecified body function group. (This enables an overview for the abnormalities. No information is lost since the original data are always available for any detailed review for an individual patient.) A Genie Score is calculated for each patient at each time point for each of the functionally related groups of parameters. Also, by making the basic unit of the Genie Score a function group, fewer tests of significance would be required if comparisons were to be made among treatment groups.

These scores can be displayed for each patient at baseline, during therapy, and at the end of therapy, thus presenting a concise view of a patient's lab abnormalities, if any. Or, at any one time point, the scores for all the patients can be ranked (by a function group); the higher the score the more severe the abnormalities that occurred within that group, thus permitting the investigator to compare the well being of his or her patients, each against the rest, throughout the course of a long-term study.

In addition to the various ways the Genie Score can be used to review, monitor, and summarize lab data, its major advantage is that it is an objective assessment. Genie Scores are all calculated by the same algorithm and require no subjective interpretation; they let the chips fall where they may. In a later section we shall illustrate how the Genie Score can be used as a statistic to compare two (or more) treatment groups in comparative clinical trials.

III.   BODY FUNCTION GROUPS USED FOR GENIE SCORE CALCULATIONS

A.   Rationale

A physician, monitoring the course of an illness in a severely ill patient usually has available the latest reading of the patient's lab measurements. In assessing patient progress, the physician usually refers not to just one of the measurements but to several of them.

Many illnesses can be diagnosed by the abnormalities they produce. Generally severe drug toxicity will manifest itself by producing abnormalities in several lab measurements, and different combinations of lab abnormalities are characteristic of different illnesses (or toxicities). Our limited knowledge has not established a unique mapping as yet, but it is almost a truism that multiple abnormalities are indicative of a potentially more serious condition than a single abnormality or none.

When the Genie Score concept was being created, one of the main objectives was to summarize lab information and provide for a meaningful display. By making the unit for calculating a Genie Score a body function group, several parameters related to a body function were grouped together, the normalized absolute deviations of the abnormalities were calculated, and they were combined to produce a Genie Score [Eq. (2)]. Where the measured value is within the reference range, the contribution to the Genie Score is zero, but the number of parameters measured within the function group is expressed by N in the calculation, so that even values within the reference range are factored into the Genie Score. The Genie Score reflects the (average) degree of lab abnormalities for that patient within the body function group being examined. A similar calculation is produced for each of the defined body function groups. Since each of the defined body function groups has a minimum of four previously defined parameters to a maximum of nine, data reduction has been achieved.

B. History

In the early evolution of the Genie Score (1983), the body function groups were selected from the usual pool of 35–40 lab parameters that were more or less routinely collected in anti-infective clinical trials. Originally there was little medical input into the original partitioning of the lab parameters. But as the idea grew more familiar (following the publication [2] in 1986), as the clinical trials became more sophisticated, as the number of lab tests expanded and science became more skilled at devising and measuring the assays, more interest was generated from the medical community in providing a carefully reasoned medical assessment for the grouping of the lab parameters.

Subsequent to the second publication [3], a series of tests were run to test the robustness of the Genie Scores with different weighting factors. The statistical conclusions were invariant, i.e., where the test showed significance with one set of weights, it showed significance with the new weights; where it was nonsignificant, it remained nonsignificant with the new weights. Since one of the experiments involved setting all the weights equal to unity, we therefore decided to take the simplest approach and have since then computed all the Genie Scores with weights equal to 1.

Figure 1 displays 10 body function groups that are presently being used to define the Genie Score. Nearly 60 parameters are identified and assigned to one of the 10 preselected body function groups. While there is no one way that this partition had to be done, this grouping does represent a reasonable and medically sound partition over which the Genie Score is calculated. All of the data used in this manuscript have been calculated using these body function groups.

By settling on the body function groups and the lab parameters contained in them, a library of Genie Scores can be established. Because Genie Scores are surrogate markers for laboratory data, and because of their compressed format, they are easy to store, manipulate, and analyze.

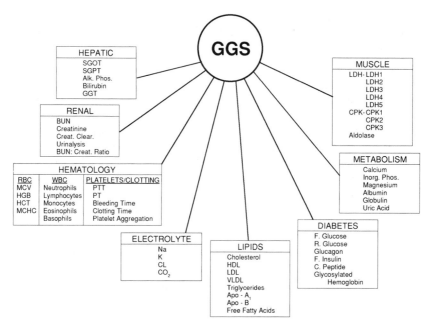

Figure 1 Body function groups used for calculating Genie Scores.

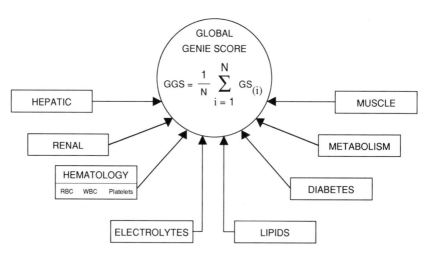

Figure 2 Body function groups used for calculating Genie Scores.

The Genie Score concept has the generality that it can evolve with science. Fig. 2 shows the Global Genie Score that is simply the average of the Genie Scores over the body function groups. The Global Genie Score is convenient for ranking the results of a full study at a given time point. By ordering the Global Genie Score from high to low (the Genie Score for each function group is carried along in the record), the most severely affected patients are easily identified. As more lab tests are created to help understand new diseases, additional function groups can be added as desired.

IV.   GENIE SCORES FOR MONITORING CLINICAL TRIALS

A.   Clinical Trials Used as Examples

To illustrate the applications of the Genie Score, data from lab measurements in two large clinical trials are used. One of the studies is a double-blind placebo-controlled study designed to assess the efficacy of an active drug as a prophylaxis against serious fungal infection in cancer patients undergoing bone marrow transplant therapy. The maximum duration of the study is 10 weeks. The second study is also double-blind but with two active drugs for a specific chronic disease. The duration of this study is up to 2 years.

For convenience in referring to the two studies, the antifungal bone marrow transplant study will be called the short-term study, whereas the chronic disease study will be called the long-term study. These studies are used only to give authenticity to the data and to illustrate facets of the Genie Score. The drugs used in the short-term study are referred to as drug X and drug Y, whereas the long-term study drugs are drug A and drug B.

B.   Ranking by Global Genie Score

Table 1 shows the Genie Scores calculated for patients in the short-term study at the third week of therapy. These scores have been ranked in descending order of the Global Genie Score (last column). Only the highest 10 and the lowest 5 Genie Scores are shown. Because these Genie Scores are calculated for seriously ill cancer patients who are recipients of bone marrow transplants, for most of the function groups (for the top 10) they are high, indicating serious lab abnormalities within the function groups. Even among the lowest five sets of scores, there is still a substantial number of abnormalities.

To put these observations in perspective, Table 2 shows the Genie Scores calculated for the patients in the long-term study. Although they have a chronic illness, they are not as sick as the cancer patients receiving transplants. This fact is reflected in the lower Genie Scores shown for the highest 10 Global Genie Scores. On the lower end of the ranking, over 50% of the patients in this chronic disease study had a Global Genie Score of zero, indicating that there were no lab

Table 1 Body Function Group Genie Scores Ranked by Global Genie Score: Time Point Third Week of Therapy, Data from Short-Term Study[a]

Patient ID number	Body function groups used to calculate Genie Scores										Global Genie Score
	Liver	Renal	RBC	WBC	Elect.	Lipid	Diabetes	Metab.	Platelet	Muscle	
A001	1067.1	195.5	0.0	36.4	3.4	—	—	—	22.4	—	220.8
A019	931.7	26.7	34.7	25.1	0.0	—	—	—	38.6	—	176.1
A042	918.5	5.2	24.0	39.5	0.0	—	—	—	27.7	—	169.1
A037	722.1	123.6	13.0	0.0	0.0	—	—	—	38.3	—	149.5
A008	480.6	355.5	17.0	0.0	0.0	—	—	—	28.4	—	146.9
A016	633.0	159.0	31.2	13.0	5.7	—	—	—	30.0	—	145.3
A011	742.2	26.3	33.1	27.0	0.9	—	—	—	34.6	—	144.0
A015	562.3	224.5	15.6	21.7	0.0	—	—	—	26.9	—	141.8
A029	661.3	36.3	29.5	28.8	1.3	—	—	—	36.6	—	132.3
A022	530.9	133.0	42.9	2.4	3.2	—	—	—	36.0	—	124.7
A041	0.0	0.0	27.8	0.0	0.0	—	—	—	0.0	—	4.6
A007	9.1	0.0	6.8	8.9	0.0	—	—	—	0.0	—	4.1
A004	0.0	0.0	19.7	0.0	4.3	—	—	—	0.0	—	4.0
A009	5.6	0.0	0.0	0.0	0.0	—	—	—	17.1	—	3.8
A032	0.0	0.0	3.4	0.0	0.0	—	—	—	9.5	—	2.2

[a]Over 350 patients in the study. Displayed are only the 10 highest, plus the 5 lowest ranked Global Genie Scores.

Table 2 Body Function Group Genie Scores Ranked by Global Genie Score: Time Point 6 Months into Therapy, Data from Long-Term Study[a]

Patient ID number	Body function groups used to calculate Genie Scores										Global Genie Score
	Liver	Renal	RBC	WBC	Elect.	Lipid	Diabetes	Metab.	Platelet	Muscle	
B001	954.0	17.0	0.0	0.0	0.0	—	—	0.0	0.0	—	138.7
B019	157.0	2.1	—	—	0.0	—	—	0.0	—	—	39.8
B005	252.3	0.0	2.6	0.0	0.0	—	—	0.0	0.0	—	36.4
B036	165.0	0.0	0.0	0.0	0.0	—	—	0.0	0.0	—	23.6
B011	30.6	0.0	44.4	0.0	0.0	—	—	17.1	15.0	—	15.3
B021	78.7	8.5	10.2	0.0	0.0	—	—	0.0	0.8	—	14.0
B001	88.7	0.0	3.4	0.0	0.0	—	—	0.0	0.0	—	13.3
B004	23.0	0.0	35.0	0.0	0.0	—	—	7.5	0.0	—	9.4
B026	65.7	0.0	0.0	0.0	0.0	—	—	0.0	0.0	—	9.4
B029	31.6	1.2	22.6	0.0	0.0	—	—	3.6	1.7	—	8.7

[a]Over 400 patients in the study. Displayed are only the 10 highest ranked Global Genie Scores. Over 50% of patients had no abnormalities at this time point; their Genie Scores are all 0.0.

Table 3A Time Sequence of Genie Scores for All Body Function Groups: Single Patient in the Bone Marrow Transplant Clinical Trial, Data from Short-Term Study

Days into study	Body function groups used to calculate Genie Scores										Global Genie Score
	Liver	Renal	RBC	WBC	Elect.	Lipid	Diabetes	Metab.	Platelet	Muscle	
0	0.0	8.8	41.0	0.0	0.4	—	—	—	0.0	—	8.4
3	4.0	6.6	38.3	0.0	0.4	—	—	—	23.8	—	12.2
5	21.1	6.6	35.1	39.1	0.0	—	—	—	37.0	—	23.2
8	56.5	28.5	9.5	40.0	0.0	—	—	—	—	—	26.9
9	34.3	48.6	51.6	37.3	0.0	—	—	—	39.0	—	35.1
10	61.6	56.4	50.0	38.2	8.9	—	—	—	33.4	—	41.4
12	237.8	40.5	34.7	35.6	0.0	—	—	—	37.6	—	64.4
14	239.3	33.7	8.9	35.6	19.5	—	—	—	37.8	—	62.5
15	468.3	32.7	0.0	35.6	8.4	—	—	—	38.2	—	97.2
16	647.6	52.2	0.0	34.7	0.0	—	—	—	29.2	—	127.3
17	741.1	110.5	3.6	32.9	1.6	—	—	—	38.6	—	154.7
18	912.2	147.7	0.0	37.3	0.0	—	—	—	37.4	—	189.1
19	509.3	172.3	0.6	37.3	0.0	—	—	—	38.8	—	126.4
21	1808.7	203.9	0.0	36.4	0.0	—	—	—	38.8	—	348.0
23	1621.6	226.6	0.0	35.6	3.4	—	—	—	37.0	—	320.7
26	1067.1	195.5	0.0	36.4	3.4	—	—	—	22.4	—	220.8

abnormalities at all among the many parameters measured at 6 months into therapy.

C. Examination of Abnormalities for Individual Patients

Having used the Global Genie Score to highlight the patients with the most extreme abnormalities, one might then want to examine the details of the abnormalities. To illustrate, Table 3A shows for the patient with the highest Global Genie Score (in the short-term study) the time sequence of Genie Scores for all the body function groups as well as the Global Genie Score. Table 3B shows the details of the liver function group for the same patient. In each of these tables, the percent deviations for the lab parameters (contained within the function group) are displayed sequentially over time. The corresponding Genie Scores, calculated from the percent deviations, are also displayed sequentially.

This display of the deviations within a function group is available for any patient in the study. It is formed as one of the substeps in the calculation of the Genie Scores. The abnormalities are expressed as percent deviations above or below the reference range. For the body function group chosen, there were no negative deviations. Had the white blood cell (WBC) group been selected, there would have been many negative deviations (i.e., deviations below the lower reference range).

Table 3B   Time Sequence of Genie Scores for Hepatic Body Function Group and % Deviations of Individual Parameters for a Single Placebo Patient in the Bone Marrow Transplant Clinical Trial, Data from Short-Term Study

Days into study	SGOT	SGPT	Alk. Phos.	Bili.	GGT	Genie Score
0	0.0	0.0	0.0	0.0	—	0.0
3	14.4	0.0	3.1	0.0	—	4.0
5	68.6	0.0	8.3	0.0	—	21.1
8	51.4	31.4	7.3	66.7	—	56.5
9	48.6	48.6	0.0	11.1	—	34.3
10	82.9	48.6	6.3	33.3	—	61.6
12	291.4	225.7	0.0	233.3	—	237.8
14	342.9	262.9	14.6	44.4	—	239.3
15	434.3	277.1	0.0	766.7	—	468.3
16	571.4	317.1	0.0	1156.0	—	647.6
17	764.7	151.4	0.0	1422.0	—	741.1
18	848.6	408.6	0.0	1622.0	—	912.2
19	—	—	—	2122.0	—	509.3
21	1028.6	528.6	11.5	3456.0	—	1808.7
23	375.1	114.3	21.9	4011.0	—	1621.6
26	100.0	0.0	0.0	3799.0	—	1067.1

D.   Quality Control Charts

While the ultimate purpose for lab safety data is to monitor for drug toxicity within individual patients, it is also possible to use these data to monitor at a glance the changes between the treatment groups. Using the Genie Scores calculated for the patients within the treatment groups, the mean Genie Score at each visit can be plotted. At baseline one would expect the scores to be close, but as the trial progresses one might expect them to differ as the therapy begins to affect the illness. If one were monitoring an ongoing trial, new points of the graph could be plotted as soon as all the data for that visit became available. In this sense, the following figures can be viewed as a type of quality control chart, which tracks the key parameters of an ongoing process.

For example, Figs. 3A–3C display the mean Genie Score for drug X and drug Y from baseline to final visit for three of the function groups. The active drug displays a pattern amazingly similar to that of the control. Note that the vertical axis in each figure represents the Genie Score for the function group specified, i.e., liver, WBC, and platelet.

Figure 4 displays the same type of chart for the long-term study. Note the 10-fold decrease in the order of magnitude of this plot relative to Fig. 3A (for the liver function group). This is in keeping with the relative severity of the illness in the patient population.

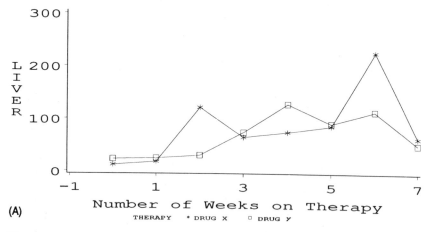

(A)

Figure 3   (A) Double-blind, placebo-controlled antifungal prophylaxis study for cancer patients undergoing bone marrow transplants, short-term study, mean Genie Score by time on therapy. (B) Double-blind, placebo-controlled antifungal prophylaxis study for cancer patients undergoing bone marrow transplants, short-term study, mean Genie Score by time on therapy. (C) Double-blind, placebo-controlled antifungal prophylaxis study for cancer patients undergoing bone marrow transplants, short-term study, mean Genie Score by time on therapy.

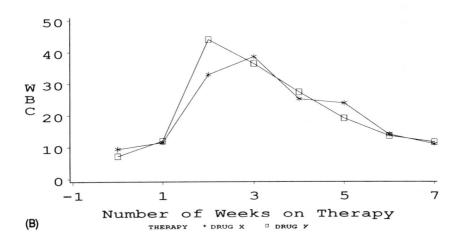

(B)

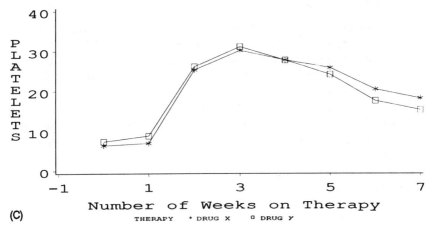

(C)

Figure 3   (*Continued*)

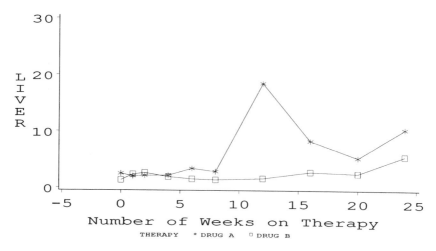

Figure 4 Double-blind, comparative study of drug A vs. drug B for patients with chronic disease, long-term study, mean Genie Score by time on therapy.

V. GENIE SCORES FOR COMPARING LABORATORY SAFETY DATA BETWEEN TREATMENT GROUPS

A. (Final–Baseline) Difference as Test Statistic

An earlier paper [3] demonstrated the use of Genie Scores as a convenient way to statistically compare the safety of treatment groups in clinical trials. The tests were performed using each patient's (final–baseline) difference (or F-B difference) in Genie Scores and then performing the Wilcoxon Rank Sum Test for each body function group.

In most new drug application (NDA) preparations, changes from baseline are used to provide a test between treatment groups using a single lab parameter at a time. While this is an accepted procedure, it has the limitation of incorporating information for only two time points. This is probably quite reasonable for a brief study of several weeks, but for long-term study lasting a year or more, we would like to examine the total experience of the entire study.

B. The Time-Averaged Genie Score (TAGS)

The Time-Averaged Genie Score (TAGS) has been developed (see Appendix 1 for the mathematical definition of the TAGS) to provide an easy and reliable method for incorporating the complete history of abnormalities.

To illustrate how nonrepresentative a final–baseline (F-B) difference can be, Fig. 5A shows the time history of one patient's Genie Score for the liver function

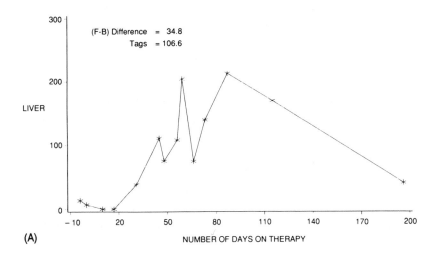

(A)

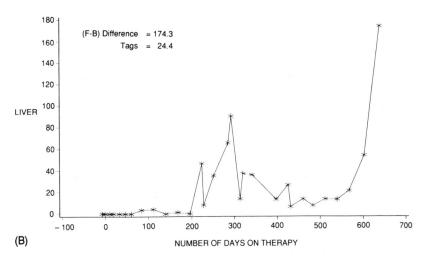

(B)

Figure 5 (A) Double-blind, comparative study of drug A vs. drug B for patients with chronic disease: Genie Scores for one patient over course of therapy, data from long-term study. (B) Double-blind, comparative study of drug A vs. drug B for patients with chronic disease: Genie Scores for one patient over course of therapy, data from long-term study. *Note*: Data in (A) and (B) based on different patients.

group. The F-B difference in Genie Score is 34.8, and the TAGS is 106.6. Judging from the figure, the TAGS conveys a more accurate assessment of this patient's liver abnormalities during the course of the study than the F-B difference.

Figure 5B illustrates another example. In this case, the patient's F-B difference is 174.3, while the TAGS is 24.4. TAGS give a more realistic representation of this patient's Genie Score liver abnormalities over the course of the study.

In addition to developing the TAGS, an area under the curve (AUC) statistic was calculated by a trapezoidal integration for the same data sets. The results were reassuringly similar.

C. Results from Long-Term and Short-Term Studies

Table 4 summarizes the results of the statistical comparison between the two treatment groups for the long-term study of chronic disease. The treatments are compared within the nine body function groups where data were collected. The F-B differences, AUC, and TAGS are compared between the two treatments.

Significant differences are noted between the two treatments for the lipid and metabolic body function groups. Using the mean rank column and noting that the lower the mean the fewer and less severe the abnormalities, one notes that drug B shows a more favorable result than drug A in the lipid group, while drug A shows a more favorable response in the metabolic body function group.

This significance is picked up by the F-B difference and the TAGS statistics. Of further note, the TAGS statistic showed an additional result (in favor of drug A) for the electrolyte body function group, illustrating again that it picks up more information from the course of the study.

Table 5 summarizes the statistical comparisons between drug X and drug Y for the short-term double-blind study of bone marrow transplant cancer patients, who are being treated with an active antifungal medicine vs. a placebo control. For the six body function groups where lab data were collected, there are no statistically significant results for either the F-B differences or the TAGS.

VI. GENIE SCORE DISTRIBUTIONS FOR VARIOUS PATIENT POPULATIONS

A. Description of the Patient Populations Used

In the future, as Genie Scores will be routinely calculated and as databases will include baseline lab information for many types of diseases, the distributions of Genie Scores (for each body function group) can be calculated and displayed as in Fig. 6 and Table 6.

Figure 6 shows the empirical cumulative distribution of baseline Genie Scores computed from the hepatic body function group for several different patient

Table 4 Double-Blind, Comparative Study of Drug A vs. Drug B for Patients with Chronic Disease: Genie Scores for Three Types of Statistical Comparison of Treatment Groups, Data from Long-Term Study

Function group	Compound (drug)	N	Baseline mean	Endpoint–baseline differences				Area under curve			Time–Averaged Genie Score		
				Mean	Median	Mean rank	p value[a]	N	Mean rank	p value[a]	N	Mean rank	p value[a]
Hepatic	A	146	1.353	1.396	0.0	214.2	0.846	147	205.6	0.098	147	209.0	0.216
	B	284	2.503	6.589	0.0	216.2		290	225.8		290	224.0	
Renal	A	145	0.241	0.607	0.0	218.0	0.420	146	209.7	0.278	146	213.7	0.576
	B	282	0.664	0.355	0.0	211.9		289	222.2		289	220.1	
RBC	A	144	1.997	1.077	0.0	217.1	0.305	146	210.1	0.350	146	212.7	0.524
	B	274	2.041	0.746	0.0	205.5		289	222.0		289	220.7	
WBC	A	144	1.370	0.320	0.0	219.3	0.191	146	226.6	0.277	146	224.6	0.394
	B	274	0.938	0.093	0.0	206.7		289	213.6		289	214.6	
Electrolytes	A	144	0.072	0.127	0.0	210.0	0.641	146	194.5	**0.004**	146	197.7	**0.011**
	B	280	0.176	0.255	0.0	213.8		289	229.8		289	228.2	
Lipids	A	33	1.297	−0.576	0.0	52.0	**0.017**	33	46.4	0.585	33	50.2	**0.089**
	B	54	1.896	−1.270	−0.2	39.1		55	43.3		55	41.1	
Diabetes	A	20	0.380	−0.140	0.0	29.2	0.753	20	24.5	0.137	20	25.9	0.311
	B	36	0.736	−0.428	0.0	28.1		36	30.7		36	29.9	
Metabolic	A	145	0.473	−0.092	0.0	193.1	**0.001**	146	176.1	**0.000**	146	175.6	**0.000**
	B	286	0.368	1.215	0.0	227.6		289	239.2		289	239.4	
Platelets	A	144	1.072	−0.163	0.0	216.8	0.246	146	222.4	0.571	146	220.2	0.772
	B	273	1.118	−0.356	0.0	204.9		289	215.8		289	216.9	
Muscle	A	0	—	—	—	—		—	—	—	—	—	
	B	0	—	—	—	—		—	—	—	—	—	
Global GS	A	147	0.898	0.626	0.0	223.8		—	—	—	—	—	
	B	290	1.086	1.282	0.0	216.6		—	—		—	—	

[a]Wilcoxon Rank Sum Test.

143

Table 5 Double-Blind, Placebo Controlled Antifungal Prophylaxis Study for Cancer Patients Undergoing Bone Marrow Transplants: Genie Scores for Three Types of Statistical Comparison of Treatment Groups, Data from Short-Term Study

Function group	Compound (drug)	N	Baseline mean	Mean	Median	Mean rank	p value[a]	N	Mean rank	p value[a]	N	Mean rank	p value[a]
				Endpoint–baseline differences				Area under curve			Time–Averaged Genie Score		
Hepatic	X	152	12.197	197.090	35.2	158.1	0.266	179	178.3	0.893	179	180.7	0.753
	Y	152	18.237	93.791	21.1	146.9		178	179.7		178	177.3	
Renal	X	153	3.732	26.958	5.9	146.4	0.156	179	174.5	0.414	179	180.7	0.753
	Y	153	3.887	35.784	8.9	160.6		178	183.5		178	177.3	
RBC	X	154	21.689	8.240	6.4	155.0	0.548	179	184.6	0.303	179	180.7	0.428
	Y	149	22.489	5.991	7.7	148.9		178	170.4		178	174.7	
WBC	X	156	8.951	12.115	14.8	152.3	0.191	179	170.3	0.277	179	168.8	0.394
	Y	149	7.444	15.008	16.7	153.8		178	186.8		178	189.3	
Electrolytes	X	152	0.654	2.766	0.9	157.0	0.362	179	181.0	0.714	179	185.3	0.248
	Y	152	0.447	2.263	0.4	148.0		178	177.0		178	172.7	
Lipids	X	0	—	—	—	—							
	Y	0	—	—	—	—							
Diabetes	X	0	—	—	—	—							
	Y	0	—	—	—	—							
Metabolic	X	0	—	—	—	—							
	Y	0	—	—	—	—							
Platelets	X	151	5.893	17.448	23.4	152.2	0.658	179	180.0	0.860	179	178.3	0.892
	Y	148	7.158	16.380	22.3	147.8		178	178.0		178	179.7	
Muscle	X	0	0.700	90.400	90.4	1.0							
	Y	0	—	—	—	—							
Global GS	X	178	8.778	41.706	17.8	185.1							
	Y	177	10.032	30.045	15.6	170.8							

[a]Wilcoxon Rank Sum Test.

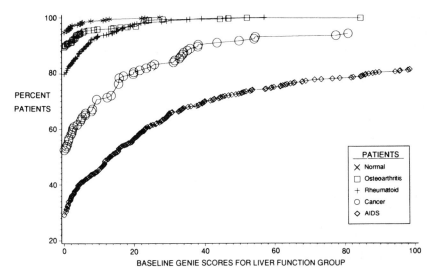

Figure 6 Empirical distribution of baseline Genie Scores for various patient populations.

Table 6 Probability Estimates of Baseline Genie Scores Exceeding X for Various Patient Populations: Hepatic Body Function Group Genie Score

Genie Score X		Patient population[a]			
	No disease (normal)	Osteo-arthritis	Rheumatoid arthritis	Cancer	AIDS
$\geq$ 0.0	0.0522	0.1055	0.2014	0.4755	0.7078
$\geq$ 2.0	0.0326	0.0892	0.1670	0.4196	0.6440
$\geq$ 5.0	0.0217	0.0568	0.1213	0.3636	0.5905
$\geq$ 10.0	0.0130	0.0423	0.0664	0.2937	0.5453
$\geq$ 15.0	0.0065	0.0385	0.0503	0.2797	0.4835
$\geq$ 20.0	0.0665	0.0345	0.0275	0.1958	0.4342
$\geq$ 30.0	0.0000	0.0081	0.0137	0.1678	0.3436
$\geq$ 40.0	0.0000	0.0081	0.0046	0.0979	0.3004
$\geq$ 50.0	0.0000	0.0041	0.0023	0.0839	0.2737
$\geq$ 60.0	0.0000	0.0020	0.0000	0.0699	0.2790
$\geq$ 80.0	0.0000	0.0000	0.0000	0.0559	0.2161
$\geq$ 100.0	0.0000	0.0000	0.0000	0.0559	0.1831

[a]Each patient population had more than 300 subjects.

populations. One is obtained from ''healthy'' subjects who participated in some phase I studies. The remaining curves are baseline scores from patients with different illnesses who are entering special studies to determine the efficacy of a drug on their particular illness.

The data are from patients who have:

Osteoarthritis
Rheumatoid arthritis
Cancer (bone marrow transplant patients)
AIDS

The curves show the differences among the distribution of Genie Scores associated with the illnesses. Data from at least 300 patients/subjects per group were used to calculate the empirical distribution. Note that the horizontal axis of Genie Scores is theoretically unbounded.

B.   Probabilistic Interpretation

One could develop a set of tables for each of the 10 body function groups and display the probabilities as is done in Table 6. These probabilities could then be used in the sense of ''life tables'' in actuarial calculations. If these tabulated results were available, they could be helpful for diagnostic discrimination and as prognostic variables related to the outcome of a course of therapy. Further research is needed to fully explore the usefulness of such approaches.

VII.   SUMMARY AND CONCLUSIONS

A.   Individual Patient Data Compression

We began this chapter with thoughts on data compression and its growing importance in areas where large amounts of data have to be digested and summarized. The preceding sections have illustrated how the Genie Score helps the clinician to digest and summarize the volumes of lab data that are routinely collected during clinical trials.

Figure 7 summarizes the data compression made possible by the Genie Score for the synopsis of an individual's lab values at one point in time. Multiply the data reduction reflected in this figure by the many lab tests each patient has during the course of therapy by the number of patients in the study and one has a quantitative value of data compressed by the Genie Scores.

Genie Scores enable a patient's entire history of lab abnormalities to be displayed in one plot (Fig. 8). This figure displays the involvement of abnormalities of one patient with AIDS and cryptococcal meningitis who was receiving amphotericin B as therapy for meningitis. The patient died shortly after 9 weeks of therapy.

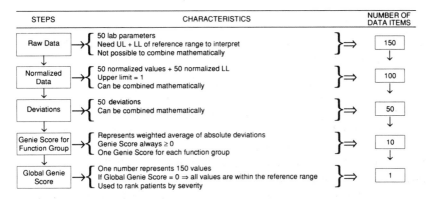

Figure 7   Data compression using the Genie Score concept, one patient at one point in time.

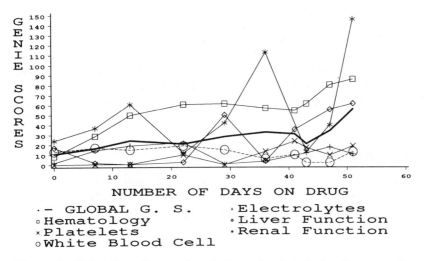

Figure 8   Global Genie Score and Genie Scores for six body function groups for one AIDS patient with active case of cryptococcal meningitis.

B.   Treatment Group Data Compression

Section V was devoted to the ways the Genie Scores could be used as a primary statistic for comparing the safety of one drug vs. other drugs when analyzing comparative trials. Two different aspects of comparison were made by using F-B differences in Genie Scores and by using the TAGS. Each statistic provides a method of summarizing safety—one by examining the scores at two time points, the other by combining the scores at all time points.

C. Conclusion

The following list highlights the major contributions of the Genie Score for assessing laboratory data:

Standardization allows parameters to be combined mathematically.
Standardization removes problems of different units.
Standardization incorporates reference range information.
Genie Score provides handle for overview of lab data for whole study.
Genie Score provides enormous data reduction.
Genie Score allows easy manipulation for a variety of statistical analyses.
Genie Score is a sensitive and consistent surrogate for lab data.
Genie Score provides a probabilistic context for assessing lab abnormalities.
Genie Score is a quantitative and objective method for comparing lab abnormalities and hence assessing safety in clinical trials.

As the need for data compression becomes increasingly urgent as more and more information must be assimilated, applying techniques such as the Genie Score will become a necessity. The Genie Score provides a summary of the laboratory experience of the patients in a clinical trial, individually or collectively. It can be used statistically to draw conclusions about the safety of an investigational drug. We do not propose that the Genie Score supplant other methods of reviewing laboratory data but rather that it be used to supplement and enhance methods currently in use.

ACKNOWLEDGMENT

The authors thank Dr. Jeffrey Lazar for sharing his medical expertise in grouping lab tests into appropriate function groups; Phillip Grzymkowski for his superb graphics; and Marjorie Dougan for her typing.

Appendix 1

Mathematical Definition of a Genie Score

Consider a group of N functionally related lab parameters with an established upper limit and lower limit of the reference range for each parameter.

Let X_i be the measurement associated with the ith lab parameter;

$X_{i(UL)}$ be the upper limit of reference range, and

$X_{i(LL)}$ be the lower limit of reference range for the ith parameter,

$i = 1, \ldots, N$.

Let $Z_i = X_i/X_{i(UL)}$ be the "normalized" value of X_i, and

$Z_{i(LL)} = X_{(iLL)}/X_{i(UL)}$ be the lower limit for Z_i, for $i = 1, \ldots, N$.

Note that $Z_{i(UL)} = 1$ for all i, $i = 1, \ldots, N$.

Let the "*normalized deviations*" be D_i, where

$$D_i = \begin{cases} Z_i - 1, & \text{if } Z_i > 1.0 \\ 0, & \text{if } Z_{i(LL)} \le Z_i \le 1.0 \\ Z_i - Z_{i(LL)}, & \text{if } Z_i < Z_{i(LL)} \end{cases} \tag{A-1}$$

for $i = 1, \ldots, N$.

Thus, if D_i is positive, the measured value is above the upper limit of reference range,

if $D_i = 0$, the measured value is within the reference range, and if D_i is negative, the measured value is below the lower limit of the reference range.

For each patient that has measurements within the function group, the Genie Score (GS) is calculated by

$$GS = K \frac{1}{N} \left[\sum_{i=1}^{N} S_i W_i \mid D_i \mid \right] \qquad (A\text{-}2)$$

where $K = k_1 * k_2$ accounts for the number of abnormal values and the number of missing values within the function group.

$k_1 = (1 + 0.2 \times NSP)$, where NSP = the number of abnormal values (out of the N parameters in the function group) observed for the patient measured.

$k_2 = [1 - (NP - NSP)\, 0.01]$, where NP = the number of parameters actually measured for the group of N specified parameters.

W_i is a weight assigned to each parameter. All W_i values are set equal to 1. S_i is a stretch factor, which equals 1 if $D_i > 0$ and equals $(2/Z_{i(LL)})$ if $D_i < 0$, for $i = 1, \ldots, N$.

The stretch factor is incorporated into the Genie Score to increase the contribution from abnormalities which are *below* the lower limit of the reference range because abnormalities below the lower reference range are bounded by zero, whereas abnormalities above the upper reference point are unbounded.

Note: Although the Genie Score can be defined in terms of the random variables X and D, as shown in Eqs. (1) and (2) of this chapter, the random variable Z, introduced in this definition, is a natural step in the transformation of the measured lab values and the reference range limits to *dimensionless normalized values*. These normalized values represent a convenient way to look for trends that might be occurring *within* the reference ranges.

Time-Averaged Genie Scores

During the course of therapy, each patient will have a set of Genie Scores for each function group where tests were done. These Genie Scores can be averaged *across time* (for each function group) to provide a set of Time-Averaged Genie Scores (TAGS) for each patient. These TAGS are single summary statistics of lab abnormalities within the function group for each patient. These TAGS can be further compressed to produce a Global TAGS, i.e., *one number per patient per study*!

Stated mathematically (for one patient):

Let

$$\text{TAGS}(i) = \frac{1}{\text{NT}} \left[\sum_{j=1}^{\text{NT}} g_i(t_j) - g_i(t_0) \right] \tag{A-3}$$

where

$g_i(t_j)$ = the Genie Score at time t_j for the ith function group
$g_i(t_0)$ = the Genie Score at baseline for the ith function group

and

$i = 1, \ldots,$ NG and NG equal the number of function groups available;
$j = 1, \ldots,$ NT(i) and NT(i) equals the number of times the Genie Score is calculated within the ith function group.

Note: if $g_i(t_0) > \sum_{j=1}^{\text{NT}} g_i(t_j)$, then TAGS($i$) = 0 $\tag{A-4}$

The Global TAGS is defined as:

$$\text{GTAGS} = \frac{1}{\text{NG}} \sum_{i=1}^{\text{NG}} \text{TAGS}(i) \tag{A-5}$$

Appendix 2

Introduction

A series of calculations is made in computing a Genie Score. Values are grouped, divided, summed, subtracted, and multiplied before a final number representing a patient's laboratory test experience is determined. (See Appendix 1 for the mathematical definitions involved in computing the Genie Score.) The purpose of this appendix is to describe and display the computer programs used to arrive at the Genie Score so that you, the reader, can implement the Genie Score system for your own use.

The programs are written in SAS Version 6.06 and run sequentially under the DEC VAX/VMS operating system. Each module performs one or two specific functions. The programs could be adapted to run in other computer languages or on other operating systems.

The output from this series of programs are two listings, one ASCII file, and several SAS datasets. One listing displays all the individual functional group scores for every patient. The second listing displays the Global Genie Scores for every patient. The ASCII file, SCORES.DAT, contains the functional groups scores and the Global Genie Scores. This ASCII file of results is suitable as input to statistical or graphics programs, such as those that produced the output shown in Table 4 and Figs. 3A–5B. Examples and further discussion of these products follow in the sections below. These displays can be either for all time points at which a patient had lab parameters measured or for just at baseline and final time points. Similarly, the ASCII file will contain multiple records per patient, in the case where lab parameters were measured at every time point, or two records per patient if only baseline and final visits are desired.

Preparing Laboratory Data (READ.SAS)

The starting point for the Genie Scores system is SAS dataset BLAB containing laboratory data. Each record in this file contains information pertaining to a single laboratory test at a single point in time. Figure A-1 in this appendix shows the records for the liver function group for a single patient. The following information is required on each record for the Genie Score programs to run:

Patient identification number
Integer time identifier: number of days since baseline
Lab test number
Lab test value
Upper limit of reference range for lab test
Lower limit of reference range for lab test

The following information is useful to have for display purposes but not critical to the Genie Scores calculations once you have the above variables:

Visit date
Visit designator
Treatment name
Treatment dose
Patient age
Patient sex

If you do not already have laboratory data stored in a SAS dataset in this format, you should preprocess the data into this form. SAS program READ.SAS reads data from several ASCII files, one for each functional group, and creates a single SAS dataset, BLAB, in the format shown above in Fig. A-1. Because of the length of this program, only the code for the liver function group is included. Code for other functional groups can be similarly written.

Assigning Lab Tests to Groups and Computing Deviations from the Reference Range (ASSGNGRP.SAS)

The first module, ASSGNGRP.SAS, assigns the lab tests to the functional groups shown in Fig. 1 and computes the deviation from reference range values. These deviations become the components of the functional group scores and the global Genie score. The deviations are computed as shown in (A-1) in Appendix 1.

BLAB SAS Data Set Records for LIVER Function Group for Patient Number C044

PAT_ID	BAS_DAYS	VISIT_ID	COL_DATE	SEX	PAT_AGE	DRG_IND	DOSE	LAB TEST*	LAB_RSLT	MIN NORM	MAX NORM
C044	-67	SB0	07JAN85	F	47.9	PRE	0	21	0.6	0	1.100
C044	0	DB0	15MAR85	F	47.9	PRE	0	21	0.6	0	1.100
C044	18	DB2	02APR85	F	47.9	YYY	d	21	0.7	0	1.100
C044	32	DB4	16APR85	F	47.9	YYY	d	21	0.6	0	1.100
C044	63	DB5	17MAY85	F	47.9	YYY	d	21	0.4	0	1.100
C044	101	DB6	24JUN85	F	47.9	YYY	d	21	0.8	0	1.100
C044	206	DB7	07OCT85	F	47.9	YYY	d	21	0.5	0	1.100
.C044	311	DB8	20JAN86	F	47.9	YYY	d	21	0.4	0	1.100
C044	395	DB9B	14APR86	F	47.9	YYY	d	21	0.5	0	1.100
C044	-67	SB0	07JAN85	F	47.9	PRE	0	28	22.0	8	20.000
C044	0	DB0	15MAR85	F	47.9	PRE	0	28	17.0	8	20.000
C044	18	DB2	02APR85	F	47.9	YYY	d	28	22.0	8	20.000
C044	32	DB4	16APR85	F	47.9	YYY	d	28	19.0	8	20.000
C044	63	DB5	17MAY85	F	47.9	YYY	d	28	28.0	8	20.000
C044	101	DB6	24JUN85	F	47.9	YYY	d	28	26.0	8	20.000
C044	206	DB7	07OCT85	F	47.9	YYY	d	28	39.0	8	20.000
C044	311	DB8	20JAN86	F	47.9	YYY	d	28	30.0	8	20.000
C044	395	DB9B	14APR86	F	47.9	YYY	d	28	45.0	8	20.000
C044	-67	SB0	07JAN85	F	47.9	PRE	0	30	19.0	9	24.000
C044	0	DB0	15MAR85	F	47.9	PRE	0	30	18.0	9	24.000
C044	18	DB2	02APR85	F	47.9	YYY	d	30	18.0	9	24.000
C044	32	DB4	16APR85	F	47.9	YYY	d	30	19.0	9	24.000
C044	63	DB5	17MAY85	F	47.9	YYY	d	30	21.0	9	24.000
C044	101	DB6	24JUN85	F	47.9	YYY	d	30	27.0	9	24.000
C044	206	DB7	07OCT85	F	47.9	YYY	d	30	37.0	9	24.000
C044	311	DB8	20JAN86	F	47.9	YYY	d	30	34.0	9	24.000
C044	395	DB9B	14APR86	F	47.9	YYY	d	30	48.0	9	24.000
C044	-67	SB0	07JAN85	F	47.9	PRE	0	35	142.0	87	250.000
C044	0	DB0	15MAR85	F	47.9	PRE	0	35	161.0	87	250.000
C044	18	DB2	02APR85	F	47.9	YYY	d	35	178.0	87	250.000
C044	32	DB4	16APR85	F	47.9	YYY	d	35	169.0	87	250.000
C044	63	DB5	17MAY85	F	47.9	YYY	d	35	157.0	87	250.000
C044	101	DB6	24JUN85	F	47.9	YYY	d	35	184.0	87	250.000
C044	206	DB7	07OCT85	F	47.9	YYY	d	35	147.0	87	250.000
C044	311	DB8	20JAN86	F	47.9	YYY	d	35	157.0	87	250.000
C044	395	DB9B	14APR86	F	47.9	YYY	d	35	148.0	87	250.000

```
*LAB TEST 21 = BILIRUBIN
 LAB TEST 28 = SGOT
 LAB TEST 30 = SGPT
 LAB TEST 35 = ALKALINE PHOSPHATASE
 LAB_TEST 31 = GGT
```

Figure A-1

Computing Functional Group Scores (COMPFCNL.SAS)

Module 2, COMPFCNL.SAS, in which the functional group scores are computed, is the most complex module. In addition to computing the functional group score for each related set of lab parameters, the number of parameters measured (NP) and the number of parameters with abnormal values, i.e., the number of significant parameters (NSP), are recorded.

To compute the functional group score, each deviation is converted to a contributing value according to the following rules:

1. If the deviation is below zero, corresponding to a lab value below the lower limit of the normal range, the contributing value is defined as

$$|DEV| * \frac{2}{MIN\_NORM/MAX\_NORM} * 100$$

where 2 is a "stretch factor";

the absolute value of the deviation is used so that the contributing values will always be positive and therefore cumulative; otherwise, a deviation below the lower limit could cancel out the effect of a deviation above the upper limit and the functional group score could be zero, which would make it appear that there were no abnormalities within this functional group when in fact there were at least two lab tests with abnormal values; and the multiplier of 100 converts values to percentages.
2.   If there is no deviation from the normal range, the contributing value is 0.
3.   If the deviation is greater than zero, the contributing factor is simply the deviation * 100.

A running total of the number of parameters measured and the number of significant parameters found is maintained. Also, the contributing factors are summed for use in determining whether all the parameters in this functional group are within the corresponding reference ranges.

When the last parameter in a functional group is encountered, the functional group score is computed. The functional group total is determined by summing the contributing factors of the parameters within the functional group, dividing by the number of parameters assigned to the group, and then multiplying by two additional factors k_1 and k_2. These factors adjust the functional group score for the number of abnormal parameters found and the number of parameters missing (see Eq. (A-2) in Appendix 1).

Finally, two output datasets are created. Dataset GROUPS contains all functional group scores and the contributing factors. Dataset ABGRPS contains just the subset of functional group scores and contributing factors that are nonzero, i.e., that contain at least one lab test with a value outside the reference range.

Computing Global Genie Scores (COMPGLBL.SAS)

The Global Genie Score is an average of the individual functional group scores. The denominator is the number of nonmissing functional group scores that are summed in the numerator. The computations are carried out in module 3, COMPGLBL.SAS. As in module 2, COMPFCNL.SAS, two datasets are created. Dataset GENIE contains all Global Genie Scores (and the functional group scores composing them). Dataset ABNORM contains just the subset of Genie Scores that are nonzero, i.e., that contain at least one functional group score with an abnormal lab test in it.

Printing Functional Group Scores (PRTFCNL.SAS)

In module 4, PRTFCNL.SAS, each functional group and its constituent normalized values are printed. For each patient, the set of records composing a functional group is labeled "Abnormal" or "All OK." This is accomplished by selecting and labeling one record per patient from the functional group with a functional group score above zero, indicating that at least one lab parameter at that particular time point had a value outside the reference range for that parameter. This subset of patient records with abnormal functional group scores is then used to label the complete set of a patient's functional group records as "All OK" or "Abnormal." Only if every parameter value is within its reference range at every time point is a set of patient records for a functional group considered "All OK." Conversely, if any functional group score at any time is greater than zero, the set of records for that functional group for that patient is considered "Abnormal." See Fig. A-2 in Appendix 2 for example output. Values for three functional groups—liver, lipid, and diabetes—are shown for two patients, 41 and 44.

The SAS Macro language is used to print the data with titles and column headings appropriate to the functional group. The output is sent to a file containing print control characters. If desired, the macro PRTGRP in this module could be modified to send the output to up to 10 different files, one for each functional group.

```
                                        FUNCTIONAL GROUP SCORES

·······························  FUNCTIONAL GROUP=LIVER PATIENT CO44 NOTE=ABNORMAL ·······························

    SINCE                                         GROUP   # SIGNIF    #                              ALK
     BL    VISIT    DATE   SEX  AGE  DRUG  DOSE    TOTAL    PARAMS   PARAMS     SGOT    SGPT    PHOS    BILI    GGT

     -67    SBO    07JAN85   F   48   PRE    0      2.3       1        4        10.0    0.0     0.0     0.0      .
       0    DBO    15MAR85   F   48   PRE    0      0.0       0        4         0.0    0.0     0.0     0.0      .
      18    DB2    02APR85   F   48   YYY    d      2.3       1        4        10.0    0.0     0.0     0.0      .
      32    DB4    16APR85   F   48   YYY    d      0.0       0        4         0.0    0.0     0.0     0.0      .
      63    DB5    17MAY85   F   48   YYY    d      9.3       1        4        40.0    0.0     0.0     0.0      .
     101    DB6    24JUN85   F   48   YYY    d     11.7       2        4        30.0   12.5     0.0     0.0      .
     206    DB7    07OCT85   F   48   YYY    d     40.9       2        4        95.0   54.2     0.0     0.0      .
     311    DB8    20JAN86   F   48   YYY    d     25.2       2        4        50.0   41.7     0.0     0.0      .
     395    DB9B   14APR86   F   48   YYY    d     61.7       2        4       125.0  100.0     0.0     0.0      .


·······························  FUNCTIONAL GROUP=LIPID PATIENT CO41 NOTE=ABNORMAL ·······························
                                                                                                            FREE
    SINCE                                    GROUP  # SIGNIF   #                                            FATTY
     BL  VISIT    DATE  SEX AGE DRUG DOSE     TOTAL  PARAMS  PARAMS   CHOLES   HDL  LDL  VLDL  TRIGLY APO A1 APO B ACIDS

       0   DBO   09JAN85   F   57  PRE   0     12.5     2       2      -19.6    .    .    .     21.8    .     .    .
     169   DB7   27JUN85   F   57  XXX   d      1.9     1       2       -5.2    .    .    .      0.0    .     .    .
     377   DB9B  21JAN86   F   57  XXX   d      8.9     2       2      -12.4    .    .    .     19.5    .     .    .


·······························  FUNCTIONAL GROUP=LIPID PATIENT CO44 NOTE=ABNORMAL ·······························

    SINCE                                    GROUP  # SIGNIF   #                                            FATTY
     BL  VISIT    DATE  SEX AGE DRUG DOSE     TOTAL  PARAMS  PARAMS   CHOLES   HDL  LDL  VLDL  TRIGLY APO A1 APO B ACIDS

       0   DBO   15MAR85   F   48  PRE   0     13.0     1       2       0.0     .    .    .     87.6    .     .    .
     206   DB7   07OCT85   F   48  YYY   d      9.2     2       2       5.7     .    .    .     47.1    .     .    .
     395   DB9B  14APR86   F   48  YYY   d     21.1     2       2      16.7     .    .    .    104.1    .     .    .


·······························  FUNCTIONAL GROUP=DIABETES PATIENT CO41 NOTE=ABNORMAL ·······························

    SINCE                                    GROUP  # SIGNIF   #                                                   GLY
     BL  VISIT    DATE  SEX AGE DRUG DOSE     TOTAL  PARAMS  PARAMS  F.GLUCOSE R.GLUCOSE GLUCAGON F.INSULIN C-PEPTIDE HGB

     -43  SB-1   26NOV84   F   57  PRE   0     23.3     1       1      116.4      .        .        .          .      .
     -42  SBO    27NOV84   F   57  PRE   0      0.0     0       1        .        .        .        .          .     0.0
       0  DBO    09JAN85   F   57  PRE   0     19.1     2       1       80.0      .        .        .          .     2.0
      16  DB2    25JAN85   F   57  XXX   d     17.3     1       1       86.4      .        .        .          .      .
      30  DB4    08FEB85   F   57  XXX   d     19.3     1       1       96.4      .        .        .          .      .
      58  DB5    08MAR85   F   57  XXX   d     26.7     1       1      133.6      .        .        .          .      .
      89  DB6    08APR85   F   57  XXX   d      0.4     1       1        1.8      .        .        .          .      .
     169  DB7    27JUN85   F   57  XXX   d      1.6     1       1        8.2      .        .        .          .      .
     268  DB8    04OCT85   F   57  XXX   d      2.8     1       1       14.0      .        .        .          .      .
     377  DB9B   21JAN86   F   57  XXX   d     21.0     1       1      105.0      .        .        .          .      .
```

Figure A-2

Printing Global Genie Scores (PRTGLBL.SAS)

Module 5, PRTGLBL.SAS, prints the Global Genie Scores for every patient and labels a patient's set of Genie Scores as "Abnormal" or "All OK." This is accomplished by selecting and labeling one record per patient from the set of records with a Genie Score above zero, indicating that at least one lab parameter at that particular time point had a value outside the reference range for that parameter. This subset of patient records with abnormal Genie Scores is then used to label the complete set of a patient's records as "All OK" or "Abnormal." Only if every parameter value is within its reference range at every time point is a set of a patient's records considered "All OK." Conversely, if any Genie Score value at any time is greater than zero, the set of records for that patient is considered "Abnormal."

Finally, the data are printed with titles, column headings, and formats in a file containing print control characters.

See Fig. A-3 in Appendix 2 for example output. It displays the entire Genie Scores history for the two patients introduced in Fig. A-2. Compare the lipid columns of Fig. A-3 with the lipid group total columns of Fig. A-2. Similarly, Fig. A-2 shows a further breakdown of the diabetes column for patient 41 and the liver column for patient 44.

GLOBAL GENIE SCORES

-------------------------------- PATIENT C041 NOTE=ABNORMAL --------------------------------

SINCE BL	VISIT	DATE	SEX	AGE	DRUG	DOSE	GENIE GRPS	LIVER	RENAL	RBC	WBC	ELECT	LIPID	DIABETES	METAB	PLATELET	MUSCLE
-43	SB-1	26NOV84	F	57	PRE	0	4.0 8	3.0	0.0	0.1	5.5	0.0	.	23.3	0.0	0.0	.
-42	SB0	27NOV84	F	57	PRE	0	0.0 1	.	.	.	.	.	.	0.0	.	.	.
0	DB0	09JAN85	F	57	PRE	0	11.8 9	1.7	0.0	1.3	71.2	0.0	12.5	19.1	0.0	0.0	.
16	DB2	25JAN85	F	57	XXX	d	11.8 8	1.7	0.0	10.8	64.4	0.0	.	17.3	0.0	0.0	.
30	DB4	08FEB85	F	57	XXX	d	3.6 8	2.8	0.0	1.4	1.9	3.3	.	19.3	0.3	0.0	.
41	UNPL	19FEB85	F	57	XXX	d	4.7 3	11.0	.	.	2.9	.	.	.	.	0.0	.
48	UNPL	26FEB85	F	57	XXX	d	4.4 3	13.2	.	.	0.0	.	.	.	.	0.0	.
58	DB5	08MAR85	F	57	XXX	d	4.4 8	8.5	0.0	0.1	0.0	0.0	.	26.7	0.0	0.0	.
89	DB6	08APR85	F	57	XXX	d	3.6 8	16.7	3.3	0.6	4.6	0.0	.	0.4	2.9	0.0	.
169	DB7	27JUN85	F	57	XXX	d	1.7 9	0.0	3.3	1.1	0.0	3.3	1.9	1.6	3.9	0.0	.
268	DB8	04OCT85	F	57	XXX	d	5.8 8	3.2	0.0	0.2	38.0	0.0	.	2.8	1.9	0.0	.
377	DB9B	21JAN86	F	57	XXX	d	4.2 9	4.6	0.0	0.0	0.0	1.6	8.9	21.0	1.6	0.0	.

-------------------------------- PATIENT C044 NOTE = ABNORMAL --------------------------------

SINCE BL	VISIT	DATE	SEX	AGE	DRUG	DOSE	GENIE GRPS	LIVER	RENAL	RBC	WBC	ELECT	LIPID	DIABETES	METAB	PLATELET	MUSCLE
-67	SB0	07JAN85	F	48	PRE	0	7.4 8	2.3	0.0	0.0	38.0	0.0	.	18.5	0.2	0.0	.
0	DB0	15MAR85	F	48	PRE	0	8.3 9	0.0	0.0	0.0	38.0	0.0	13.0	23.5	0.0	0.0	.
18	DB2	02APR85	F	48	YYY	d	7.2 8	2.3	0.0	0.4	38.0	0.0	.	16.5	0.0	0.0	.
32	DB4	16APR85	F	48	YYY	d	6.8 8	0.0	0.0	0.0	38.0	0.0	.	16.0	0.0	0.0	.
63	DB5	17MAY85	F	48	YYY	d	3.8 8	9.3	0.0	0.0	0.0	0.0	.	21.5	0.0	0.0	.
101	DB6	24JUN85	F	48	YYY	d	9.7 8	11.7	0.0	0.0	38.0	0.0	.	27.8	0.2	0.0	.
206	DB7	07OCT85	F	48	YYY	d	10.9 9	40.9	0.0	0.0	38.0	0.0	9.2	7.4	2.3	0.0	.
311	DB8	20JAN86	F	48	YYY	d	4.6 8	25.2	0.0	0.0	0.0	0.0	.	11.8	0.2	0.0	.
395	DB9B	14APR86	F	48	YYY	d	15.2 9	61.7	0.0	0.0	38.0	0.0	21.1	12.6	3.6	0.0	.

Figure A-3

Creating the File SCORES.DAT Containing Functional Group Scores and Global Genie Scores (WRITE.SAS)

Module 6, WRITE.SAS, produces a "flat" or ASCII file called SCORES.DAT from the output of module 3, COMPGLBL.SAS. This file contains both functional group scores and Global Genie Scores, along with identifying information such as patient identification number, visit date, age, sex, drug, and dose, and is formatted for input to statistical and graphics programs. See Fig. A-4 for an example file and Fig. A-5 for the format of this file. Module 6, WRITE.SAS, outputs in fixed-column format the information stored in permanent SAS dataset GENIE. Missing values are simply left blank.

Summary

We have described a set of computer programs used to compute and output Genie Scores for further computation, review, analysis, summary, and presentation of laboratory data. Possible modifications and enhancements to the system as described include a menu-driven structure to allow users easy access to the programs, facilities for limiting computation of Genie Scores to subsets of the input dataset, and the creation of standard programs to compute statistics and graph results.

Example SCORES.DAT File

```
C041  57.4 F SB-1  26NOV84  -43 PRE   0   3.0   0.0   0 1   5.5   0.0          21.3   0.0   0.0   8   4.0
C041  57.4 F SB0   27NOV84   42 PRE   0                                         0.0                   1   0.0
C041  57.4 F DB0   09JAN85    0 PRE   0   1.7   0.0   1.3  71.2   0.0  12.5  19.1   0.0   0.0   9  11.8
C041  57.4 F DB2   25JAN85   16 XXX   d   1.7   0.0  10.8  64.4   0.0        17.3   0.0   0.0   8  11.8
C041  57.4 F DB4   08FEB85   30 XXX   d   2.8   0.0   1.4   1.9   3.3        19.3   0.3   0.0   8   3.6
C041  57.4 F UP    19FEB85   41 XXX   d  11.0                     2.9                      0.0   3   4.7
C041  57.4 F UP    26FEB85   48 XXX   d  13.2                     0.0                      0.0   3   4.4
C041  57.4 F DB5   08MAR85   58 XXX   d   8.5   0.0   0 1   0.0   0.0        26.7   0.0   0.0   8   4.4
C041  57.4 F DB6   08APR85   89 XXX   d  16.7   3.3   0.6   4.6   0.0         0.4   2.9   0.0   8   3.6
C041  57.4 F DB7   27JUN85  169 XXX   d   0.0   3.3   1.1   0.0   3.3   1.9   1.6   3.9   0.0   9   1.7
C041  57.4 F DB8   04OCT85  268 XXX   d   3.2   0.0   0.2  38.0   0.0         2.8   1.9   0.0   8   5.8
C041  57.4 F DB9B  21JAN86  377 XXX   d   4.6   0.0   0.0   0.0   1.6   8.9  21.0   1.6   0.0   9   4.2
C042  44.4 M SB0   22AUG84 -141 PRE   0   0.0   2.5   8.5   0.0   0.0        24.7   0.0   0.0   8   4.5
C042  44.4 M SB1   09JAN85   -1 PRE   0                                         5.9                   1   5.9
C042  44.4 M DB0   10JAN85    0 PRE   0   5.8   7.5  21.9  38.0   0.0   0.0   7.3   0.0   0.0   9   8.9
C042  44.4 M DB2   30JAN85   20 XXX   d   0.0  12.5  27.9   0.0   0.0        31.5   0.0   0.0   8   9.0
C042  44.4 M DB4   13FEB85   34 XXX   d   0.0  10.0  34.1   0.0   0.0         0.6   0.0   0.0   8   5.6
C042  44.4 M DB5   18MAR85   67 XXX   d   7.0   7.5  23.0   0.0   2.5        26.7   0.0   0.0   8   7.7
C042  44.4 M DB6   05APR85   85 XXX   d   5.8  12.5  22.0  38.0   0.0        17.3   0.0   0.0   8  12.0
C042  44.4 M DB7   19JUL85  190 XXX   d   0.0  10.0  21.7   0.0   0.0   0.0  25.5   0.0   0.0   9   4.4
C042  44.4 M DB8   22OCT85  285 XXX   d   0.0   5.0  25.0   0.0   0.0        18.0   0.0   0.0   8   6.0
C042  44.4 M DB9B  14JAN86  369 XXX   d   2.2  17.5   9.8   2.2   0.0   2.0   0.0   0.0   0.0   9   3.7
C044  47.9 F SB0   07JAN85  -67 PRE   0   2.3   0.0   0.0  38.0   0.0        18.5   0.2   0.0   8   7.4
C044  47.9 F DB0   15MAR85    0 PRE   0   0.0   0.0   0.0  38.0   0.0  13.0  23.5   0.0   0.0   9   8.3
C044  47.9 F DB2   02APR85   18 YYY   d   2.3   0.0   0.4  38.0   0.0        16.5   0.0   0.0   8   7.2
C044  47.9 F DB4   16APR85   32 YYY   d   0.0   0.0   0.0  38.0   0.0        16.0   0.0   0.0   8   6.8
C044  47.9 F DB5   17MAY85   63 YYY   d   9.3   0.0   0.0   0.0   0.0        21.5   0.0   0.0   8   3.8
C044  47.9 F DB6   24JUN85  101 YYY   d  11.7   0.0   0.0  38.0   0.0        27.8   0.2   0.0   8   9.7
C044  47.9 F DB7   07OCT85  206 YYY   d  40.9   0.0   0.0  38.0   0.0   9.2   7.4   2.3   0.0   9  10.9
C044  47.9 F DB8   20JAN86  311 YYY   d  25.2   0.0   0.0   0.0   0.0        11.8   0.2   0.0   8   4.6
C044  47.9 F DB9B  14APR86  395 YYY   d  61.7   0.0   0.0  38.0   0.0  21.1  12.6   3.6   0.0   9  15.2
C045  46.1 M SB0   23JAN85  -29 PRE   0   4.7   0.0   0.6  38.0   0.0         6.0  17.1   0.0   8   8.3
C045  46.1 M DB0   21FEB85    0 PRE   0   0.0   0.0   0.0  38.0   0.0   7.4  61.4  17.1   0.0   9  11.8
C045  46.1 M DB2   13MAR85   20 YYY   d   0.0   0.0   0.4   0.0   0.0        24.2  19.9   0.0   8   5.6
C045  46.1 M DB4   27MAR85   34 YYY   d   0.0   0.0   3.1   0.0   0.0        50.9  18.0   0.0   8   9.0
C045  46.1 M DB5   24APR85   62 YYY   d   0.0   0.0   0.0   0.0   0.0        22.2  22.6   0.0   8   5.6
C045  46.1 M DB6   05JUN85  104 YYY   d   4.7   0.0   0.4   0.0   0.0        24.4  21.7   0.0   8   6.4
C045  46.1 M DB7   11SEP85  202 YYY   d   0.0   0.0   5.2  38.0   0.0  19.1  19.8  18.9   0.0   9  11.2
C045  46.1 M DB8   04DEC85  286 YYY   d   4.7   0.0   0.0   0.0   0.0         1.0  18.0   0.0   8   3.0
C045  46.1 M DB9B  11MAR86  383 YYY   d   0.0   0.0   2.9  38.0   0.0  15.3  18.6  21.7   0.0   9  10.7
```

Figure A-4

```
                         Format of SCORES.DAT File
Variable Description                        Columns          Format
--------------------                        -------          ------
Patient Identification Number                1-11            11 characters
Patient Age                                  12-16           5.1
Patient Sex                                  18              1 character (M/F)
Visit Designator                             20-24           5 characters
Visit Date                                   26-32           DDMONYY
Number of Days Since Baseline                33-37           integer
Drug                                         39-43           5 characters
Dose                                         45-52           real
LIVER Function Group Score                   53-58           6.1
RENAL Function Group Score                   60-65           6.1
RBC Function Group Score                     67-72           6.1
WBC Function Group Score                     74-79           6.1
ELECT Function Group Score                   81-86           6.1
LIPID Function Group Score                   88-93           6.1
DIABETES Function Group Score                95-100          6.1
METAB Function Group Score                   102-107         6.1
PLATELET Function Group Score                109-114         6.1
MUSCLE Function Group Score                  116-121         6.1
Number of Non-Missing Groups                 123-124         integer
Global Genie Score                           126-131         6.1
```

Figure A-5

The system as currently implemented is flexible, allowing changes to be easily made in the list of lab tests included in each functional group, the weights assigned to those parameters, and the order in which the parameters are displayed.

The use of computer programs to calculate and display the Genie Scores makes the employment of Genie Scores in monitoring and analyzing clinical trials a powerful tool for the pharmaceutical research scientists.

```
************************************************************************
* Functional Group scores and Overall Genie scores ...                *
*                                                                      *
* READ.SAS - This program reads in data from ASCII files and creates  *
* (Module     an output SAS data set with one record per lab test per *
*   0.5)      patient per date, with normal range attached.           *
*                                                                      *
* Input:   LIVER.DAT - ASCII FILE OF LIVER FUNCTION TESTS             *
*          RENAL.DAT - ASCII FILE OF RENAL FUNCTION TESTS             *
*          RBC.DAT - ASCII FILE OF RED BLOOD CELL TESTS               *
*          WBC.DAT - ASCII FILE OF WHITE BLOOD COUNT TESTS            *
*          ELECT.DAT - ASCII FILE OF ELECTROLYTE TESTS                *
*          LIPID.DAT - ASCII FILE OF LIPID TESTS                      *
*          DIABETES.DAT - ASCII FILE OF DIABETES-RELATED TESTS        *
*          METAB.DAT - ASCII FILE OF METABOLISM TESTS                 *
*          PLATELET.DAT - ASCII FILE OF PLATELET TESTS                *
*          MUSCLE.DAT - ASCII FILE OF MUSCLE TESTS                    *
*                                                                      *
* Output: NORM.BLAB - SAS data set with "normalized" lab test values, *
*                     upper weights, lower weights, and functional    *
*                     group numbers (and demographic information).    *
************************************************************************;

OPTIONS PAGESIZE=62 LINESIZE=80;

FILENAME LIVER     'LIVER.DAT';          /*  Input files of data, one per */
FILENAME RENAL     'RENAL.DAT';          /*    function group.            */
FILENAME RBC       'RBC.DAT';            /*                               */
FILENAME WBC       'WBC.DAT';            /*                               */
FILENAME ELECT     'ELECT.DAT';          /*                               */
FILENAME LIPID     'LIPID.DAT';          /*                               */
FILENAME DIABETES  'DIABETES.DAT';       /*                               */
FILENAME METAB     'METAB.DAT';          /*                               */
FILENAME PLATELET  'PLATELET.DAT';       /*                               */
FILENAME MUSCLE    'MUSCLE.DAT';         /*                               */

LIBNAME NORM '[]';

DATA LIVER;
  LENGTH LAB_RSLT 4;
  INFILE LIVER;
  INPUT PAT_ID $   1-11     BAS_DAYS 12-18    DRG_IND 19-25
        RSLT1 $   26-32    LLN1      33-39   ULN1   40-46   TEST1   47-49
        RSLT2 $   50-56    LLN2      57-63   ULN2   64-70   TEST2   71-73
        RSLT3 $   74-80    LLN3      81-87   ULN3   88-94   TEST3   95-97
        RSLT4 $   98-104   LLN4     105-111  ULN4  112-118  TEST4 119-121
        RSLT5 $  122-128   LLN5     129-135  ULN5  136-142  TEST5 143-145
        RSLT6 $  146-152   LLN6     153-159  ULN6  160-166  TEST6 167-169;
```

* If Laboratory Results are NORMAL or Within Normal Limits, use the Lower
  Limit of the Normal (reference) range for the value of this lab test. This
  is arbitrary -- the Upper Limit of the Normal range could also be used, as
  could any value within the reference range. Any of these values will result
  in a deviation = 0.;
* If the Laboratory Result is Not Done or Chemistry is Not Done, use a missing
  value for the value of this lab test.;

```
        IF RSLT1 = 'NORM' OR RSLT1 = 'norm' OR RSLT1 = 'WNL' THEN RSLT1 = LLN1;
   ELSE IF RSLT1='ND' OR RSLT1='nd' OR RSLT1='C-ND' OR RSLT1='C ND' THEN RSLT1=.;
        IF RSLT2 = 'NORM' OR RSLT2 = 'norm' OR RSLT2 = 'WNL' THEN RSLT2 = LLN2;
   ELSE IF RSLT2='ND' OR RSLT2='nd' OR RSLT2='C-ND' OR RSLT2='C ND' THEN RSLT2=.;
        IF RSLT3 = 'NORM' OR RSLT3 = 'norm' OR RSLT3 = 'WNL' THEN RSLT3 = LLN3;
   ELSE IF RSLT3='ND' OR RSLT3='nd' OR RSLT3='C-ND' OR RSLT3='C ND' THEN RSLT3=.;
        IF RSLT4 = 'NORM' OR RSLT4 = 'norm' OR RSLT4 = 'WNL' THEN RSLT4 = LLN4;
```

```
ELSE IF RSLT4='ND' OR RSLT4='nd' OR RSLT4='C-ND' OR RSLT4='C ND' THEN RSLT4=.;
    IF RSLT5 = 'NORM' OR RSLT5 = 'norm' OR RSLT5 = 'WNL' THEN RSLT5 = LLN5;
ELSE IF RSLT5='ND' OR RSLT5='nd' OR RSLT5='C-ND' OR RSLT5='C ND' THEN RSLT5=.;
    IF RSLT6 = 'NORM' OR RSLT6 = 'norm' OR RSLT6 = 'WNL' THEN RSLT6 = LLN6;
ELSE IF RSLT6='ND' OR RSLT6='nd' OR RSLT6='C-ND' OR RSLT6='C ND' THEN RSLT6=.;

DOSE     = .;        /* If you wanted to print these values on your  */
PAT_AGE  = .;        /* reports, you can include them in the input   */
SEX      = ' ';      /* files and add columns to the INPUT statement */
COL_DATE = .;        /* above, or attach them later to the BLAB data */
VISIT_ID = ' ';      /* set.                                         */

IF RSLT1 NE . THEN DO;
   LAB_TEST = TEST1;  LAB_RSLT = RSLT1;  MIN_NORM = LLN1;  MAX_NORM = ULN1;
   OUTPUT;                /* Output one record per lab test per pt per date*/
END;
IF RSLT2 NE . THEN DO;
   LAB_TEST = TEST2;  LAB_RSLT = RSLT2;  MIN_NORM = LLN2;  MAX_NORM = ULN2;
   OUTPUT;
END;
IF RSLT3 NE . THEN DO;
   LAB_TEST = TEST3;  LAB_RSLT = RSLT3;  MIN_NORM = LLN3;  MAX_NORM = ULN3;
   OUTPUT;
END;
IF RSLT4 NE . THEN DO;
   LAB_TEST = TEST4;  LAB_RSLT = RSLT4;  MIN_NORM = LLN4;  MAX_NORM = ULN4;
   OUTPUT;
END;
IF RSLT5 NE . THEN DO;
   LAB_TEST = TEST5;  LAB_RSLT = RSLT5;  MIN_NORM = LLN5;  MAX_NORM = ULN5;
   OUTPUT;
END;
IF RSLT6 NE . THEN DO;
   LAB_TEST = TEST6;  LAB_RSLT = RSLT6;  MIN_NORM = LLN6;  MAX_NORM = ULN6;
   OUTPUT;
END;

KEEP PAT_ID PAT_AGE SEX DRG_IND DOSE COL_DATE VISIT_ID BAS_DAYS
     LAB_TEST LAB_RSLT MIN_NORM MAX_NORM;

DATA RENAL;
   .
   .
   .

DATA RBC;
   .
   .
   .

DATA WBC;
   .
   .
   .

DATA ELECT;
   .
   .
   .

DATA LIPID;
```

```
       .
 DATA DIABETES;
       .
       .
       .
 DATA METAB;
       .
       .
       .
 DATA PLATELET;
       .
       .
       .
 DATA MUSCLE;
       .
       .
       .
 DATA BLAB;                  /* Combine all function group data sets into one. */
   SET LIVER RENAL RBC WBC ELECT LIPID DIABETES METAB PLATELET MUSCLE;

 PROC SORT DATA=BLAB OUT=NORM.BLAB;
   BY PAT_ID BAS_DAYS LAB_TEST;

 ********************************************************************************
 * Functional Group scores and Global Genie scores ...                         *
 *                                                                             *
 * ASSGNGRP.SAS - This program assigns functional group numbers to the         *
 * (Module 1/6) lab parameters of interest.                                    *
 *                                                                             *
 * Input:  BLAB.SSD - SAS data set with one record per lab test per            *
 *                    patient per date, with normal range attached.            *
 *                                                                             *
 * Output: NORM.INDIV - SAS data set with "normalized" lab test values         *
 *                    and functional group numbers (and demographic            *
 *                    information).                                            *
 ********************************************************************************;

 OPTIONS PAGESIZE=62 LINESIZE=80;

 LIBNAME OUTPUT V606 '[]';
 LIBNAME NORM V5 '[]';

 DATA INDIV;
   SET NORM.BLAB;
   IF MAX_NORM = 0 THEN DEV = LAB_RSLT;    /*If normal range 0-0, any value  */
   ELSE DO;                                /*   at all is a deviation.       */
     NORMVAL = LAB_RSLT / MAX_NORM;        /*"Normalize" each lab test value.*/
     IF LAB_RSLT < MIN_NORM THEN DEV = NORMVAL - MIN_NORM/MAX_NORM;
       ELSE IF 0 <= NORMVAL <= 1 THEN DEV = 0;   /*Find the deviation*/
       ELSE DEV = NORMVAL - 1;
   END;

       IF LAB_TEST = 21 THEN DO;           /* 1st lab test */
         FCNL = 1;                         /* assign functional group */
         WU = 1.0;               /* assign weight if abnorm above upper limit */
         WL = 1.0;               /* assign weight if abnorm below lower limit */
       END;
   %MACRO ASSIGN(T,F,U,L);
   ELSE IF LAB_TEST = &T THEN DO;          /* all other lab tests */
     FCNL = &F;                            /* assign functional group */
     WU = &U;                   /* assign weight if abnorm above upper limit */
     WL = &L;                   /* assign weight if abnorm below lower limit */
   END;
   %MEND ASSIGN;
```

```
%ASSIGN (   28,1,1.0,1.0)
%ASSIGN (   30,1,1.0,1.0)
%ASSIGN (   31,1,1.0,1.0)
%ASSIGN (   35,1,1.0,1.0)
%ASSIGN (   44,2,1.0,1.0)
%ASSIGN (   47,2,1.0,1.0)
%ASSIGN (   48,2,1.0,1.0)
%ASSIGN (   49,2,1.0,1.0)
%ASSIGN (    1,3,1.0,1.0)
%ASSIGN (    2,3,1.0,1.0)
%ASSIGN (   15,3,1.0,1.0)
%ASSIGN (   17,3,1.0,1.0)
%ASSIGN (    7,4,1.0,1.0)
%ASSIGN (  608,4,1.0,1.0)
%ASSIGN (  609,4,1.0,1.0)
%ASSIGN (  610,4,1.0,1.0)
%ASSIGN (  611,4,1.0,1.0)
%ASSIGN (  612,4,1.0,1.0)
%ASSIGN (   54,5,1.0,1.0)
%ASSIGN (   55,5,1.0,1.0)
%ASSIGN (   56,5,1.0,1.0)
%ASSIGN (   57,5,1.0,1.0)
%ASSIGN (   63,6,1.0,1.0)
%ASSIGN (   64,6,1.0,1.0)
%ASSIGN (   65,6,1.0,1.0)
%ASSIGN (  171,6,1.0,1.0)
%ASSIGN (  172,6,1.0,1.0)
%ASSIGN (  173,6,1.0,1.0)
%ASSIGN (  276,6,1.0,1.0)
%ASSIGN (  312,6,1.0,1.0)
%ASSIGN (   67,7,1.0,1.0)
%ASSIGN (   68,7,1.0,1.0)
%ASSIGN (  131,7,1.0,1.0)
%ASSIGN (  190,7,1.0,1.0)
%ASSIGN (  191,7,1.0,1.0)
%ASSIGN (  229,7,1.0,1.0)
%ASSIGN (   25,8,1.0,1.0)
%ASSIGN (   26,8,1.0,1.0)
%ASSIGN (   50,8,1.0,1.0)
%ASSIGN (   58,8,1.0,1.0)
%ASSIGN (   59,8,1.0,1.0)
%ASSIGN (  199,8,1.0,1.0)
%ASSIGN (    5,9,1.0,1.0)
%ASSIGN (   19,9,1.0,1.0)
%ASSIGN (  122,9,1.0,1.0)
%ASSIGN (  123,9,1.0,1.0)
%ASSIGN (  126,9,1.0,1.0)
%ASSIGN (  129,9,1.0,1.0)
%ASSIGN (   32,10,1.0,1.0)
%ASSIGN (  151,10,1.0,1.0)
%ASSIGN (  152,10,1.0,1.0)
%ASSIGN (  153,10,1.0,1.0)
%ASSIGN (  154,10,1.0,1.0)
%ASSIGN (  155,10,1.0,1.0)
%ASSIGN (  156,10,1.0,1.0)
%ASSIGN (  157,10,1.0,1.0)
%ASSIGN (  158,10,1.0,1.0)
%ASSIGN (  205,10,1.0,1.0)
%ASSIGN (  415,10,1.0,1.0)


KEEP PAT_ID PAT_AGE SEX DRG_IND DOSE COL_DATE VISIT_ID BAS_DAYS
    LAB_TEST LAB_RSLT FCNL WU WL MIN_NORM MAX_NORM DEV;


PROC SORT DATA=INDIV OUT=OUTPUT.INDIV;
  BY PAT_ID BAS_DAYS FCNL;
```

```
***********************************************************************
* Functional Group scores and Global Genie scores...                 *
*                                                                     *
* COMPFCNL.SAS - This program computes the FUNCTIONAL GROUP scores.   *
* (Module 2/6)                                                        *
*                                                                     *
* Input:  NORM.INDIV - SAS data set from ASSGNGRP.SAS with "normalized"*
*                      lab test values and functional group numbers.  *
*                                                                     *
* Output: NORM.GROUPS - SAS data set with one record per patient per  *
*                       functional group.  Each record contains the   *
*                       Functional Group score and a value for each   *
*                       parameter in the Functional Group.            *
*          NORM.ABGRPS - SAS data set which contains one record per    *
*                       patient per functional group if the Functional *
*                       Group score is non-zero--that is, if there is  *
*                       at least one parameter with a value outside the*
*                       normal range.                                 *
***********************************************************************;


OPTIONS PAGESIZE=62 LINESIZE=132 CENTER;

LIBNAME NORM '[]';

DATA NORM.GROUPS NORM.ABGRPS;
  SET NORM.INDIV;
  BY PAT_ID BAS_DAYS FCNL;
  RETAIN COMP1-COMP11 CONT1-CONT11 NP NSP CHECK LABTST1-LABTST11;
  ARRAY C (I) COMP1-COMP11;        /*components -- raw devns from normal*/
  ARRAY CT (I) CONT1-CONT11;       /*contributing factors -- devn x wt  */
  ARRAY LT (I) LABTST1-LABTST11;   /*lab test values                    */
  IF FIRST.FCNL THEN DO;           /*Initialize arrays and counters.    */
      DO OVER C;
          C = .;
      END;
      DO OVER CT;
          CT = .;
      END;
      DO OVER LT;
          LT = .;
      END;
      CHECK = 0;
      NP = 0;                           /*number of parameters measured      */
      NSP = 0;          /*number of significant parameters -- ie devn NE 0*/
  END;
  %MACRO GROUPS(GRP,HOWMANY,P1,P2,P3,P4,P5,P6,P7,P8,P9,P10,P11); /*Compute */
      IF FCNL = &GRP THEN DO;                      /*FUNCTIONAL GROUP scores */
          IF LAB_TEST = &P1 THEN DO;       /*First parameter in fcnl grp*/
              LABTST1 = LAB_RSLT;
              COMP1 = DEV * 100;
              NP = NP + 1;


              IF DEV < 0 THEN DO;
                  CONT1 = ABS(DEV) * WL * 2/(MIN_NORM/MAX_NORM) * 100;
                                                      /*Include stretch    */
                  CHECK = CHECK + CONT1;              /*factor for value   */
                  NSP = NSP + 1;                      /*below lower limit*/
              END;                                    /*of normal          */
              ELSE IF DEV = 0 THEN CONT1 = 0;
              ELSE DO;
                  CONT1 = DEV * WU * 100;
                  CHECK = CHECK + CONT1;
                  NSP = NSP + 1;
              END;
          END;
```

```
      %MACRO INDIV(K);                      /*All other parameters in */
      ELSE IF LAB_TEST = &&P&K THEN DO; /*functional group         */
               LABTST&K = LAB_RSLT;
               COMP&K = DEV * 100;
               NP = NP + 1;
               IF DEV < 0 THEN DO;
                  CONT&K = ABS(DEV) * WL * 2/(MIN_NORM/MAX_NORM) * 100;
                  CHECK = CHECK + CONT&K;
                  NSP = NSP + 1;
               END;
               ELSE IF DEV = 0 THEN CONT&K = 0;
               ELSE DO;
                  CONT&K = DEV * WU * 100;
                  CHECK = CHECK + CONT&K;
                  NSP = NSP + 1;
               END;
      END;
      %MEND INDIV;
      %DO J = 2 %TO &HOWMANY;
         %INDIV(&J)
      %END;
      IF LAST.FCNL THEN DO;
         GRPTOTAL = (1 + .2 * NSP) * (1 - .01 * (NP-NSP)) *
            SUM(CONT1,CONT2,CONT3,CONT4,CONT5,CONT6,CONT7,CONT8,CONT9,CONT10,
            CONT11) / &HOWMANY;
         IF CHECK = 0 THEN STATUS='    OK';
         ELSE DO;
            STATUS='NOT OK';
            OUTPUT NORM.ABGRPS;   /*keep track of a record with a non-0*/
         END;                     /*functional group score             */
         OUTPUT NORM.GROUPS;
      END;
   END;
%MEND GROUPS;
%GROUPS(1,5,28,30,35,21,31)
%GROUPS(2,4,47,48,49,44)
%GROUPS(3,4,15,1,2,17)
%GROUPS(4,6,7,608,611,612,609,610)
%GROUPS(5,4,54,55,56,57)
%GROUPS(6,8,63,173,172,171,64,276,312,65)
%GROUPS(7,6,67,68,190,191,229,131)
%GROUPS(8,6,58,59,199,25,26,50)
%GROUPS(9,6,5,122,19,123,129,126)
%GROUPS(10,11,32,151,152,153,154,155,205,156,157,158,415)
DROP LAB_TEST LAB_RSLT MIN_NORM MAX_NORM I WU WL CHECK;



*******************************************************************
* Functional Group scores and Global Genie scores...            *
*                                                               *
* COMPOVG.SAS - This program computes Global Genie scores, counts the *
* (Module 3/6)  number of functional groups which contribute to the  *
*               Global Genie score, counts the number of functional  *
*               groups with any lab test values outside the normal   *
*               range, and keeps track of records with a non-zero    *
*               Global Genie score.                             *
*                                                               *
* Input:  NORM.GROUPS - SAS data set from COMPFCNL.SAS with one record *
*                        per patient per functional group.      *
*                                                               *
* Output: NORM.GENIE - SAS data set with one record per patient per *
*                       date.  contains Global Genie score and  *
*                       contributing Functional Group scores.   *
*         NORM.ABNORM - SAS data set with one record per patient per *
*                        date if the Global Genie score is non-zero-- *
*                        that is, if at least one of the Functional *
*                        Group scores is non-zero.              *
*******************************************************************;
```

```
OPTIONS PAGESIZE=62 LINESIZE=132 CENTER;

LIBNAME NORM '[]';

DATA NORM.GENIE NORM.ABNORM;
   SET NORM.GROUPS;
   BY PAT_ID BAS_DAYS;
   RETAIN GEN1-GEN10 NG CHECK;
   ARRAY G (I) GEN1-GEN10;
   IF FIRST.BAS_DAYS THEN DO;
      DO OVER G;
         G = .;
      END;
      CHECK = 0;
      NG = 0;
   END;
   DO J = 1 TO 10;
      IF FCNL = J THEN DO;
         I = J;
         G = GRPTOTAL;
         CHECK = CHECK + GRPTOTAL;
         NG = NG + 1;
      END;
   END;
   IF LAST.BAS_DAYS THEN DO;
      GENIE = SUM(GEN1,GEN2,GEN3,GEN4,GEN5,GEN6,GEN7,GEN8,GEN9,GEN10) /
                 N(GEN1,GEN2,GEN3,GEN4,GEN5,GEN6,GEN7,GEN8,GEN9,GEN10);
      IF CHECK = 0 THEN STATUS = '    OK';
      ELSE DO;
         STATUS = 'NOT OK';
         OUTPUT NORM.ABNORM;
      END;
      OUTPUT NORM.GENIE;
   END;

TITLE2 "FUNCTIONAL GROUP SCORES";
TITLE3 " ";

******************************************************************************
* Functional Group scores and Global Genie scores...                        *
*                                                                            *
* PRTFCNL.SAS - This program identifies patients with ALL OK values of      *
* (Module 4/6)  Functional Group scores and prints a listing of             *
*               Functional Group scores by FCNL PAT_ID DATE.                 *
*                                                                            *
* Input:  NORM.GROUPS - SAS data set from COMPFCNL.SAS with one record       *
*                       per Functional Group per patient per date.           *
*         NORM.ABGRPS - SAS data set from COMPFCNL.SAS with one record       *
*                       per Functional Group per patient per date if         *
*                       the Functional Group score is non-zero.              *
*                                                                            *
* Output:  PRTFCNL.LIS - Listing of Functional Group scores and             *
*                        contributing parameter values by Functional         *
*                        Group, patient, and date.                           *
******************************************************************************;


OPTIONS PAGESIZE=62 LINESIZE=132 CENTER;

LIBNAME NORM '[]';

PROC SORT DATA=NORM.GROUPS OUT=GROUPS;
   BY FCNL PAT_ID BAS_DAYS;

PROC SORT DATA=NORM.ABGRPS OUT=ABGRPS;
   BY FCNL PAT_ID BAS_DAYS;

PROC FORMAT;
   VALUE FCNLGRP  1='LIVER' 2='RENAL'    3='RBC'       4='WBC'       5='ELECT'
                  6='LIPID' 7='DIABETES' 8='METABOLIC' 9='PLATELET' 10='MUSCLE';
```

```
DATA ABGRPS2;
  SET ABGRPS;
  BY FCNL PAT_ID;
  IF FIRST.PAT_ID;            /*Mark patient records where functional */
  NOTE = 'ABNORMAL';          /*group scores are not zero.  Keep only */
  KEEP FCNL PAT_ID NOTE;      /*one record per patient.               */

DATA LIVER RENAL RBC WBC ELECT LIPID DIABETES METABOL PLATELET MUSCLE;
  MERGE GROUPS ABGRPS2;
  BY FCNL PAT_ID;
  FORMAT FCNL FCNLGRP.;


  IF NOTE = ' ' THEN NOTE = "ALL OK";
       IF FCNL = 1 THEN OUTPUT LIVER;
  ELSE IF FCNL = 2 THEN OUTPUT RENAL;
  ELSE IF FCNL = 3 THEN OUTPUT RBC;
  ELSE IF FCNL = 4 THEN OUTPUT WBC;
  ELSE IF FCNL = 5 THEN OUTPUT ELECT;
  ELSE IF FCNL = 6 THEN OUTPUT LIPID;
  ELSE IF FCNL = 7 THEN OUTPUT DIABETES;
  ELSE IF FCNL = 8 THEN OUTPUT METABOL;
  ELSE IF FCNL = 9 THEN OUTPUT PLATELET;
  ELSE IF FCNL = 10 THEN OUTPUT MUSCLE;

%MACRO PRTGRP (GRPTSTN,HOWMANY,TSTN1,TSTN2,TSTN3,TSTN4,TSTN5,TSTN6,TSTN7,
                              TSTN8,TSTN9,TSTN10,TSTN11);
 PROC PRINT DATA = &GRPTSTN UNIFORM LABEL;
  BY FCNL PAT_ID NOTE NOTSORTED;
  ID BAS_DAYS;
  VAR VISIT_ID COL_DATE SEX PAT_AGE DRG_IND DOSE GRPTOTAL NSP NP
      COMP1-COMP&HOWMANY;
  FORMAT VISIT_ID $4. COL_DATE DATE7. SEX $1. PAT_AGE 3.0


        DOSE 3.0 GRPTOTAL COMP1 10.1 COMP2-COMP&HOWMANY 5.1 NSP NP 2.0;
  LABEL  FCNL = 'FUNCTIONAL GROUP'  PAT_ID = 'PATIENT ID'
         BAS_DAYS = 'SINCE BL'  VISIT_ID = 'VISIT'
         COL_DATE = 'DATE'  PAT_AGE = 'AGE'  DRG_IND = 'DRUG'
         GRPTOTAL = 'GROUP TOTAL'  NSP = '# SIGNIF PARAMS'  NP = '# PARAMS'
         COMP1 = "&TSTN1"  COMP2 = "&TSTN2"  COMP3 = "&TSTN3"  COMP4 = "&TSTN4"
         COMP5 = "&TSTN5"  COMP6 = "&TSTN6"  COMP7 = "&TSTN7"  COMP8 = "&TSTN8"
         COMP9 = "&TSTN9"  COMP10 = "&TSTN10"  COMP11 = "&TSTN11";
%MEND PRTGRP;

%PRTGRP (LIVER,    5, SGOT,SGPT,ALK PHOS,BILI,GGT)
%PRTGRP (RENAL,    4, BUN,CREAT,CR CL,BUN/CREAT)
%PRTGRP (RBC,      4, MCV,HGB,HMCT,MCHC)
%PRTGRP (WBC,      6, WBC,NEUTR,LYMPH,MONO,EOSIN,BASO)
%PRTGRP (ELECT,    4, SODIUM,POTASS,CHLOR,CO2)
%PRTGRP (LIPID,    8, CHOLES,HDL,LDL,VLDL,TRIGLY,APO-A1,APO-B,FREE FATTY ACIDS)
%PRTGRP (DIABETES, 6, F.GLUCOSE,R.GLUCOSE,GLUCAGON,F.INSULIN,C-PEPTIDE,GLY HGB)
%PRTGRP (METABOL,  6, CALCIUM,INOR.PHOS,MAGNES,ALBUMIN,GLOBULIN,URIC ACID)
%PRTGRP (PLATELET, 6, PLATE,PTT,PT,BLEED TIME,CLOT TIME,PLATE AGG)
%PRTGRP (MUSCLE,  11, LDH,LDH1,LDH2,LDH3,LDH4,LDH5,CPK,CPK1,CPK2,CPK3,ALDOLASE)
```

```
TITLE2 "GLOBAL GENIE SCORES";
TITLE3 " ";

****************************************************************************
* Functional Group scores and Global Genie scores...                      *
*                                                                          *
* PRTGLBL.SAS - This program identifies patients with ALL OK values of     *
* (Module 5/6) the Global Genie scores and prints a listing of Global      *
*              Genie scores by PAT_ID DATE.                                 *
*                                                                          *
* Input:  NORM.ABNORM - SAS data set from COMPGLBL.SAS with one record     *
*                       per patient per date if the Global Genie score     *
*                       is non-zero.                                        *
*         NORM.GENIE  - SAS data set from COMPGLBL.SAS with one record      *
*                       per patient per date.                               *
*                                                                          *
* Output: PRTGLBL.LIS - Listing of Global Genie scores and                 *
*                       contributing Functional Group scores by            *
*                       patient and date.                                   *
****************************************************************************;

OPTIONS PAGESIZE=62 LINESIZE=132 CENTER;

LIBNAME NORM '[]';

DATA ABNORM2;
  SET NORM.ABNORM;
  BY PAT_ID;
  IF FIRST.PAT_ID;
  NOTE = 'ABNORMAL';
  KEEP PAT_ID NOTE;

DATA NOTE;
  MERGE NORM.GENIE ABNORM2;
  BY PAT_ID;
  IF NOTE = ' ' THEN NOTE = ' ALL OK ';

PROC SORT DATA = NOTE OUT = NORM.NOTE;
  BY PAT_ID NOTE BAS_DAYS;

PROC PRINT DATA = NORM.NOTE UNIFORM LABEL;
  BY PAT_ID NOTE;
  ID BAS_DAYS;
  VAR VISIT_ID COL_DATE SEX PAT_AGE DRG_IND DOSE GENIE NG GEN1-GEN10;
  LABEL BAS_DAYS = 'SINCE BL'  VISIT_ID = 'VISIT'   COL_DATE = 'DATE'
        PAT_AGE = 'AGE'   DRG_IND = 'DRUG'   NG = '# GRPS'
        GEN1 = 'LIVER'   GEN2 = 'RENAL'   GEN3 = 'RBC'   GEN4 = 'WBC'
        GEN5 = 'ELECT'   GEN6 = 'LIPID'   GEN7 = 'DIABETES'   GEN8 = 'METAB'
        GEN9 = 'PLATELET'   GEN10 = 'MUSCLE';
  FORMAT COL_DATE DATE7. VISIT_ID $4. SEX $1. PAT_AGE 3.0 DRG_IND $4.
         DOSE 4.0 GENIE GEN1 9.1 GEN2-GEN10 6.1 NG 2.0;
```

```
*******************************************************************************
* Functional Group scores and Global Genie scores ...                         *
*                                                                             *
* WRITE.SAS -  This program writes out data to an ASCII file from             *
* (Module 6/6) SAS data set NORM.GENIE, creating one record per patient       *
*              per day containing PAT_ID, PAT_AGE, SEX, DAY, DRUG, DOSE,       *
*              10 GROUP SCORES, GENIE SCORE                                    *
*                                                                             *
* Input:  NORM.GENIE                                                          *
*                                                                             *
* Output: SCORES.DAT - ASCII file as described above                          *
*******************************************************************************;

OPTIONS MISSING = ' ';

LIBNAME NORM '[]';

DATA _NULL_;
  SET NORM.GENIE;
  FILE SCORES;
  PUT  PAT_ID 1-11  PAT_AGE 12-16 .1  SEX 18  VISIT_ID 20-24
       @26 COL_DATE DATE7.  BAS_DAYS 33-37  DRG_IND 39-43  DOSE 45-52
       GEN1 53-58 .1  GEN2 60-65 .1  GEN3 67-72 .1  GEN4 74-79 .1  GEN5 81-86 .1
       GEN6 88-93 .1  GEN7 95-100 .1  GEN8 102-107 .1  GEN9 109-114 .1
       GEN10 116-121 .1  NG 123-124  GENIE 126-131 .1;
```

REFERENCES

1. Lewis TA. *Challenges for the '90s*. Special publication of the American Statistical Association; 1990.
2. Sogliero-Gilbert G, Mosher K, Zubkoff L. A procedure for the simplification and assessment of lab parameters in clinical trials. *Drug Inf J*. 1986;20:279–286.
3. Gilbert GS, Ting N, Zubkoff LA. A statistical comparison of drug safety in controlled clinical trials: the Genie Score as an objective measure of lab abnormalities. *Drug Inf J*. 1991;25:81–96.

8

Laboratory Parameters and Drug Safety

Norman E. Pitts*

Pfizer Inc.
Groton, Connecticut

Laboratory parameters play a key role in the monitoring of drug effects. According to the desirability of the drug effect produced, these tests are commonly categorized as efficacy parameters or safety parameters. With regard to efficacy, laboratory parameter(s) may provide a true, direct measure of the desired therapeutic effect (e.g., blood glucose) or, alternatively, they may represent surrogate or indirect end point(s) of a beneficial therapeutic effect (e.g., CD4 counts). The validity of these surrogate parameters as a true measure of therapeutic benefit is directly proportional to the strength of the correlation that exists between change in the surrogate end point and the ultimate therapeutic effect desired.

However, classifications that seek to differentiate laboratory parameters on the basis of efficacy or safety are clearly artifactual since the effect on a given parameter is not necessarily restricted to either a beneficial or a toxic effect. In many instances the distinction is quantitative rather than qualitative. It may be only the magnitude or direction of change in a particular laboratory parameter that distinguishes a toxic from a beneficial effect. For instance, in the clinical trial of a hypoglycemic agent a drug-induced decline in blood sugar, which is within reasonable limits, represents a direct end point of therapeutic effect. On the other hand, a drug-induced decline of some considerable magnitude to hypoglycemic levels represents an adverse safety reaction. Implicit within this seemingly simplistic illustration is a more subtle and fundamental message regarding the approach to safety evaluation.

---

*Retired.

It underscores a fundamental difference in approach to efficacy and safety analysis in clinical research. Efficacy is addressed by an analysis of the behavior of patients as a group in a controlled setting. The sine qua non of acceptable efficacy and a therapeutically useful drug is a predictable pharmacological effect. Ideally the pharmacological effects that are the basis of a drug's therapeutic effect should be present fairly universally across the particular patient population exposed. This makes it possible to satisfy appropriate statistical standards within the framework of research studies that are logistically feasible in terms of their size.

The position with respect to safety evaluation on the other hand shows some unique differences. Safety events, especially the more serious, are quite commonly manifest as relatively infrequent events in the patient population exposed. As a consequence, the contribution that statistical methodology can make to safety analysis is frequently curtailed by the limitations imposed by the pathological mechanism of the toxicity and its mode of clinical presentation. Adequate statistical standards may only be achievable in controlled studies whose size exceeds the practical capabilities of the research phase or even, in some instances, the postmarketing phase also. Inevitably, therefore, safety analysis is often and sometimes exclusively an evaluation of individual patient response carried out in an uncontrolled setting. This dictates a fundamental shift in emphasis regarding the analytical methodology utilized for safety evaluation as compared with that for efficacy evaluation. Any meaningful and comprehensive approach to safety evaluation must reflect this difference in emphasis.

The fundamental criterion for an efficacious drug always favors the application of statistical methodology, whereas the pathological characteristics of significant safety events often militate against its application. This fundamental concept as it affects the optimum approach to safety evaluation will be explored in greater detail.

I. MECHANISMS OF DRUG-INDUCED TOXICITY

The pathological mechanism underlying a particular expression of drug-induced toxicity plays an important role in determining how this toxicity presents clinically. This in turn has implications with respect to devising effective approaches for the detection of toxicity as well as to an understanding of the strengths and weaknesses of the different analytical approaches available.

From a mechanistic point of view drug toxicity may be classified into several broad categories. These categories are as follows:

1. Primary pharmacological effects of the drug
2. Secondary pharmacological effects
3. Intrinsic toxic effects
4. Idiosyncratic host response

5. Immune-based reactions
6. Drug interactions

While this classification is applicable to drug toxicity in general, it has particular relevance to drug-induced toxicity as manifested by abnormalities in laboratory parameters.

A. Primary Pharmacological Effects

Toxicity of this type results from an augmentation or exaggeration of the primary pharmacological effects of the drug. These are the pharmacological actions that serve as a basis for the beneficial therapeutic effect of the drug. Since these effects are the basis of the drug's therapeutic activity a dose–response relationship may usually be demonstrated and the effects are observed in the majority of patients exposed to adequate doses. This form of toxicity is most commonly seen with overdosage, intentional or accidental. This is particularly likely to occur in early studies when drug dosage has inadvertently been set too high.

In other situations it may represent an exaggerated response as a result pharmacodynamic sensitivity or susceptibility. This is well illustrated by the sulfonylureas. Certain underlying conditions may render the patient particularly susceptible to the glucose-lowering and hypoglycemic effects of these drugs. Another example is provided by antihypertensive agents such as prazosin and terazosin in which the therapeutic effect is mediated by presynaptic α blockade. Syncope due to postural hypotensive effects is commonly observed if dosage recommendations are exceeded. However, this same phenomenon may also be present in approximately 1% of patients who receive the recommended initial starting dose, an occurrence that is presumably related to an increased individual susceptibility to drug. This type of pharmacological response in a small number of individuals following normal or inordinately small doses is often termed *idiosyncrasy*. However, such patients are better classified as hyperresponders and the term idiosyncrasy reserved for those situations in which the reactions are not related to the known pharmacology of the drug and their pathogenesis poorly understood (vide infra).

While excessive effects in individual patients is certainly a function of the dose administered, it should be remembered that a variety of genetic and environmental factors may be responsible for significant interpatient differences in drug metabolism and therapeutic response. Although this increased susceptibility to drug may exist as an individual phenomenon and occur sporadically in certain individuals, it may also manifest as a group phenomenon involving discrete patient populations, e.g., the elderly. In the elderly age group such differential effects may arise as a result of differences in pharmacodynamic sensitivity or metabolic handling and pharmacokinetics or perhaps a combination of these factors. In this age group it is not uncommon for decreased renal function (reduced creatinine clearance) to exist and operate to alter the dose–response relationships with respect to optimum drug effects.

In those situations in which drug toxicity is manifest as an extension of the drug's primary pharmacological activity, there is usually little difficulty in its detection.

B. Secondary Pharmacological Effects

The term *secondary pharmacological effects* is not strictly accurate since this category actually comprises two different types of situation, only one of which is most appropriately described by this term. For instance, there are those situations in which the pharmacological effects responsible for the toxicity are basically of a different type from those mediating the primary therapeutic effect. These pharmacological effects are appropriately described as secondary effects since they do not form the basis of the drug's primary therapeutic effect. Examples would include the hypotensive effects of the phenothiazines as a result of their α-adrenergic blocking potential and the effect of the tricyclic antidepressants on the eye and alimentary tract as a result of their anticholinergic effects.

But also included in this category are those types of situation in which the basic pharmacological mechanism involved in the adverse reaction is the same as that responsible for the primary therapeutic effect. However, this pharmacological activity is being manifested in a different target organ and thereby producing an unwanted or adverse effect. These latter situations are more accurately described as *secondary pharmacodynamic effects*. Two examples may serve to illustrate this point.

The nonsteroidal anti-inflammatory drugs (NSAIDs) are generally thought to exert their beneficial effect in the arthritides by an inhibition of prostaglandin biosynthetase in the joint. However, this same pharmacological mechanism is also manifest in other target organs, e.g., gastrointestinal tract and kidney, thereby producing unwanted adverse effects. Since this chapter is concerned with laboratory parameters and drug safety, the kidney provides a particularly relevant example. NSAID-induced inhibition of renal prostaglandin biosynthetase impacts adversely upon prostaglandin-regulated medullary and deep cortical circulation with a resulting decrease in renal blood flow. This pharmacophysiological effect produces a reduction in glomerular filtration rate (GFR), which in turn results in an increase in blood urea nitrogen (BUN). Although this occurs in the majority of patients exposed to this class of drug, it may not be clinically apparent since qualitatively the effect may be quite subtle. The BUN deviations from baseline may be exceedingly small and only represent movement within the normal range which does not exceed the upper limit of normal. In such cases the changes may escape detection clinically and appropriate statistical analysis is required for their demonstration (Fig. 1). These BUN changes are fully reversible on discontinuation of drug and although clearly adverse they do not generally have toxicity implications. However, in isolated cases, when this effect is

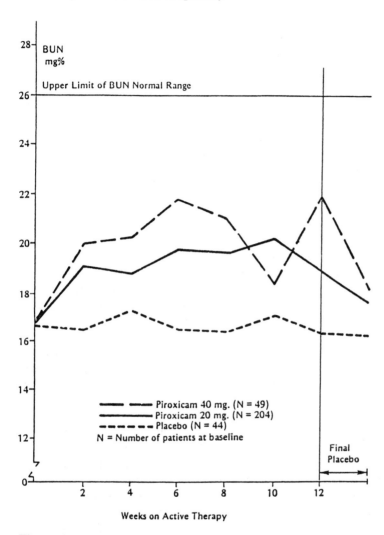

Figure 1 Average BUN vs. time on drug.

manifest in the presence of preexisting renal function impairment, it may rise to the level of a true toxicity. It may unmask previously unsuspected renal disease or lead to further significant deterioration of renal impairment already known to exist.

Mechanistically cancer chemotherapy agents present an analogous situation. Here again the drug effects that underly the primary therapeutic effect are being manifest in other target organs. However, in this instance they much more frequently present as overt clinical toxicity. These agents owe their therapeutic utility to their ability to inhibit tumor cell proliferation either by their ability to damage DNA (cyclophosphamide) or by an impairment of purine and pyrimidine metabolism (5-fluorouracil). However, this effect is not confined exclusively to tumor cells but is also manifest in normal cells undergoing active proliferation, e.g., hemopoietic stem cell proliferation. Like the primary therapeutic effect, the toxic effect on the bone marrow is seen across the entire patient population exposed to drug and it is dose-related. In the doses used clinically the effect is anything but subtle and is apparent from clinical observation. In the case of the chemotherapeutic agent mithramycin, the cytotoxic effects extend beyond the bone marrow and are also exerted on the actively proliferating bone osteoclast with a resulting impact on serum calcium levels. This has also led to the experimental use of this agent in Paget's disease.

C. Intrinsic Toxicity

In some instances the mechanism by which a drug produces its adverse effect is an intrinsic toxicity that is quite separate and distinct from its known pharmacological effects. True intrinsic toxicity possesses certain characteristics that differentiate it from the two most common mechanisms of serious drug-induced toxicity encountered clinically: idiosyncrasy and hypersensitivity (vide infra). Perhaps one of the most important characteristics of this type of toxicity is its reproducibility in the experimental animal. The direct corollary of this absence of species specificity is an ability to reliably predict human safety experience from the animal toxicology studies. This clearly has important implications for clinical research.

However, this type of toxicity also possesses other characteristics that tend to favor rather than impede its detection in the clinic. Implicit in the mechanism of this particular form of toxicity is the fact that it will manifest in most of the patients exposed to drug, assuming that the dose is appropriate. Characteristically it occurs in a consistent, predictable, and dose-related fashion, usually but not always after fairly brief exposure to drug. By its very nature this type of toxicity commonly precludes development of the drug and its acceptance into broad therapeutic use, unless there are other factors that impact favorably on the benefit-to-risk calculus.

The antimetabolite group of drugs used in cancer chemotherapy are indiscriminately toxic to a variety of proliferating normal tissues in addition to neoplastic tissue. However, the nature of the disease being treated, the options available and their therapeutic utility all combine to greatly outweigh the potential risk. The dose-related nature of the toxicity permits careful dose adjustment to avoid serious toxicity developing. As indicated above, these drugs are probably better classified under "Secondary Pharmacological Effects."

A more appropriate example of intrinsic toxicity is provided by the widely used drug acetaminophen (paracetamol), which displays an intrinsic toxicity with respect to the liver. In this instance it is the unique characteristics of the dose–response relationship of the hepatotoxicity that permits its widespread use as a harmless, safe analgesic. It has been estimated that a single dose of 15 g is required to produce hepatotoxic effects in a 70-kg human, as compared with a maximum single therapeutic dose of 1000 mg [1]. This difference between therapeutic and toxic doses is so wide that hepatotoxic doses are not encountered except with overdosage as a suicide attempt. Mechanistically the toxicity is thought to be due to a highly reactive metabolite of acetaminophen. This metabolite is only produced in trace amounts when normal therapeutic doses are administered and is therefore readily inactivated by conjugation with glutathione. When very large doses are ingested glutathione is depleted and the capacity of the liver to conjugate the metabolite effectively is overwhelmed. The end result is hepatotoxicity and hepatic cell necrosis as a consequence of the unconjugated and highly reactive metabolite binding covalently to hepatic cell macromolecules. As would be anticipated from the mechanism of this toxicity, the hepatotoxicity is reproducible in animals although there are considerable interspecies differences. These differences most probably have a pharmacokinetic/metabolic basis and are a function of differing dose–response relationships.

Although the fundamental characteristic of intrinsic toxicity is its universality in all patients exposed to drug, one should nevertheless note that in some instances it may only manifest in a small defined segment of the total population exposed. For instance, in order for the intrinsic hematological toxicity of oxidant drugs to manifest there must be a preexisting hereditary abnormality present, e.g., glucose-6-phosphate dehydrogenase (G-6-PD) deficiency. This fact would seem to blur the lines of distinction between the intrinsic toxicity category and the idiosyncratic toxicity category. It may well be that the allocation a drug to one or another category is artifactual and depends entirely on whether or not the metabolic aberration responsible has been identified. This point is discussed more fully below.

D. Idiosyncrasy

This and the following category of immune-based toxic reactions constitute the most common underlying mechanisms for the more serious toxic drug reactions encountered in clinical practice. Their importance is underscored by the fact that they possess certain characteristics that can give rise to significant diagnostic difficulties during the clinical research program. These difficulties concern not only the initial recognition of a potential toxicity but also the establishment of a relationship to drug once the possible toxicity is detected. Indeed, it may well be that on occasion toxicities of this type may not manifest or may not be recognized until the drug is on the market.

The actual mechanism of this type of toxic reaction is unknown but it is certainly considerably different from toxicity due to the known pharmacological effects of the drug. Host idiosyncrasy would appear to be the most tenable hypothesis and mechanistically the toxicity results from some metabolic aberration in the specific patient. The hepatotoxic potential of the NSAIDs and the myelotoxic potential of phenylbutazone and chloramphenicol are considered to be instances of such idiosyncratic effects. Typically this type of toxicity occurs in an unpredictable and sporadic fashion and is of low incidence. Unlike intrinsic toxicity it does not have the characteristics of a dose-related toxic response manifest in patients as a group. Rather, it is a unique reaction occurring infrequently in isolated discrete individuals and usually with no clear dose–response relationships. The characteristics of the individual host are thought to be of prime importance in determining the occurrence of this form of toxicity. Generally it is not reproducible in the experimental animal and animal toxicology studies therefore provide little guidance with respect to the toxicity that might be encountered in the clinic. There are however some isolated instances in which it has been possible to produce lesions in animal species. Nevertheless, this has not been within the context of formal animal toxicology studies but in special experimental models involving metabolic manipulation, e.g., isoniazid. Clinically the toxicity does not show a clear dose–response relationship and the duration of exposure prior to its appearance can vary from a few weeks to many months.

A pharmacogenetically determined metabolic idiosyncrasy in some individuals has been postulated and certainly the few known mechanisms would appear to give credence to this particular view. In this connection one might cite the prolonged apnea due to succinylcholine administration in susceptible patients. This results from a qualitative defect in plasma pseudocholinesterase and the familial occurrence of the phenomenon suggests a genetic defect. Another example is provided by the genetically determined deficiency of G-6-PD. The deficiency of this enzyme in the erythrocyte results in oxidized glutathione accumulation following the administration of oxidant drugs. The glutathione accumulation then leads to erythrocyte membrane disruption and hemolysis.

The unique toxicity of oxidant drugs, such as primaquine and sulfonamides, in the presence of G-6-PD deficiency is important in another respect. It serves to emphasize the fact that the distinction between the different types of toxicity can be blurred. Acetaminophen-induced hepatic toxicity is a metabolically mediated intrinsic toxicity that is manifested by all exposed patients who are given an adequate dose of drug. On the other hand, the hemolytic anemia due to G-6-PD deficiency will vary in frequency depending on the incidence of the underlying enzymatic defect. This can be as low as <1 in 1000 in Caucasians, 11% in African-Americans, or as high as 50% in certain Kurdish populations.

If an underlying metabolic aberration is the mechanism of the drug toxicity, then these two examples would appear to suggest that it is simply the frequency of its occurrence in the population that determines whether the effect is ultimately classified as intrinsic or idiosyncratic toxicity. Furthermore the more ubiquitous the defect, e.g., acetaminophen, the more likely that it will not be limited to the human species but seen also in the animal.

E. Hypersensitivity

In a pragmatic sense this mechanism may also be regarded as a manifestation of host idiosyncrasy. However, it may be differentiated from the idiosyncratic reactions already discussed, in which a metabolic etiology is probable, by the fact that there is clinical and other evidence to suggest a hypersensitivity or immune-based reaction. This type of toxicity is attributed to the intact drug or a metabolite functioning as a hapten and the hypothesis has been advanced as the mechanism for the hemopoietic and hepatic toxicity of a number of drugs. There is little in the way of direct evidence to support this hypothesis and efforts to demonstrate cell-mediated immunity as a mechanism for hemopoietic and hepatic injury have produced variable results. Such evidence as does exist derives primarily from the collateral features suggesting hypersensitivity which accompany certain drug-induced hepatotoxicities. These may include such manifestations as fever, eosinophilia, lymph node enlargement, lymphocytosis, and biopsy material from the involved organ showing eosinophils as a prominent component of the inflammatory infiltrate present.

Overall the clinical presentation of hypersensitivity-mediated toxicity resembles that seen with idiosyncrasy. The events occur sporadically and unpredictably and are most typically of low incidence. The incidence varies between a fraction of 1% and 1 or 2%, but may in some instances be higher. It tends to manifest early in the first few weeks of therapy and is not related to size of dose. There is a prompt reappearance of the injury on rechallenge. In common with the idiosyncratic type of reaction it is not reproducible in the animal and animal toxicology provides no warning of its possible occurrence.

Clinically there is the same blurring of the line of distinction between idiosyncratic and hypersensitivity toxicity as exists mechanistically between intrinsic toxicity and idiosyncratic toxicity. Not unexpectedly, therefore, considerable debate may occur between different authorities with regard to the exact mechanism of toxicity of a particular drug. Isoniazid hepatotoxicity is generally concluded to be due to a metabolic idiosyncrasy but some workers, based on the occasional occurrence of chills, fever, and eosinophilia accompanying the hepatotoxicity, regard it as a hypersensitivity mechanism [2].

There is one clinical characteristic that can be of great practical importance in the detection of both idiosyncratic and hypersensitivity reactions. Certain drugs that are accompanied by a low incidence of overt organ toxicity of idiosyncratic or hypersensitivity origin may also cause abnormalities of the relevant laboratory parameters in a much higher percentage of patients. However, these abnormalities do not progress further to the point of overt toxicity.

For instance, the administration of chlorpromazine or erythromycin estolate is accompanied by a 1–2% incidence of clinically manifest hepatotoxicity. But abnormal liver function parameters (serum transaminases), in the absence of overt toxicity, are observed in a much higher proportion of patients (13–50%) [3]. A similar phenomenon is seen in association with isoniazid therapy. This drug characteristically manifests a low-incidence (1%) idiosyncratic hepatotoxicity due to reactive metabolite formation but is also accompanied by a 10–20% incidence of SGPT and serum glutamic oxaloacetic transaminase (SGOT) abnormalities that do not progress to true hepatotoxicity. One explanation for this phenomenon is that mechanistically it is a completely separate effect from the low-incidence hepatotoxicity resulting from a hypersensitivity or idiosyncratic reaction. Components of both a direct intrinsic toxicity and a hypersensitivity/idiosyncratic toxicity are present in the same molecule.

An somewhat analogous situation exists with respect to the myelotoxicity of chloramphenicol. This drug is responsible for a very low incidence (1 in 24,000–40,000) [4] delayed type of myelotoxic reaction, probably idiosyncratic, which results in an irreversible pancytopenia. It may occur after a single dose or after prolonged therapy, and in some instances it may only appear after drug discontinuation. It is not dose-related and appears to be caused by a genetically determined biochemical or metabolic difference rather than a hypersensitivity reaction such as quinacrine-induced aplastic anemia [5]. There is also another type of chloramphenicol-induced myelotoxic reaction. This is a dose-related immediate type of reaction, and one that is observed much more frequently than the idiosyncratic reaction. This is not a prodrome of the low-incidence aplastic anemia seen with chloramphenicol. It is a direct toxic effect and appears to be related to an inhibition of mitochondrial protein synthesis. The reaction occurs to some extent in all patients exposed to the drug but may be severe in some subjects. It is a dose-related suppression of marrow function that is progressive with time on drug but will promptly reverse upon discontinuation of therapy. Whilst its effects are most evident in the erythroid series, there may also be an effect on granulocytes and platelets. The reaction is accompanied by an increase in serum iron, a decrease in reticulocyte count, and a vacuolization of bone marrow cells.

The possible existence of such dual effects suggests a useful approach to the evaluation of potential low-incidence organ toxicity. This is an approach that may assist in establishing causality. Whenever a suspected instance of drug-induced organ toxicity occurs, e.g., bone marrow, liver, and kidney, careful clinical assessment and evaluation of the individual patient must be the first priority. Frequently this is the only way in which a relationship to drug may be substantiated. But, as a standard routine, whenever such isolated incidents occur one should always reexamine the total database for evidence of a broader incidence of asymptomatic and possibly minimal elevations of the relevant laboratory parameters, e.g., WBC, granulocyte count, transaminases. Such elevations, if present, may be apparent clinically. Alternatively, when the effects are more subtle and limited to movement within the normal range, or when the same changes in laboratory parameters may occur in association with the primary disease, concomitant therapy, or coexisting pathology, statistical analytical techniques may be required for their detection.

If a broader incidence of such elevations is in fact shown to be present it may constitute important supportive evidence of a drug-induced etiology for the toxicity observed in the individual patient. However, if these changes are absent it does not exclude the possibility.

Clearly the mechanisms of drug toxicity can have important implications for the whole process of safety monitoring as well as the optimum approach to laboratory parameter evaluation.

II. FACTORS CONFOUNDING SAFETY EVALUATION

There are a number of factors that collectively or individually have the potential to impact adversely on the process of safety data generation, the identification of toxic events, and the assessment of causality. Some of these exert a subtle but nevertheless important influence on safety evaluation and are most appropriately categorized as attitudinal factors. Others are a function of the pathological basis and mode of clinical presentation of the toxic event and raise problems of detection and causality attribution. It is important that due recognition be accorded all of these factors when formulating an approach to safety evaluation in order that steps may be taken to minimize their potential for confounding the collection and interpretation of data.

A. Attitudinal Factors

Attitudinal factors play an important role in influencing the approach of the physician investigator to the patient who experiences a serious adverse event. The attitudinal characteristics of a physician primarily oriented toward patient care are quite different from those that motivate the physician who is primarily oriented toward research. These attitudinal factors can have a significant effect on the nature and extent of the data collected thereby potentially impacting the quality of any causality judgment. The importance of this observation lies in the fact that a large number of clinical investigators are primarily and predominantly involved in patient care and they may carry the attitudinal characteristics of medical practice over into their research studies.

The physician engaged in patient care is exclusively "treatment outcome"–oriented in his or her approach to patients. The primary focus is the individual patient and not data derived from a group of patients to answer a research question. The interest in clinical observations and data acquisition is important only insofar as it serves the narrow purpose of the treatment outcome and treatment decisions with respect to the individual patient.

By contrast, the physician who is predominantly involved in research tends to be more "data generation"–oriented. His or her interest in clinical observations and data acquisition has broader horizons and places emphasis on the potential importance of the data with respect to the overall research objectives, regardless of whether the data collected may be strictly relevant to the treatment objectives of a particular patient.

For this reason the data collected by the research-oriented physician with respect to suspected drug toxicity will often go beyond that which is reasonably required to constitute optimum medical care of that specific patient. In sharp contradistinction the treatment outcome approach of the practicing physician will often lead to data which, while perfectly adequate for proper treatment care of the patient, are deficient in certain respects relative to the overall research objectives of the study. This is not to say that accurate clinical information is not important for proper diagnosis and treatment decisions in the course of routine patient care. What it does say is that the level of data acquisition sufficient to ensure optimum patient care and treatment outcome is often inadequate for the precise causality assessments that are required for research purposes and that may be regarded as unnecessarily burdensome on the patient by the treating physician.

These attitudinal differences tend to be of degree rather than absolute and the extent to which the practicing physician can, albeit temporarily, assume the attitudinal characteristics of the research physician will be of pivotal importance in determining the quality of his or her clinical research study.

The possible impact of these attitudinal differences is well illustrated if one considers the hypothetical situation of a patient developing evidence of significant hepatic dysfunction during the course of investigational drug administration in a clinical research setting. In such a case both the data generation approach of the research physician and the treatment outcome approach of the practicing physician will lead to prompt discontinuation of the investigational drug. The differences contingent on attitudinal orientation emerge in what happens subsequently.

The research-oriented clinician, while having concern for the individual patient, will be intent on gathering every piece of data that might possibly be relevant to an accurate assessment of causality. The treatment outcome approach, on the other hand, will probably focus on whether the abnormalities of liver function subside spontaneously following drug withdrawal and, if so, what alternative therapy may be substituted. These considerations, and not research objectives, will be the driving force determining what data are collected. If the abnormalities are subsiding, comprehensive evaluation to definitively establish causation will probably be regarded as having little practical relevance to treatment care. The most important consideration now becomes the issue of alternative therapy. If, however, the abnormalities do not subside upon drug withdrawal, then causality will be pursued more aggressively. Indeed, the appropriate alternative treatment options may be contingent on such knowledge. The additional data now possess treatment relevance for the patient as opposed to a strictly research relevance.

One may move from this purely hypothetical situation to the practical reality of a case that arose within the writer's own experience. It serves to add further emphasis to these seemingly theoretical observations. A 700-patient database, free of serious toxicity, was already available for a drug in phase II evaluation when several patients in one specific study developed abnormalities of liver function. This was the only study being conducted in this particular geographic location and public health epidemiological data indicated an increased incidence of viral hepatitis in the area at that particular time. There was also evidence suggesting the possible exposure of these particular patients.

The hepatic abnormalities did not progress following drug withdrawal and over a period of time slowly subsided. The treating physician, as well as a local gastroenterologist who saw the patients, concluded that viral hepatitis was responsible and that the events were not causally related to the drug. Based on these views, and in the absence of the serology available today, the treating physician did not consider that expert evaluation of a liver biopsy was essential to treatment of these patients. Notwithstanding this view and motivated by a research interest this issue was pursued. A hepatologist, expert in drug-induced lesions, concluded from the histological appearances of the liver biopsies that two of the six events were in fact drug-induced [6]. The subsequent course of the clinical program provided ample confirmation of the existence of drug-induced hepatotoxicity. This experience illustrates very well the tensions that may arise between research attitudes and treatment-oriented attitudes. Certainly expert evaluation of a liver biopsy proved to be a critical determinative factor. However, given the circumstances, a strong case could certainly be made for a treating physician's view that the additional information was not essential to the proper treatment of the patients.

As already noted, the pragmatic implication of these observations arises from the fact that clinical research programs must necessarily involve a whole spectrum of physicians. Some will be experienced research physicians but others will be predominantly engaged in medical practice and have less or possibly no prior research experience. It is therefore mandatory that monitoring approaches be adopted that seek to guard against the possible loss of data for these reasons. Measures must be adopted to ensure that all the appropriate investigations are performed, and in a timely fashion.

B. Mode of Clinical Presentation

There is yet another source of potential problems that may operate to confound safety evaluation. This may arise from the fact that frequently the clinical manifestations of a particular manifestation of drug toxicity are very similar, if not indistinguishable, from clinical syndromes that may arise not as a result of the investigational drug but from other sources. These sources include concomitant therapy, intercurrent pathology, or possibly the actual disease state under study.

Confusion with other pathologies is particularly likely to occur with respect to drug-induced abnormalities of liver function. The liver, by virtue of its central metabolic role, is potentially at risk of injury from any absorbed drug or its metabolites. Therefore it is not unexpected to find that hepatic injury constitutes one of the commoner modes of presentation of serious drug-induced toxicity. However, its recognition it complicated by the fact that hepatic injury also arises from a variety of other pathologies. A further complication is that the liver possesses only a limited capacity to manifest such injury clinically. It therefore tends to respond in a stereotyped fashion with respect to the clinical evidence of dysfunction regardless of the exact etiology. As a consequence the standard laboratory parameters of liver function (LFT) have their main utility in detecting hepatic dysfunction and cannot be relied on for assistance in establishing its exact etiology, drug-induced or otherwise. While the pattern of LFT change can certainly be of help in identifying the clinical syndrome of hepatotoxicity presenting, e.g., hepatocellular damage or cholestasis, there is no parameter that is pathognomonic of drug-induced injury. Each of these syndromes has a variety of other possible etiologies, and an alteration in LFT is only diagnostic of liver injury per se and not pathognomonic of the exact etiology of that injury. A proper definition of etiology will probably necessitate other additional nonroutine tests—if indeed such exist, which is not necessarily the case.

In this context recent advances in viral serology have greatly improved the diagnostic precision of drug-induced hepatic injury. Viral hepatitis was formerly a source of considerable diagnostic difficulty when knowledge of this disease was confined to the entity now identified as hepatitis A and appropriate serology had not been developed. This confusion was compounded by the fact that in that same era the potential of certain procedures to transmit viral hepatitis was not recognized and no standard procedures were employed to avoid this possibility. It has been suggested, for instance, that some of the cases of gold-induced hepatitis during this early period may in fact have been instances of needle-transmitted viral hepatitis [7]. It is more than likely that the apparent discrepancy between the incidence figures quoted in many of the earlier reports may have resulted from such diagnostic confusion. Some early reports placed the incidence of hepatotoxicity due to gold as high as 9.4% [8]. The subsequent identification of the causal virus and the availability of diagnostic serology for hepatitis A and B, and more recently hepatitis C (non-A, non-B) has greatly improved the ability to differentiate drug-induced injury from viral hepatitis. However, it has not entirely eliminated the problem.

Viral hepatitis, identified as hepatitis B or C, is not uncommon in any given cross-section of the population and provides a background noise from which it may be difficult to distinguish true drug-induced injury. The possible confounding effects of hepatitis B infection on the diagnosis of drug-induced hepatotoxicity recently acquired added importance in clinical research. The prevalence of this disease now extends beyond a circumscribed group of high-risk individuals such as prisoners, illegal drug users, and homosexuals to the population at large. To an increasing extent it is involving patient populations that are very likely to be involved in clinical studies. The prevalence rate of 7–10% which is given for the United States overall can seriously compound the difficulties of detecting a 1% or less incidence of drug-induced hepatotoxicity if patient monitoring and assessment does not reach the highest standards. Similar considerations hold true for other manifestations of drug-induced toxicity, e.g., hemopoietic in which the etiological basis may be other than the investigational drug under study.

The ability to recognize drug-induced toxicity simulating other pathologies is further complicated by the fact that quite frequently serious drug-induced injury tends to be an unpredictable event of low incidence. The opportunity to make those observations that are critical and relevant to the detection of drug toxicity and accurate causality attribution will only occur infrequently and sporadically. It is absolutely essential that the maximum information be derived from each case in a timely manner as and when it occurs. The process of data generation must emphasize constant vigilance for the prompt recognition of any possible low-incidence drug-induced toxicity that may occur suddenly and unexpectedly during the clinical program. This vigilance cannot be relaxed even after many hundreds or a thousand or more patients have been studied uneventfully because of the probability of occurrence when very low-incidence toxicities are involved. Prompt recognition coupled with thorough and comprehensive clinical evaluation to establish causality is essential. If a case is missed or the data are valueless, in a diagnostic sense, because of inadequate evaluation or a lack of timely observations, it may be a considerable time before the opportunity for accurate assessment of the potential toxicity again presents itself with the occurrence of another instance. An important opportunity will have been lost for a timely causality assessment, something that is not in the best interests of the safety of patients who are being exposed to the drug. Until such time as another toxic event occurs and is recognized, patients will continue to be exposed without being able to identify or quantify the potential risk for their benefit and in the interests of an adequate informed consent.

III. IMPACT ON SAFETY MONITORING

Although there are several different pathological mechanisms of drug-induced toxicity, their mode of clinical presentation may be conveniently separated into two main types of clinical picture. The mode of clinical presentation in turn determines the most effective approach to safety assessment.

On the one hand, the toxicity may present as consistent, dose-related effects that occur with reasonable frequency in the greater proportion of individuals exposed. When such effects are manifest as significant deviations from the normal range, they are readily apparent and easily detectable clinically. This is true, for instance, of the myelosuppression induced by cytotoxic agents. However, since drug toxicity of this type is frequently dose-related, it is possible that the doses of the investigational drug employed in the clinic are only on the threshold of toxicity. The manifestations of toxicity may therefore be minimal, representing, in some instances, nothing more than a consistent rise within the normal range. Minimal changes such as this will probably escape clinical detection and require statistical techniques for their demonstration. It is in this particular clinical manifestation of drug toxicity that statistical methodology has its most important application. The use of statistical methodology to detect the subtle effects of NSAIDs on BUN (vide supra) provides an excellent example, although in this instance the drug effect is a secondary pharmacological effect as opposed to an true toxic effect. In analytical terms there is a close analogy between the approach to drug toxicity presenting in this manner and that employed for efficacy parameters. Analysis seeks to define group effects, i.e., the behavior of patients as a group rather than as individuals.

On the other hand, the clinical presentation of drug toxicity may be that which occurs in the form of sporadic, unpredictable, low-incidence events. This category is extremely important for two reasons. First, the more serious forms of drug-induced organ toxicity, those that provide the greatest diagnostic challenge, tend to fall into this category. Second, the unpredictable sporadic nature and low incidence further compound the difficulties of detection. These factors combine to create a situation in which safety assessment techniques must place primary reliance on the clinical evaluation of individual patients. Therefore careful monitoring of studies to detect events, and competent clinical evaluation when detected, is critical to success.

The well-controlled study that is fundamental to efficacy evaluation is unable to make the same valuable contribution to this type of safety problem. Absolute numbers of patients exposed to drug is more critical to the detection of this type of toxicity than study design.

In most cases the clinical research program undertaken to support marketing approval of a new drug comprises several thousand patients. A figure of 3000 patients would be representative of the average number of patients exposed to the experimental drug in such a program. These patients are derived in the main from a series of randomized controlled efficacy studies.

In an average program the number of patients per group in any one controlled study does not commonly exceed a maximum of 300 and in many programs study numbers will be considerably smaller. While this number of patients may provide adequate power to detect clinically and statistically meaningful inter-group differences in various efficacy parameters, its potential contribution to safety analysis is much more limited. The numbers may be adequate to compare and contrast subjective side effect profiles between treatment groups but they will usually be inadequate for comparisons involving the more serious forms of low-incidence organ toxicity. Differences between treatment groups for such safety events will inevitably rest on clinical judgments unsupported by statistical confirmation.

For instance, in a study involving 300 patients per treatment group (Table 1) the difference between the treatment group and the control group only reaches statistical significance if the events occur in the treatment group with a frequency of 1.3% or higher. If the events occur with a frequency less than 1.3%, then the differentiation between groups must rest solely on clinical assessment and statistical confirmation is lacking. The quality of the clinical evaluation is therefore critical most especially if a definitive test for a drug-induced etiology is not available.

A further difficulty may be introduced by the fact that the clinical presentation of the toxicity may resemble, or be identical with, the clinical manifestations of an event that may occur spontaneously in the control population for reasons unrelated to drug. When this occurs the ability to distinguish statistically between

Table 1 Comparison of Two Groups of 300 Patients

Observed incidence (%)		Number of events		Statistical significance
Treated	Controls	Treated	Controls	
1.3	0	4	0	$\leq.05$
1.7	0	5	0	$\leq.05$
2.0	0	6	0	$\leq.05$
2.3	0	7	0	$\leq.05$
2.7	0	8	0	$\leq.01$
2.3	0.3	7	1	$\leq.05$
2.7	0.3	8	1	$\leq.05$
3.0	0.3	9	1	$\leq.05$
3.3	0.3	10	1	$\leq.05$
3.7	0.3	11	1	$\leq.01$
3.7	0.7	11	2	$\leq.05$

groups becomes even further compromised. The presence of even minimal background noise in the control group (Table 1) means that the incidence of suspected drug toxicity in the treatment group must now exceed 2% before the intergroup differences between investigational drug and control reach statistical significance.

If a toxic event has an incidence of 1% then there is a 95% probability that at least one event will occur if 300 patients are exposed to drug (Table 2). However, as already noted, a controlled study of 300 patients per group possesses very little power to detect statistically significant differences between groups with low-incidence toxicity. Therefore, if the objective is to explore low-incidence toxicities the potential return from 600 patients exposed to the investigational drug in an open uncontrolled study is far greater than that from 300 patients per group in a controlled study.

Given these limitations, it is clear that the total number of patients exposed to the investigational drug in the total clinical program has more relevance for the detection of low-incidence toxicity than individual controlled studies. But even though the total numbers of patients exposed in clinical research programs are commonly in the thousands, there are still significant limitations on the ability to detect infrequently occurring toxicity. If the true underlying incidence of a toxic event is 0.1%, then 3000 patients exposed to drug provides a 95% probability of seeing at least one event (Table 2). This is not to say that an event with a frequency of 0.1% may not in fact be seen in the first 10–20 patients exposed to drug. The true import of these observations is that one cannot have reasonable confidence that a toxicity of the order of 0.1% does not exist until at least 3000 patients have been exposed. The data in Table 2 serve to make some very important points with respect to safety evaluation. First, they emphasize the limited opportunity to detect drug-induced toxicity during a clinical research program when it is present in an incidence of less than 1%. As a logical corollary of this it is exceedingly important to ensure that possible toxic events are not missed and that they receive careful and comprehensive clinical evaluation. Opportunities for accurately profiling the drug's safety may be few and far

Table 2 Sample Size Required For 95% Chance Of Observing at Least One Toxic Event

Observation	Probability of side effect	Number
1	.10000	28.43
2	.01000	298.07
3	.00100	2,994.23
4	.00010	29,995.82
5	.00001	299,571.73

between and should not be lost. Nevertheless, some toxicities of a low frequency may simply not manifest themselves during the course of the clinical research program. This is a matter of probabilities as a function of the incidence of the toxicity and is the basis for a postmarketing surveillance requirement.

IV. FAILURE TO DETECT LOW-INCIDENCE TOXICITY

The consequences of a failure to promptly detect low-incidence toxicity, or to correctly attribute the adverse events to drug, once identified, can be quite serious. The upper confidence bound (95%) for an observed incidence of 0.1% in 3000 patients is 0.21%. This means that based on the incidence observed in the clinical research program the true incidence in the population at large could possibly be as high as 0.21%.

Suppose for instance that three drug-induced hepatotoxic events occur in a clinical research program involving 3000 patients but the true significance of the events has been missed. They have occurred in a geographic area in which there have been a number of reports of viral hepatitis to local health authorities. This fact together with poor clinical evaluation and diagnostic skills has led to the events being erroneously attributed to viral hepatitis. If, following approval, the drug has an "explosive" entry onto the market, as indeed some drugs do, then as many as 1.5 million patients may be exposed to drug in the first year of use. In such an eventuality, given that the 95% upper confidence bound indicates that the true incidence of hepatotoxicity could be as high as 0.21%, as many as 3000 patients could manifest hepatotoxicity in the first year of marketing.

V. EVALUATION OF LABORATORY PARAMETERS

Drug safety monitoring and evaluation with respect to laboratory parameters has two components, both of which are essential to its success. These are data generation and data evaluation. The two areas are closely correlated. Any measure that seeks to improve the quality of data generation will inevitably improve the quality of data evaluation and safety assessment. Conversely, anything that tends to detract from the quality of the data generated will adversely impact on the reliability of the safety assessment and causality judgment. Data generation issues assume even greater importance when dealing with infrequent and unanticipated toxicity. The safety evaluation section of study protocols cannot reasonably be expected to anticipate all the testing that may be required for any unexpected toxicity that may present. Accordingly, measures must be taken to minimize the potential loss of important data, data that may have a bearing on the causality assessment.

A. Data Generation

There are a variety of measures, over and above a well-designed protocol, that may be taken to ensure the prompt and timely acquisition of all relevant data at the time the toxicity manifests.

A protocol for a well-designed study will set forth in specific detail the laboratory parameters that are to be monitored for safety purposes and the frequency with which such monitoring is to be carried out.

The phase I studies present some unique problems when compared with the clinical studies conducted in the later phases of clinical research and development program (phases II, III, and IV). At this early time there is no prior human experience on which to draw for guidance, no experience that might serve to raise the index of suspicion for the possible occurrence of specific toxic manifestations in the trials. Certainly there will always be a body of preclinical animal toxocology available which has been developed with the sole purpose of supporting these initial human phase I studies. If the primary purpose of this animal testing is to characterize, qualitatively and quantitatively, the potential morbid histological and toxic effects of the drug, it follows that the animal results should be extrapolatable to humans. Unfortunately, while such studies may indeed provide valuable advanced warning of potential human toxicity, all too frequently the animal findings, as a predictor of human toxicity, prove to be spurious both in a positive and a negative sense.

In a positive sense significant toxicity may be observed in animal toxicology studies, which prompts a need for further work. In many such cases, after further studies, intensive scientific debate, and the passage of time, the drug is finally administered to humans with the result that the animal toxicity is not relevant to humans. This is not necessarily surprising in view of the historical record. A number of valuable and long established drugs are still on the market today that would probably not be able to survive contemporary toxicology requirements and reach the initial phases of human study. It would seem that the ability to devise ever increasing animal toxicology requirements far exceeds the ability to understand and interpret the data with respect to their relevance for humans. The very extent of the animal testing required may represent a subconscious attempt to compensate for this deficiency.

In a negative sense some serious toxicities, which are not infrequently associated with drug therapy, do not have their counterpart in a reliable animal model. It is important to recognize this fact and the limitation it places on any extrapolations from the animal results to human experience [9,10]. It may well be that metabolic differences, presently unknown, may exist between species and be determinative of the validity of such extrapolations.

Certain mechanisms of toxicity that are extremely important in the context of human drug toxicity do not appear to have their counterpart in the experimental animal. This is particularly true of hypersensitivity and most idiosyncratic mechanisms that commonly underly serious hemopoietic and hepatic toxicities in humans. They are rarely reproducible in, or predictable from, the animal studies [11,12]. This is particularly unfortunate given the importance of these serious organ toxicities as drug safety problems in humans. It is in these particular types of drug toxicity that a reliable animal model is badly needed—a need that is underscored by the serious nature of this type of toxicity and the fact that its rare and sporadic occurrence poses significant problems with respect to early detection.

When viewed objectively the formal requirement for the routine performance of specific animal studies of different durations in certain species represents, at best, a somewhat simplistic administrative solution to an exceedingly complex scientific problem. For the present the only reliable predictor for humans is the species at risk, i.e., man himself. This places an added emphasis on formulating an effective approach to safety evaluation.

Phase I studies are the first of a long series of studies designed to define the safety profile of the drug in humans. As such care must be taken to ensure that conditions are appropriate for the early recognition and precise quantification of any adverse drug effect that may present, whether predicted or unpredicted. The normal volunteers selected for phase I studies should be free from concomitant pathology, the use or abuse of drugs or alcohol, and any other factors likely to confound the interpretation of test results. Regardless of whether normal subjects or patient volunteers with the target disease are utilized for phase I, efforts should be made to ensure that the baseline values for the laboratory parameters to be monitored are stable and within normal range. To this end, the laboratory test battery should be performed as a screening procedure for the inclusion or exclusion of potential study participants approximately 1 week prior to the actual commencement of the study. The laboratory test battery should then be repeated in close proximity to the first administration of drug (24 hr before is a convenient time). It is this latter set of values that will determine the patients' inclusion in the study and provide the baseline against which to assess any subsequent drug-induced effects.

A large number of options are available with regard to the laboratory parameters that may be monitored and the approach should be to employ, as a routine, a standard minimum battery of laboratory tests. This should include the commonly used parameters of hemopoietic function, hepatic function, renal function, metabolic function, and blood chemistries. This approach provides broad coverage of the more likely manifestations of drug-induced toxicity. For the initial phase I studies drug-induced end-organ toxicity, present in the preclinical animal toxicology studies, may suggest additional specific laboratory parameters or an increase in testing frequency of the customary parameters. As the clinical studies progress beyond the phase I stage, accumulating experience with the drug in humans will best serve to indicate the extent to which this standard battery needs to be modified or supplemented with additional tests.

The standard test battery employed is essentially a compromise. There is no means of predicting with any degree of certainty exactly what type of toxicity may occur. Likewise, there can be no assurance that any significant low-incidence toxicity associated with the drug will actually manifest early, if at all, during the clinical research program. A compromise must be reached between the large number of laboratory parameters potentially available, what it is practical and reasonable to do, and what constitutes reasonable coverage of possible toxicity. The aim is to have available, as a minimum, some ability to detect early warning signals of toxicity in all of the various organ systems potentially at risk. Once a safety problem manifests there will be an opportunity to reassess the situation and to introduce any additional and more specific parameters now deemed appropriate.

Not uncommonly, the exploration of a specific toxicity issue in an individual patient during the course of a study may require the use of additional parameters over and above those included in the standard battery. In such cases the absence of a baseline value can introduce difficulties in the interpretation of the test results. For this reason, and certainly initially while the drug's human safety profile remains relatively unexplored, it is a wise policy to take an additional aliquot of blood at the same time blood is drawn for the baseline laboratory test battery. This duplicate specimen may then be banked and stored for possible future use. It may subsequently prove invaluable as a source of vital baseline data for evaluating possible toxicity occurring during the study. In any routine laboratory test battery it is logistically impossible to provide for every conceivable parameter that might ultimately prove to be relevant and this approach can help obviate potential problems arising from a failure to anticipate the need for a particular parameter.

Reference has already been made to the need to differentiate viral hepatitis from drug-induced liver damage. This is a problem to be confronted in clinical studies at any stage of the clinical research program. One response to this is to include an HB_sAg test in the standard laboratory test battery performed at baseline. The availability of this information at baseline has two potential uses. It will serve to identify the patient who is incubating hepatitis B at the time of initial screening for inclusion in the study or, alternatively, it will identify the patient who may be a chronic carrier. In either event, if the positive result is not actually used to exclude the patient from the study, the finding can assist in clarifying the situation should the patient subsequently develop LFT abnormalities. A patient, presently asymptomatic with normal liver function parameters, who is being considered for inclusion in a study may conceivably be incubating hepatitis B or have a chronic infection. Such a patient, recruited into a study, could subsequently cause diagnostic problems with respect to causality assessment and the differentiation of drug-induced liver injury from concomitant disease. The inclusion of HB$_s$Ag in the baseline battery of laboratory tests would be of assistance in making this differentiation.

B. Serious Event Reporting

The federal regulations are quite explicit in defining those safety events encountered during a study that must be reported promptly [13]. One of the most important aspects of study monitoring is for the study monitor to remind the study personnel of their obligations with respect to the prompt reporting of serious safety events in compliance with federal regulations. Instructions regarding these requirements are given to the investigator and staff by the monitor during the site visit prior to initiation of the study and on subsequent interval monitoring visits. However, in view of the key role of the investigator in channeling this information to the sponsor in a timely fashion, the study protocol should also contain a section that specifically delineates his or her responsibilities and the different types of event that are subject to this reporting requirement (Appendix 1). Essentially the use of this protocol section provides a mechanism for ensuring continuing interval reinforcement of the monitor's instructions between visits. This approach is of particular importance in the effort to obtain the compliance of investigators in countries whose national regulatory authorities do not have such reporting requirements, and who are not therefore as familiar with this procedure as U.S. investigators.

Prompt notification of significant safety events to the clinical monitor is important in that it permits his or her intimate involvement in considering the steps to be taken in evaluating the event. This is important for two reasons. First, it provides added assurance that all the appropriate measures to determine causation are taken in a timely fashion. In this context the experience of the clinical monitor in such matters can be of critical importance, especially with the less experienced investigator. This is particularly relevant to the comments made earlier with respect to the research-oriented physician as opposed to the treatment-oriented physician. In addition, the monitor may have ready access to expert opinion in this particular area of drug toxicity.

Second, the clinical monitor is able to provide a perspective that derives from his familiarity with the total database, a perspective that may be particularly relevant with regard to a determination of causality. For instance, if a case of suspected drug-induced hepatotoxicity is reported, then the possible causal relationship to drug may be clarified if the monitor is aware that a low incidence of transaminase elevations is being seen in the total database.

From time to time, depending on the feedback from the clinical program, it may be desirable to extend the breadth of the immediate reporting requirement beyond that required by federal regulation. The purpose of this is to more fully explore the significance of a safety event and to do this in a manner that provides a greater assurance of patient safety. For instance, if the possibility of drug-induced agranulocytosis is suspected, then as a conservative measure this section may be modified to require the immediate reporting of all patients whose granulocyte count falls, not to the levels that would mandate drug discontinuation and prompt notification, but to levels sufficient to raise an index of suspicion, say, 3000/mm^3, i.e., levels that ordinarily would not be immediately reportable but may nevertheless have relevance if occurring in a significant number of patients. This ensures much closer monitoring of a potential toxicity problem and makes the maximum provision possible for patient safety until such time as the true toxicity profile is better defined.

C. The Central Clinical Laboratory

The total database for any clinical research program is composed of data drawn from a large number of clinical studies. When each individual study site uses its own clinical pathology laboratory, attempts to combine laboratory parameter data across studies may fail for any of a number of reasons. One of the most important obstacles to pooling data from different studies lies in the fact that each laboratory will have established its own normal ranges for reference purposes. There is also the possibility that the units of measurement may differ between laboratories for some parameters. From a purely analytical perspective one solution to this problem is to "normalize" the laboratory values and various techniques are available to accomplish this.

Certainly normalization addresses the problem inherent in different laboratories using different normal ranges. But there are other considerations. A number of other variables can impact the validity of data pooling across laboratories. These include differences relating to the actual test performance, the standardization of techniques, and the existence of laboratory or instrument error. But there is a consideration of even greater importance. Ideally the approach used to facilitate data pooling for purposes of formal analysis should also facilitate the visual review of laboratory data by the clinical research associate (CRA) or physician for purposes of clinical evaluation and safety monitoring. The optimum approach should be one that enhances the efficiency of the CRA in the day-to-day monitoring of laboratory safety data across the entire program. It would require that this individual only carry in mind, and be thoroughly familiar with, one set of normal ranges and units of measurement. As a consequence the CRA would readily be able to scan laboratory data by study or across the entire database, detect abnormalities, obtain an instant appreciation for the degree of abnormality existing, and readily be able to visually compare laboratory values between patients in different studies. This entire spectrum of needs is most conveniently addressed by the use of one central laboratory to process all the laboratory specimens arising during the course of the clinical research program. In fact, of all the various approaches to this problem the use of the central laboratory is the only one that benefits each of the two essential, and complementary, approaches to laboratory parameter safety analysis: clinical evaluation of the individual patient and formal statistical analysis of group changes. This is an extremely important consideration given the fact that clinical evaluation of the individual patient is always important in safety assessment but in many instances formal statistical approaches are impotent and noncontributory.

The important contributions that the use of a central laboratory makes to efficient safety monitoring are best considered under the following headings: (a) routine ongoing review of laboratory safety data and (b) response to specific abnormalities.

1. Routine Ongoing Review of Laboratory Safety Data

Available technology with respect to data transfer allows the central laboratory to make the laboratory data immediately available to the sponsor on line, for prompt and current review of any abnormalities by the CRA. Simultaneously it allows for the expeditious input into the accumulating clinical trial database of all the laboratory values generated, both abnormal and normal. Under this approach, not only are significant abnormalities available for immediate clinical evaluation and follow-up by the CRA or physician, but the most current total laboratory database possible is also immediately available for clinical review or more formal analysis.

Agreement is reached with the central laboratory regarding the threshold values for each parameter that must be exceeded in order for the value to be regarded as significantly abnormal. All values that exceed this threshold level will be flagged by the central laboratory. The investigator is notified immediately by telephone from the central laboratory of all such flagged values so that any further action on his part may be promptly instituted. In addition, arrangements are made for these same abnormalities to be flagged on the terminal output available simultaneously at the sponsor company's research center. The complete laboratory test batteries are sent to the investigator as and when all tests are completed. The sponsor will receive the full laboratory data on line in a continuing fashion for entry into the clinical trial database.

The prompt receipt of flagged abnormalities at the sponsor site means that the CRA and the investigator become aware of the abnormal findings simultaneously, thus greatly enhancing the efficiency of safety monitoring by the CRA. The CRA, supported by the project physician, is able to monitor the laboratory safety data by study and across the entire clinical program in an efficient and ongoing manner. He or she is as current with the laboratory data as the investigator is, receiving the results as they are generated. This significantly enhances his or her ability to identify a possible safety incident promptly and respond appropriately. The CRA is in a position to contact the investigator immediately to ensure that all appropriate measures for patient evaluation and causality assessment are taken in a timely fashion (vide infra). This central laboratory approach probably represents the most efficient way of minimizing the risk that essential elements of patient evaluation may not be done promptly and at the appropriate time. When combined with the more recent approach of remote data entry (RDE) for demographic, efficacy, and side effect data it provides the most current and comprehensive monitoring approach possible.

The use of a central laboratory serves another useful purpose in that it enables the monitor to perform his safety-monitoring duties in a manner that goes well beyond the identification of sporadic abnormalities. It provides the monitor with the capability for concurrent electronic monitoring of the total clinical trial database of laboratory parameters for whatever assistance this might provide in interpreting the significance of a reported abnormality. Indeed, the availability of this functionality can play an extremely important role in assessing the significance of an abnormal event since it may uncover valuable evidence supportive of a causal relationship to drug. With the assistance of appropriately designed software, the CRA or project physician can scan the data, study-by-study or across the entire database, constructing to his or her own design a variety of customized displays or scatterplots.

If, for instance, a patient is discovered to have developed an agranulocytosis and causality is at issue the CRA may wish to scan the database for other evidence of an effect on granulocytes. The database could be searched for a hitherto unsuspected and wider incidence of a much more subtle effect on granulocytes. If present this could provide valuable presumptive evidence for a drug-induced etiology. In these circumstances, it would be useful to scan the database for patients who had at least one value of $< 3000/mm^3$ while on drug, or one or more values while on drug, i.e., changes that had not been of a magnitude sufficient to cause discontinuation of drug or attract the attention of the investigator.

Similarly, if an instance of severe hepatic dysfunction occurs a search may be made for evidence of transaminasemia in the database. Experience with such drugs as erythromycin estolate, with components of a hypersensitivity mechanism and a direct intrinsic toxicity, has shown that this can provide valuable corroborative evidence for the existence of drug-induced hepatotoxicity. Furthermore, it is well documented that patients may react to drugs that manifest idiosyncratic hepatotoxicity by initially developing an increase in transaminases which then subsides and does not progress to frank hepatotoxicity. Therefore if the LFTs return to normal with continued therapy this cannot be regarded as excluding a drug-induced hepatotoxicity. Accordingly, any search for evidence of a previously unsuspected and subtle transaminasemia must include both patients whose increased levels persist and those whose levels subside with continued therapy. A transaminasemia that appears to be limited to one study or certain specific studies may raise the question of whether the changes may be attributable to causes other than drug and prompt a review of the patient population and other circumstances surrounding the study.

In addition, the database may be searched for patients showing abnormalities in two or more correlated liver function parameters that may not previously have attracted attention but in the light of the current incident may assume added meaning. Such searches can be progressively focused by changing the specified threshold level that must be exceeded for the patient to appear in the display.

Finally, in addition to customized scatterplots and similar displays of the accumulating database, the CRA may utilize one or more of the various LAB-CAT tabular displays to obtain a more informative categorization of the abnormalities being seen (vide infra).

Clearly, the central laboratory concept, when combined with current technology for data transfer and functionality for easy data manipulation and display by the CRA, greatly enhances the CRA's ability to closely follow and monitor the laboratory safety parameters across the entire program. The CRA can follow the laboratory safety data in the closest approximation to a real-time mode possible thereby minimizing the possibility that significant data will be missed and ensuring a prompt response to problems as and when they arise.

However, from the perspective of the physician-investigator there would appear to be a very real and significant negative to this approach. The question that will inevitably arise is whether or not the central laboratory approach will compromise the efficient and prompt care of the patient who develops a serious toxicity. In the event that a patient develops a significant laboratory abnormality the investigator will almost certainly want the assurance and benefit of immediate feedback from his or her own hospital laboratory. But these needs are quite compatible with the use of a central laboratory and can be addressed in a way that further improves the efficiency of the system as a whole. In such situations, the investigator will be asked as a standard routine to split the blood specimens withdrawn. One set of specimens will be sent to the local hospital laboratory for immediate testing and the duplicate set will be forwarded in the usual manner to the central laboratory.

This approach serves at least four important objectives. First, it completely eliminates any possibility that proper patient care is being compromised by the use of the central laboratory, always a first priority. Second, by assuring the investigator that patient care is not prejudiced it gives him or her greater peace of mind regarding participation in the central laboratory approach. Third, it preserves intact the concept of a uniform database from one central laboratory and ensures that this concept is not disrupted by the occurrence of the event, even though specimens are being sent to the local hospital laboratory during this period. Finally, and most importantly, experience teaches that on occasion there may be an added benefit, in that the duplication of specimens may serve to highlight a spurious abnormality due to laboratory error that would otherwise have gone undetected.

2. Response to Specific Abnormalities

Whenever there is a failure on the part of the investigator to respond appropriately to abnormal laboratory parameters as possible warning signals of drug-induced toxicity, important information may be lost. This loss may be irretrievable because essential additional tests were either not carried out or were carried out too late. The protocol section relating to serious event reporting (Appendix 1) and the use of a central laboratory are both intended to address this problem but they are not infallible. They do, after all, still depend to some extent on the human factor, whether it be the investigator or the CRA or both. For certain specific situations the contribution of this human factor can be further reduced by two additional steps that tend to make the evaluation process largely mechanical and automatic. One of these involves a further elaboration of the central laboratory approach and the other the use of specific safety evaluation protocols as appendices to the study protocol.

With regard to the former, a procedure may be established whereby the central laboratory will routinely and automatically, without any request being made, conduct certain additional specified tests on the available blood specimen whenever certain threshold levels of abnormality are exceeded for designated parameters. For instance, whenever an elevated alkaline phosphatase level is detected isoenzyme fractionation will be carried out routinely by the central laboratory on the available blood specimen to establish an osseous or hepatic origin. If there is an isolated serum glutamic oxaloacetic transaminase (SGOT) elevation or an SGOT elevation accompanied by an increase in lactic dehydrogenase (LDH), a creatinine phosphokinase (CPK) estimation will be routinely performed to differentiate a hepatic from a muscle origin for the enzyme elevations. An elevated CPK or LDH will always call for the performance of electrophoretic isoenzyme separation to determine the origin of the enzyme, whether skeletal or myocardial muscle, and in the case of LDH to also exclude a hepatic origin.

This procedure offers a great deal of flexibility and the examples cited by no means exhaust the possibilities. It constitutes a somewhat mechanical approach to ensuring that some possibly important tests are not omitted.

3. Safety Evaluation Protocols

The importance of attitudinal factors on the part of the physician has already been stressed as a possible reason for the failure to collect important information relative to potential drug toxicity. Various approaches to minimizing the impact of this have already been mentioned. These include the serious adverse event reporting section of the protocol, and the various benefits that derive from the use of a central laboratory to conduct the laboratory testing for all studies in the clinical research program.

Even with frequent monitoring there is a very real probability that safety events are going to arise at times remote from actual monitoring visits. With the use of a central laboratory it is anticipated that the CRA will be on top of the situation and ensure that the necessary and appropriate follow-up is carried out, but the human factor may nevertheless intrude and vital tests may be omitted. It is of little value to discover that an event occurred a month previously and that, although drug was discontinued, certain tests essential to causality attribution were not performed at the time and it is now too late. Frequently such omissions are not remediable by post hoc actions.

The use of safety evaluation protocols represents one final measure in attempts to ensure that this does not happen. This approach complements that of requiring the central laboratory to conduct specified additional tests whenever abnormalities occur in certain parameters. The difference is that the central laboratory approach relates to specific individual parameters whereas the safety evaluation protocol approach relates to the total evaluation of the patient for a specific organ toxicity.

Under this approach a safety evaluation protocol is attached as an appendix to each study protocol. It details the exact steps to be followed in the event that evidence of different types of organ toxicity occur that may be related to drug. They are designed to guide the investigator, and CRA, through certain basic essential steps that should be carried out in the evaluation of this type of organ toxicity. Their purpose is not to anticipate every eventuality but rather to ensure that the minimum required for the efficient evaluation of this type of toxicity is in fact done. They reflect a concern that vital information may be irretrievably lost if certain essential tests are not carried out at the appropriate time.

As a minimum these protocols deal with the occurrence of events suggesting hepatic, hemopoietic, or renal toxicity. The first two are of particular importance in view of their frequency as manifestations of serious drug-induced toxicity. A specimen safety evaluation protocol for the evaluation of possible hepatic toxicity is provided in Appendix 2 following this chapter. It outlines precisely the steps to be followed and the tests to be carried out in the event of hepatic toxicity occurring. It can never substitute completely for careful clinical reasoning and evaluation of the specific situation presenting. But it does serve to ensure that at least a minimum of the essential tests for this type of toxicity are in fact carried out, and in a timely manner. If other types of toxicity become apparent or are suspected during the clinical program, e.g., renal toxicity, then a protocol appendix addressing this particular toxicity is constructed and attached to the protocol.

VI. LABORATORY PARAMETER EVALUATION

The different ways in which the various types of drug-induced toxicity, especially the more serious forms, may present clinically mandates a different approach to safety evaluation as compared to that adopted for efficacy analysis. The primary focus is different. Safety assessment is more frequently a question of the response of patients as individuals whereas efficacy evaluation is a question of the response of patients as a group. Safety evaluation must always proceed on the assumption that drug-induced toxicity, often serious, may only manifest as low-incidence sporadic events.

Statistical analysis can contribute little to safety evaluation in such situations since the events are only detectable clinically. If one patient in a 100-patient controlled study develops evidence of hepatic dysfunction that is missed clinically, it cannot be discovered by routine statistical analysis of laboratory parameters, e.g., baseline/final group mean changes, trend analysis, etc. Therefore safety evaluation must always stress the early clinical identification and causality assessment of potential drug toxicities, as and when they occur, in individual patients. Statistical approaches must always be used with a full awareness of their possible limitations.

Safety assessment is therefore primarily a clinical exercise and only secondarily statistical. This is in the sense that, although precise clinical observations are fundamental to the evaluation of efficacy, appropriate statistical techniques are required to determine whether any meaningful conclusions may be drawn from the observations relative to efficacy. Safety evaluation, on the other hand, may be viewed as beginning and frequently remaining entirely a clinical judgment. In efficacy analysis the statistician tells the physician what has been found, but in safety evaluation only the physician knows what has been found. This is clearly a gross oversimplification but it nevertheless serves to make a very important point.

The difference between safety and efficacy evaluation is not entirely one of focus; there is also an important temporal element. Apart from those specific instances in which a sequential design is used or the study protocol calls for an interim analysis, formal efficacy analysis is usually carried out at the end of a study. However, safety evaluation is inevitably a continuous ongoing exercise throughout the course of the study or the clinical program as a whole. It is not, and by its very nature cannot be, an exercise confined to the end of the study.

The primary objective of safety monitoring is to define drug safety in a continuing ongoing fashion as the database accumulates. If this objective has been realized, then safety analysis conducted at the end of study, or an entire program, should primarily serve a confirmatory purpose. It should reaffirm the safety assessment, made as data accumulated, rather than function as a safety analysis de novo. It provides final verification that nothing has been missed during the course of the study.

It is therefore necessary to adopt a two-pronged approach to the analysis of laboratory safety parameters to comprehensively address the various ways in which drug toxicity may manifest. These two approaches are, in order of emphasis:

1. Clinical evaluation of individual patients with significant abnormalities
2. Statistical analytical techniques applied to group changes

Only clinical evaluation will be discussed in this chapter.

A. Clinical Evaluation

An average new drug application may contain data relating to at least 25,000–50,000 measurements for each individual laboratory parameter. The final clinical review and evaluation of such large volumes of laboratory safety data presents a very substantial workload for the physicians. This problem might be considered academic if sole reliance could be placed on formal statistical analysis of the data. The analytical task would then become entirely a mathematical exercise, one that could be automated and greatly facilitated by available computer-based technology.

The question therefore naturally arises as to whether computer technology can also be utilized to ease the burden on the clinician for safety evaluation purposes when the primary emphasis is on clinical review and judgment. And if this can be accomplished, there is the second-order question of whether this can be accomplished in a manner that does not simultaneously detract from the reliability of the whole process. Clearly these are relevant questions since the burden presented by this type of data review can only be expected to escalate as clinical programs increase in size.

In recognition of this methodology was developed some 15 years ago that sought to reduce the review burden on the clinical monitor by utilizing a form of "computer-assisted clinician review" of safety data. Clinical algorithms were developed that simulated the process of laboratory data review by the clinician. These algorithms permit computer-generated identification and preliminary categorization of laboratory abnormalities. These laboratory categorization systems (LABCATS) were originally written in a third-generation language (FORTRAN) but the programming was subsequently rewritten, over the course of time, in SAS [14]. Although SAS is primarily known for its statistical analytical capability it also provides excellent data manipulation functionality that make it ideally suited to this purpose. The programs are self-documenting and easy to maintain.

LABCATS functions as an artificial clinical intelligence simulating the logic employed by the clinician who is evaluating laboratory data in order to assess its possible relevance to drug safety. This computerized categorization process generates a preliminary clinical sorting of the data and leaves the physician with a much reduced data load of prescreened possibly drug-related abnormalities for detailed review.

A further advantage of the LABCATS system, particularly in view of the ongoing nature of safety assessment, is that it is ideally suited both to the ongoing review of an accumulating database by the CRA and to the final summarization of completed studies. When combined with the advantages of the central laboratory approach and the current electronic transfer of laboratory data to the sponsor it provides additional functionality to assist the CRA in his monitoring efforts (vide supra).

VII. LABORATORY CATEGORIZATION SYSTEM (LABCATS)

LABCATS reviews all the laboratory parameters from the entire database and separates the data into two distinct groupings depending on whether or not a laboratory abnormality occurred during drug administration (Appendix 3).

One of these groupings (category N) contains all those patients in whom the baseline may have been normal, abnormal, or missing but all subsequent laboratory values on therapy were normal. When this output is used with the second grouping of abnormal values it serves a useful verification and quality assurance purpose, as opposed to a review purpose. It serves as a check to ensure that all patients in the database with laboratory data are accounted for in the safety review. It also ensures that the denominator used for incidence calculations is correct.

The second grouping comprises all patients in whom an abnormality was encountered during therapy. These abnormalities are then categorized according to the computer-generated algorithm. The definition of an abnormality for any of the various parameters tested is determined with reference to the central pathology laboratory's current normal ranges. A conservative approach is adopted for those patients in whom the baseline value is missing. In such cases the baseline is arbitrarily presumed to be within the normal range for purposes of deciding whether or not an abnormality is present.

For each laboratory parameter a threshold value is defined that must be exceeded before any deviation is considered clinically significant and abnormal (Appendix 4). The assigning of these threshold values takes cognizance of the fact that some laboratory parameters such as electrolytes, e.g., serum sodium or potassium, are subject to much tighter homeostatic control than others such as the serum chemistries, e.g., SGPT and SGOT. Other parameters such as those reflecting metabolic breakdown tend to occupy a somewhat intermediate position. Another factor to be taken into consideration is the characteristic distribution of normal values for that parameter. The distribution may be symmetrical or skewed and this will impact on the likelihood for values that are nevertheless normal to lie outside the commonly accepted normal range.

The definition of an abnormal value will also differ depending on whether or not the baseline value is abnormal. In some instances more stringent criteria are applied for the definition of an abnormality during therapy when this occurs against the background of an abnormal baseline, e.g., hemoglobin and hematocrit. Other parameters are allowed a greater deviation with respect to an abnormal baseline value before being classified as abnormal, e.g., SGOT and SGPT (Appendix 5).

A preferred approach to estimates of what constitutes a clinically significant elevation of a given laboratory parameter would be provided by an analysis of the values obtained during the prestudy placebo run-in period. However, this period is customarily of the order of 1 or 2 weeks and rarely exceeds 4 weeks, and this may not provide sufficient data over a sufficient period of time to permit a true appreciation of the extent of the temporal variation and periodicity of the parameter. Furthermore, a prestudy placebo run-in period is not invariable in all studies.

Based on these predetermined criteria of what constitutes a clinically significant abnormality with respect to baseline for the various laboratory parameters, LABCATS initially assigns all laboratory abnormalities occurring during therapy to one of five categories (Appendix 3). Categories 1–4 of LABCATS comprise those abnormalities which, without more, are not considered to have a causal relationship to drug.

Categories 1 and 2 are those instances in which the deviation from the normal range (or baseline abnormal value) does not exceed the predetermined threshold value. The abnormality is therefore regarded as being so small as to be clinically insignificant. Category 3 represents abnormalities that are clinically significant relative to the normal range or to an abnormal baseline value. However, these abnormalities only occur as single, isolated, and unconfirmed abnormalities that cannot be replicated and that return to baseline or within the normal range on continued therapy. Category 4 abnormalities, on the other hand, are those instances in which an abnormality exceeding the stated threshold is sustained for two or more values only to return to the normal range and remain there with continued therapy. For patients in whom the baseline value was abnormal the abnormality is required to fall to or below the baseline value.

Allocation to category 4 makes an initial, provisional assumption that sustained abnormalities that return to normal with continued therapy are not drug-related. While this may be a useful starting position to adopt, it is not necessarily true. It can represent evidence of toxicity and other factors may arise that prompt a need to look more closely at the patients in this category for evidence supporting drug-induced toxicity. Such would arise, for instance, if the category

4 abnormalities were not confined to one parameter, e.g., SGOT, but occurred in two or more correlated liver function parameters, e.g., SGPT, SGOT, and alkaline phosphatase. But even if confined to one parameter the index of suspicion would be raised if the investigational drug group contained an excess of category 4 abnormalities compared with the incidence in the control group(s).

Category 4 abnormalities of a particular parameter are also subject to mandatory reappraisal if a true drug-induced toxicity, manifested by that particular parameter(s), is documented during the course of the clinical research program. For instance, if one or more isolated episodes of possible drug-induced hepatotoxicity have occurred, then category 4 should be reexamined both with respect to the individual parameters and groups of correlated parameters. If present, it is likely that these transient elevations also represent a drug-induced effect, the return to normal with continued therapy notwithstanding. The incidence of category 4 abnormalities with the investigational drug should also be compared with the incidence in the control groups. The impressions gained may serve to alter one's perception of the potential risk.

The fifth category of abnormality in this initial computer output is most conveniently described as "provisional category 9." It comprises all the abnormalities that do not fall within categories 1–4 and therefore are more likely to be related to drug. This category is subjected to detailed review by the physician and the abnormalities in this category are finally and definitively assigned to one or other of categories 5–9.

During this process some abnormalities will be retained as category 9 and regarded as possibly related to drug. Others may be reassigned, based on physician review, to category 5 (documented laboratory error), category 6 (likely to be due to coexisting disease), category 7 (likely to be due to concomitant therapy), or category 8. This latter category comprises those situations in which the abnormality exceeds the threshold value but does not appear to be due to laboratory error, coexisting disease, or concomitant therapy. Nevertheless the reviewing physician does not consider the abnormality to be clinically significant or related to drug. This category is primarily intended to provide for those situations in which the abnormalities only exceed the stated threshold value for an abnormality by one or two units.

Category 8 also serves another purpose. Physician review of the provisional category 9 patients should be performed blind in order to make the process of final categorization as objective and unbiased as possible. In those instances in which physician evaluation is not conducted on a blind basis, or when more than one person is involved in the categorization, the number of abnormalities allocated to category 8 can provide a useful check both on the objectivity and impartiality of the process and on interreviewer variability. If there is one unblinded reviewer is there an apparent excess of category 8 classifications? Or if there is more than one reviewer in a program is there evidence of a reporting bias as indicated by their respective assignments to category 8.

A. Individual Patient Review

Individual patient review must be completed before any form of summary review can be carried out. One approach would be to defer this process, for the majority of patients, until the completion of the study or the entire clinical program. If this approach is followed the only exception would be for those patients manifesting evidence of possible drug toxicity who required prompt evaluation and causality attribution at the time of the event.

The preferred approach, however, is to categorize patients in an ongoing fashion, as and when individual patients complete therapy and the data are available in the database. This approach fully capitalizes on the benefits accruing from the use of a central laboratory and the ability to have laboratory parameter data in the clinical trial database fairly promptly and in as close an approximation to a real-time mode as possible. It is therefore consistent with the need to conduct safety monitoring on the most current basis possible during the program and can significantly contribute to this process. For instance, LABCATS can generate interim summary displays of abnormality categories as a means of reviewing the developing database and assisting in the interpretation of potential toxicities as they arise. And finally there is a very real logistic advantage in that this approach distributes the burden on the reviewing clinician(s) more evenly over time.

If the preferred sequential approach is followed the laboratory data review at the completion of the study or the clinical program constitutes a final quality assurance check on the validity of the conclusions drawn as the database accumulated. However, regardless of whether the review is done on a continuing basis or at the completion of the program, the approach to categorization is the same.

The computer output provided to the clinician for this purpose is in two forms, the laboratory categorization listing (LCL) and the patient laboratory profile (PLP). The LCL lists each completed patient who has developed an abnormality of any parameter during therapy and gives the abnormality category assigned and certain other key units of data (Appendix 6). For each abnormal value the LCL lists certain units of information essential to proper identification. These include the patient ID, which identifies both the patient and the study involved, sex, age, specimen collection date, and the laboratory parameter. In addition, information is provided with respect to the upper and lower limits of the normal range for that parameter for the reporting laboratory, the baseline value, the most abnormal value during therapy, the dose of drug associated with the abnormality, and the category to which that abnormality has been assigned by the computer algorithm. Provision is made for information regarding the identity of study drug(s) and dosage information to be removed in the interests of preserving the blind for categorization purposes. The categories initially assigned by computer are categories 1–4 and the provisional category 9 to which reference has already been made. For the convenience of the physician reviewer the abnormalities are also flagged as being high (H) or low (L).

Each provisional category 9 abnormality in the LCL is next reviewed and evaluated by the physician in order to make the final definitive assignment of these abnormalities to one or other of categories 5, 6, 7, 8, or 9. Once this assignment has been made the provisional category 9 for each abnormality is changed to the final category in the database. To assist the physician in categorizing the abnormalities he is provided with a patient laboratory profile (PLP) for each individual patient with an abnormality (Appendix 7).

Drug-induced toxicity is not a static phenomenon but a dynamic process that evolves over time. Therefore the pattern of change occurring in the relevant laboratory parameters must also be carefully evaluated over time, together with the movement of any other correlated parameters. Note must be taken of the time relationship of other events to the occurrence of the abnormality and a possible contributory role. For instance, it is particularly important to take into consideration the possible role of coexisting pathology or concomitant therapy either as the primary factor or based on some interaction with the investigational drug. The PLP provides a chronology of all this essential information in a concise, easily assimilable format.

It lists for each patient the values for all laboratory parameters across time during the course of the study, including the predrug period, the period of drug administration and any postdrug period. Study drug dosage and change of dose is identified for each time period during the study. For convenience of review the upper and lower limits of the normal range are listed for each parameter and all values falling above or below the normal range are clearly flagged. The computer assigned category is also listed for each abnormality. The degree of abnormality of the baseline value and the most abnormal value on treatment is indicated by an appropriate notation, using an arbitrary 5-point scale of severity. Additional information that may be relevant to the safety review and a meaningful causality judgment is also included on the patient profile. For instance, in addition to patient demographic data, information on primary and secondary disease and the use and timing of any concomitant therapy is also included.

The use of the PLP allows the reviewing physician to factor in the possible contribution of other pathology and concomitant medication and also to take into consideration changes occurring in other correlated parameters when categorizing an abnormality. The clinician's assignment of each provisional category 9 abnormality to one or another of categories 5, 6, 7, 8, or 9 is then entered into the computer as the final definitive categorization. This provides the basis of the final version of the LCL, which is then used for safety review, analysis, and use in regulatory submissions if indicated.

The clinician reviewing these data for final definitive categorization should preferably remain blind as to the identity (investigational drug, comparative agent, or placebo) of the therapy being administered and associated with the abnormality. This is essential in order to eliminate personal bias in arriving at a causality judgment and assigning a category. The system therefore allows for the deletion of drug name and any information, including dosage information, which might lead to breaking of the blind. If more than one reviewer is utilized, then a comparison of the proportions of patients in categories 5–9 may provide evidence of an inconsistent approach or bias in categorization. While the number of abnormalities categorized by two reviewers may be comparable one may have allocated a greater proportion to category 9 (Possibly drug-related) and the other to category 6 (Coexisting disease), category 7 (Concomitant therapy), or category 8 (Regarded as clinically insignificant). A preponderance of patients in category 8 rather than category 9 must carry with it a presumption of assignment bias, possibly due to unblinded review. This would be particularly true if this distribution pattern was distinctive of the investigational drug group as compared with the control groups.

Provision may be made for the categorization process to be done interactively at a terminal rather than by a review of printouts. Interactive use of the system is particularly appropriate to the use of the LABCATS system as a tool for safety monitoring as well as for data summarization. Under this approach the current LCL could be periodically called up on the screen and the list scanned for completed patients with a provisional category 9 abnormality who had accumulated since the last review of the LCL. The relevant PLP could then be retrieved on the screen and final category assignments made. In addition, as and when instances of documented laboratory error were encountered during the course of the program, the LCL and PLP would be retrieved and the abnormality assigned to category 5.

B. Summary Review

Once the process of individual patient review has been completed the LABCATS system lends itself to various formats of summary review and data display based on the final version of the laboratory categorization listing (LCL). If the final categorization is being made more or less contemporaneously with individual patients completing therapy such summary reviews may be undertaken sequentially over time as the database gradually accumulates as well as at the termination of the whole program when the entire database is available.

If the sequential categorization approach is adopted LABCATS can function both as an important component of the normal safety monitoring process and for data summarization at the completion of the program and in anticipation of regulatory filing. In such cases the final summarization serves the twin purposes of substantiating the safety conclusions developed over time and verification that safety events have not been missed.

If, however, final categorization is deferred until the end of the program it will impact the detail rather than the scope of LABCATS application to safety evaluation. On the one hand, its contribution to final safety data review and display in preparation for regulatory filing will be undiminished. But for interim summary safety data displays during the course of the program there will be a limitation with respect to the level of detail to which these may be taken. They will only be able to use the categories listed on the preliminary LCL, categories N, 1, 2, 3, 4, and provisional category 9. While this may still provide useful data, some critical information may nevertheless be lost or, at least, not currently available.

A popular approach to the display of laboratory parameter findings, either for the total database, a particular data subset, or an individual study, is to plot the baseline value for the parameter against a subsequent value, most commonly the final value on therapy. While this type of display is useful and instructive, it does have important limitations.

It may be characterized as being static and mathematical rather than dynamic and clinical. By its very design it only depicts changes at one fixed point in time subsequent to baseline. But drug-induced toxicity is inherently dynamic and evolving over time, and an examination of the time course of the effects on the different parameters is often critical to a proper assessment of the existence of toxicity. This type of graphic display is simply not responsive to the changes in laboratory parameters that may be occurring during therapy as a result of drug or some other influence.

In spite of these criticisms it remains a common form of presentation for laboratory data summarization. If a central laboratory is used and the appropriate functionality is provided to the CRA, this type of graphic display can also be used to monitor the developing database interactively.

Figure 2 shows typical plots of baseline vs. final value for SGPT and SGOT values from the pooled data from a number of controlled studies comparing the investigational drug drug A with the standard control drug B. The plots do not appear to indicate any difference between the two drugs with respect to an effect on transaminases. However, Table 3 shows the data tabulation from these same studies based on categorization by the LABCATS system. This type of display can be produced from LABCATS during the summarization phase at the completion of the program, or while the studies are in progress if patients are categorized as they complete therapy. It will instantly be appreciated that the laboratory categorization display suggests a different interpretation of the data from that obtained from the baseline/final graphic display of transaminase values.

For drug A and the control drug B there are a few category 9 (possibly due to drug) abnormalities for each of the four liver function parameters (LFTs), but with respect to the effect of drug B on transaminases there is little difference between the number of category 9 values and the category 6 (likely due to other disease). Unlike the impression gained from the plots of transaminase values the effect of drug A on LFT can be distinguished from that of the control drug. There

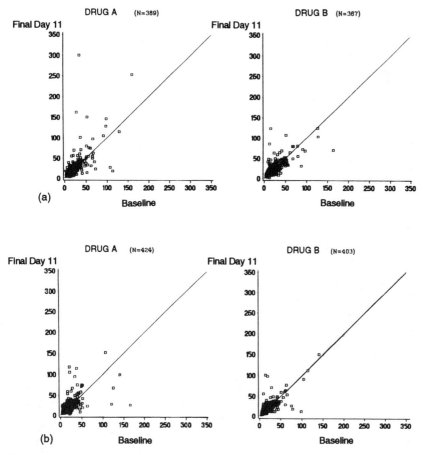

Figure 2 (a) Plot of baseline and day 11 values: SGPT (IU/L). Comparative studies of drug A and drug B. (b) Plot of baseline and day 11 values SGOT (IU/L). Comparative studies of drug A and drug B.

is an excess of category 9 abnormalities compared with the control and in addition there is also an excess of patients showing a sustained elevation of transaminases that then return to normal (category 4). This latter finding would appear to suggest that drug A has a true effect on hepatic function and is supportive of the category 9 findings representing a drug-induced hepatic toxicity.

If laboratory categorization is not carried out sequentially as patients complete therapy during the program the amount of information available in LABCATS tabular displays is curtailed to some extent. It may nevertheless still provide some valuable insight into possible drug toxicity. For instance, Fig. 3 displays

Table 3 Number of Patients with Hepatic Enzyme Abnormalities According to Laboratory Categorization

	Drug A				Drug B			
	SGOT (IU/L)	SGPT (IU/L)	Alk. Ph (IU/L)	T. bili (mg/dl)	SGOT (IU/L)	SGPT (IU/L)	Alk. Ph (IU/L)	T. bili (mg/dl)
Total number tested	477	441	479	480	458	419	460	458
Number with any category of abnormality	68	72	46	27	55	58	45	37
Category N: The baseline value was normal, abnormal, or missing and all values during therapy were normal.	409	369	433	453	403	361	415	421
Category 1: The baseline value was abnormal and the deviation of the most abnormal value from baseline during therapy was so small as to be clinically insignificant.	9	17	22	7	19	22	19	7
Category 2: The baseline value was normal or missing and the deviation of the most abnormal value during therapy was so small as to be clinically insignificant.	14	9	8	3	7	9	8	4
Category 3: The baseline value was normal or missing and there was a single clinically significant abnormal value during therapy which returned to normal during continued therapy.	4	1	7	11	17	10	5	14

The baseline value was abnormal and there was a single divergent value that differed significantly from baseline but returned to within baseline limits during therapy.

Category 4:	The baseline value was normal or missing and there were two or three significant abnormal values within a 6-week period that all lay on the same side of the normal range; no value reached the level of marked abnormality and the last two values during therapy were within normal limits.	17	15	1	0	0	0	0	0
	The baseline value was abnormal and there were two or more significant abnormal values compared to baseline within a 6-week period that lay on the same side of the normal range as the baseline; the last two values during therapy did not differ significantly from baseline. The abnormal values were consecutive, or they differed significantly from baseline and were interspersed with values differing less than the insignificant percent from baseline.								
Category 5:	Documented laboratory error.	0	0	0	0	0	0	0	0
Category 6:	The abnormality appeared likely to be due to the primary disease or to a coexisting disease process.	5	8	1	0	4	4	1	0
Category 7:	The abnormality appeared likely to be due to concomitant drug therapy.	0	0	0	0	0	0	1	0
Category 8:	The abnormality was considered to be clinically insignificant or not due to therapy upon review by a physician.	8	7	5	2	3	6	6	3
Category 9:	The abnormality was possibly related to study drug therapy.	11	15	2	4	5	7	5	9

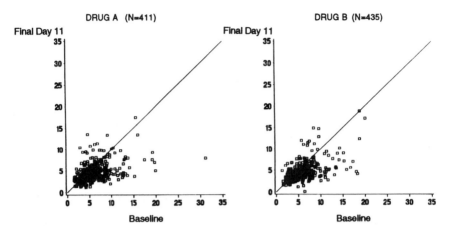

Figure 3 Plots of baseline and day 11 values: neutrophils ($10^3/\mu$l). Comparative studies of drug X and drug Y.

plots of baseline/final absolute neutrophil counts from comparative studies comparing the investigational drug X with the standard control drug Y. Earlier in the program there had been an instance of agranulocytosis associated with drug X. However, a causal relationship to the investigational drug was uncertain in view of concomitant therapy with a marketed drug known to have this propensity, albeit of very low incidence. Against this background the plot does not appear to show any effect of drug X on neutrophils. In fact there is a close similarity between the two drugs and no suggestion of any differential effect with respect to neutrophils. However, even though full categorization has not been carried out the LABCATS display nevertheless provides some interesting information (Table 4) that is not evident from the plots. The provisional category 9 abnormalities are similar between the two drugs, although it is possible that ultimately with final assignment of the provisional category 9 abnormalities to categories 5–9 a difference will be discerned. However, even with this curtailed display there is a clear excess of patients in the drug X group showing a sustained effect on neutrophils that nevertheless returns to normal with continued therapy (category 4). This is suggestive of drug effect and suggests that the original incident was causally related to drug.

Both of these examples are illustrative of a point made earlier. Graphic displays of the data such as those described above are only able to capture one fixed point in time. Evidence of drug-induced toxicity most commonly derives from the evolving pattern of laboratory parameter changes over time and may easily be missed by graphic displays of one time point. It is for this reason that clinical evaluation is so important in safety assessment since it is able to appreciate this dimension. The data displays derived from the LABCATS system approximate closer to the ideal of clinical evaluation than the graphic displays and make an important contribution to the evaluation of drug safety.

A comparison of data bases in terms of laboratory categorization can also serve other useful purposes in the evaluation of the database. It may be used to compare the laboratory profile of various patient subsets, e.g., the elderly, with that seen in the database as a whole or with other subsets. When the total database is drawn from two different geographic locations, e.g., studies from a U.S. clinical program and a non-U.S. clinical program, the laboratory categorization profile may be employed as a convenient means of comparing and contrasting the two databases. This may be undertaken in order to justify the pooling of data from these two sources to produce an overall safety profile in terms of laboratory parameters.

VIII. ADDITIONAL OUTPUT

Various forms of additional of output may be provided to further enhance the utility of the LABCATS system to assist physician review of laboratory data. Perhaps the most useful of these relates to the display of clusters of correlated laboratory parameters. Quite commonly an important indicator of drug-induced toxicity is the existence of a change in two or more correlated laboratory parameters rather than a change in a single isolated parameter. This is particularly relevant when the increase in the single parameter is not marked. A mild to moderate increase in SGPT probably has greater relevance if accompanied by similar elevations in one or more other LFTs.

The importance of other related parameters relative to causality judgments is recognized in the LABCATS system by providing the physician with the complete patient profile of laboratory data to assist in categorizing the abnormalities in the LCL. But even though the movement of other related parameters is factored into the categorization decision with respect to any given parameter, the final categories are still assigned to single parameters. The displays do not differentiate between the category 9 SGPT elevation, which involves only that parameter, and the category 9 SGPT elevation, which is also accompanied by elevations in two or three other LFT.

However, this weakness is not confined to the LABCATS system but is a feature of all the conventional modes of presentation of laboratory data. For display purposes they all focus on the incidence of abnormality in terms of single parameters and ignore the concomitant changes in other correlated parameters. Conventional tabular displays of the incidence of laboratory abnormalities always show the percent incidence of abnormalities for the individual parameters. This can be misleading. A 1% incidence of SGPT abnormalities has quite a different meaning if each abnormality was associated with abnormalities of one or more other LFTs and does not represent isolated abnormalities of that parame-

Table 4 Provisional Categorization of Neutrophil (1000/ul) Abnormalities

	Drug X (neutros 1000/ul)	Drug Y (neutros 1000/ul)
Total number tested	452	476
Number with any category of abnormality	82	85
Category N: The baseline value was normal, abnormal, or missing and all values during therapy were normal.	371	391
Category 1: The baseline value was abnormal and the deviation of the most abnormal value from baseline during therapy was so small as to be clinically insignificant.	30	27
Category 2: The baseline value was normal or missing and the deviation of the most abnormal value during therapy was so small as to be clinically insignificant.	14	15
Category 3: The baseline value was normal or missing and there was a single clinically significant abnormal value during therapy which returned to normal during continued therapy.	1	26
The baseline value was abnormal and there was a single divergent value that differed significantly from baseline but returned to within baseline limits during therapy.		
Category 4: The baseline value was normal or missing and there were two or three significant abnormal values within a 6-week period that all lay on the same side of the normal range; no value reached the level of marked abnormality and the last two values during therapy were within normal limits.	18	0
The baseline value was abnormal and there were two or more significant abnormal values compared to baseline within a 6-week period that lay on the same side of the normal range as the baseline; the last two values during the therapy did not differ significantly from baseline. The abnormal values were consecutive, or they differed significantly from baseline and were interspersed with values differing less than the insignificant percent from baseline.		
Provisional Category 9: Abnormality is considered to be drug related subject to review by a clinician.	19	17

ter alone. This could be addressed in the LABCATS system by further programming designed to further subdivide category 4 and provisional category 9 (and ultimately category 9) listings depending on whether the abnormality consists of one or two or more related parameters.

During the course of any clinical research program the normal safety-monitoring process may identify documented laboratory errors. Whenever this occurs an appropriate notation to that effect will be made in the relevant laboratory record in the database. All documented laboratory errors thus identified will appear on the initial LCL output as category 5. Other laboratory errors that go undetected at the time must be identified retrospectively by the physician, if indeed that it possible. In this context this process may be assisted by computer-generated flagging of possible instances of hemolysed specimens in the provisonal category 9 output.

The algorithm for this programming is based on the fact that a hemolysed specimen will invalidate certain laboratory parameter determinations as a result of the release of erythrocyte contents. The color change resulting from hemolysis can also invalidate assays that involve photometric measurements utilizing the shorter wavelengths of the visible spectrum. Hemolysis of a blood specimen can therefore lead to spurious values for serum potassium, lactic dehydrogenase, SGOT, or acid phosphatase. Bilirubin levels may also be increased. This arises because the released hemoglobin can interfere with certain specific chemical reactions, in this cases the diazotization reaction used for bilirubin determination. Provisional category 9 abnormalities would be flagged to bring them to the physician's attention if an abnormality of serum potassium is associated with an abnormality of one or more of the other parameters characteristically affected by hemolysis.

IX. SUMMARY

Drug-induced toxicity may arise by a variety of different mechanisms and these in turn play an important part in influencing the manner in which the toxicity presents clinically. The clinical presentation may vary from sporadic, isolated events of low incidence to dose-related consistent effects seen with much greater frequency across the exposed patient population. This requires an approach to safety assessment that is significantly different from that adopted for efficacy analysis.

Statistical methodology occupies a pivotal role in efficacy analysis. It may also play a similar role in safety analysis but, quite frequently, it is unable to make an important contribution because of the mechanism and clinical presentation of the toxicity. For this reason clinical evaluation remains the only viable approach to the detection of many forms of drug-induced toxicity. It is therefore essential that methodologies seeking to maximize the efficiency of the clinical approach to safety evaluation be made available.

Appendix 1

Protocol Section For Serious Event Reporting

Immediate Reporting of Significant Adverse Experience

All deaths, serious adverse experiences, and study drug discontinuations whether due to adverse experience or concomitant disease occurring during the study period or the posttherapy period must be reported immediately. Such reports will be made regardless of treatment group or suspected relationship to drug.

All reports will be made by telephone to the Clinical Monitor, Dr. _____ at the following location, Tel. _____

Such serious adverse experience includes but is not restricted to the following events:

1. Fatal events.
2. Life-threatening or potentially life-threatening events.
3. Permanently disabling events.
4. An event requiring inpatient hospitalization.
5. Congenital anomaly, cancer, or the effects of drug overdose.

It should be emphasized that, regardless of the above criteria, any additional adverse experience which the investigator considers significant enough to merit immediate reporting should be so treated.

Special Reporting Requirements

For this particular compound all instances of the following type should be reported immediately even though they do not fall within the definitions given above, regardless of whether or not they result in drug discontinuation.

_____

_____

Appendix 2

Protocol for Hepatic Safety Evaluation

Baseline Requirements

Before inclusion in a clinical study a patient must satisfy the following requirements:

1. A negative hepatitis B surface antigen test (HBsAg).
2. No biochemical evidence of hepatic disease. Values for SGPT (ALT), SGOT (AST), alkaline phosphatase (AP), and total serum bilirubin (SBR) must not exceed levels of greater than 10% above the upper limit of normal.
3. Patients may be admitted with values above these threshold levels if the protocol so allows. Such exceptions may be made for studies specifically addressed to patients with hepatic dysfunction and in study populations in which such abnormalities are likely to be found as part of the disease process.
4. If a patient has already commenced study therapy prior to the availability of baseline liver function tests, treatment should be discontinued immediately if repeat testing confirms the abnormality. The patient should then be followed as for minimial or marked abnormality (see below).

Liver Function Abnormalities Arising During the Trial

If a laboratory value is obtained during the trial which is $> 20\%$ above the upper limit of normal for AP or SBR, or $> 50\%$ above the upper limit of normal for SGPT (ALT) or SGOT (AST), the abnormal parameter(s) should be repeated as soon as possible and preferably within 72 hours. When a central laboratory is being used the local hospital laboratory may be used to follow the patient during the reaction, providing duplicate specimens are drawn on each occasion and forwarded to the central laboratory. This ensures complete uniformity of the source of all laboratory data in this particular patient. This, in turn, serves to facilitate comparison of the laboratory record during this period with the prior experience in this patient, as well as with other patients in this study and across the entire program. An ability to accomplish this can be particularly valuable if the event occurs in a subset of patients who are only represented in any appreciable number across the entire clinical program.

Upon repeating the laboratory parameter(s) to confirm the abnormality the following additional tests should be performed:

1. If the SGOT > SGPT a creatine phosphokinase with isoenzyme fractionation should be obtained.
2. If AP is elevated an AP fractionation and γ-glutamyltransferase should be obtained.
3. If SBR is elevated direct and indirect bilirubin determinations, a Coomb's test and a reticulocyte count should be obtained.

If the initial abnormalities are confirmed on repeat testing and the data obtained support a probable hepatic origin for the abnormality, the patient will be categorized as showing a minimal or marked abnormality and monitored accordingly.

Marked Abnormality

Marked abnormality is defined as those patients showing an SGOT or SGPT > 3 times the upper limit of normal, and/or an AP > 1.5 times the upper limit of normal, and/or an SBR > 2 times the upper limit of normal. Such patients will be immediately discontinued from therapy and the company clinical monitor notified by telephone.

The laboratory studies required include: HBsAg, Anti-Hbc, Anti-HAV (IgM and IgG), SGOT, SGPT, AP (and isoenzyme fractionation), SBR (direct and indirect), CBC, one-stage prothrombin time, serum proteins. If the clinical index of suspicion warrants their performance then cytomegalovirus, heterophile antibody titers and toxoplasma will be included. The patient will be followed by liver function tests and CBC at weekly intervals.

Arrangements will be made for an appropriate gastrointestinal consultation as soon as possible. A liver biopsy is desirable as an aid to identifying the etiology of the hepatic dysfunction and providing definitive information on the drug's safety profile. If a liver biopsy is performed the slides and a tissue block will be supplied to the company in order to facilitate expert pathological opinion.

Rechallenge will not be embarked on without due consideration of the type of liver injury manifest and the associated risk of rechallenge. If conducted it will be regarded as a separate clinical trial and will require both informed consent and institutional review board approval.

Minimal Abnormality

Minimal abnormality is defined as those patients with an SGPT or SGOT > 1.5 times the upper limit of normal and/or an AP or SBR > 1.2 times the upper limit of normal but not meeting the requirements for a marked abnormality. Such patients will be followed at weekly intervals and SGPT, SGOT, AP (with fractionation), SBR, and CBC.

Trial medication will be discontinued if the liver function tests progress to marked abnormality or there is cause for clinical concern, e.g., an abnormality of one parameter progresses to include several parameters. In such instances the full workup described under ''Marked Abnormality'' will be instituted.

Appendix 3

Definitions for Laboratory Parameter Categorization

Category N   The baseline was normal, abnormal, or missing and all values during therapy were within the normal range. This category is included for quality assurance purposes in order to provide verification that all patients have been accounted for.

Category 1   The baseline value was abnormal (outside the normal range) and the deviation of the most abnormal value from baseline during therapy was so small as to be clinically insignificant.

Category 2   The baseline value was normal (within the normal range) or missing and the deviation of the most abnormal value from the normal range during therapy was so small as to be clinically insignificant.

Category 3   The baseline value was normal (within the normal range) or missing and there was a single, clinically significant abnormal value which returned to normal during therapy. *Or* the baseline value was abnormal (outside the normal range) and there was a single divergent value that differed significantly from the baseline value but returned to the baseline value or below during therapy.

Category 4   The baseline value was normal (within the normal range) or missing and there were two or three significant abnormal values within a 6-week period which all lie on the same side of the normal range. No value reached the level of marked abnormality and the last two values during therapy were within normal limits.

The abnormal values were consecutive or interspersed with normal values. *Or* the baseline value was abnormal (outside the normal range) and there were two or more significant abnormal values compared to baseline within a 6-week period and all lie on the same side of the normal range as the baseline. The last two values during therapy did not differ significantly from baseline. The abnormal values were consecutive, or there were abnormal values differing significantly from baseline interspersed with values representing insignificant increases beyond the normal range.

Category 5* There was a documented laboratory error.

Category 6* The abnormality appeared likely to be due to the primary disease or to a coexisting disease process.

Category 7* The abnormality appeared likely to be due to concomitant drug therapy.

Category 8* The abnormality was considered to be clinically insignificant or not due to therapy upon review by the physician.

Category 9* The abnormality is considered to be possibly related to drug therapy.

---

* These categories are not assigned by computer. The initial computer output groups all of these abnormalities together as ''Provisional Category 9''. Assignment to categories 5 to 9 as appropriate is made by the physician after review of the patient.

Appendix 4

Definition of Abnormal Test Values When Baseline Value Was Normal or Missing

Laboratory test	Clinically relevant direction[a]	Abnormality (%)	Marked abnormality (%)
HGB	Decrease	10	25
HCT	Decrease	10	25
RBC	Either	10	25
Platelets	Decrease	10	25
WBC	Either	10	25
Neutros (ABS)	Either	10	25
Eos (ABS)	Increase	25	50
Basos (ABS)	Increase	25	50
Lymphs (ABS)	Either	10	25
Monos (ABS)	Increase	25	50
Bands (ABS)	Increase	10	25
Total bilirubin	Increase	10	50
Direct bilirubin	Increase	10	50
Indirect bilirubin	Increase	10	50
Total protein	Either	5	25
Serum albumin	Either	5	25
Serum globulin	Either	10	50
SGOT	Increase	10	50
CPK	Increase	10	50
SGPT	Increase	10	50

Appendix 4   (*Continued*)

Laboratory test	Clinically relevant direction[a]	Abnormality (%)	Marked abnormality (%)
GGT	Increase	10	50
LDH	Increase	10	50
Alkaline phosphatase	Increase	10	50
Blood urea	Either	10	50
BUN	Increase	10	50
Creatinine	Increase	10	50
Uric acid	Increase	10	50
Sodium	Either	5	25
Potassium	Either	5	25
Chloride	Either	5	25
CO_2	Either	5	25
Calcium	Either	5	25
Inorganic phosphorus	Either	5	25
Glucose, fasting	Either	10	50
Glucose, random	Either	10	50

[a]Only clinically relevant direction of abnormality considered and percent limits applied to the limit on normal range closest to that abnormality.

Appendix 5

Definition of Abnormal Test Values When Baseline Value Was Abnormal

Laboratory test	Clinically relevant direction[a]	Abnormality (%)	Marked abnormality (%)
HGB	Decrease	5	10
HCT	Decrease	5	10
RBC	Either	5	10
Platelets	Decrease	10	25
WBC	Either	20	50
Neutros (ABS)	Either	10	25
Eos (ABS)	Increase	25	50
Basos (ABS)	Increase	25	50
Lymphs (ABS)	Either	10	25
Monos (ABS)	Increase	25	50
Bands (ABS)	Increase	10	25
Total bilirubin	Increase	10	50
Direct bilirubin	Increase	10	50
Indirect bilirubin	Increase	10	50
Total protein	Either	5	25
Serum albumin	Either	5	25
Serum globulin	Either	10	50
SGOT	Increase	20	50
CPK	Increase	20	50
SGPT	Increase	20	50
GGT	Increase	20	50
LDH	Increase	20	50
Alkaline phosphatase	Increase	20	50
Blood urea	Either	10	50
BUN	Increase	10	50
Creatinine	Increase	10	50
Uric acid	Increase	10	50
Sodium	Either	5	25
Potassium	Either	5	25
Chloride	Either	5	25
CO_2	Either	5	25
Calcium	Either	5	25
Inorganic phosphorus	Either	5	25
Glucose, fasting	Either	20	50
Glucose, random	Either	20	50

[a]Only clinically relevant direction of abnormality considered and percent limits applied to the change from abnormal baseline.

Appendix 6
Laboratory Categorization Listing

Drug Treatment Drug X

Patient ID	Sex	Age	Collection date	Laboratory parameter	Low normal	High normal	Baseline value	Most divergent value	Flag	Dose	Category
104A1160003	M	68	020785	Gluc, random	80.00	160.00	267.00	188.00	H	125	1
104A1160003	M	68	021485	RBC	4.70	6.10	4.75	4.57	L	125	2
104A1160003	M	68	021485	HCT	42.00	52.00	39.60	37.70	L	125	1
104A1160003	M	68	022885	HGB	14.00	18.00	13.20	12.20	L	125	9
104A1160003	M	68	031985	Eos(ABS)	0.00	0.43	0.00	0.70	H	125	9
104A1160003	M	68	031985	WBC	4.80	10.80	12.00	14.10	H	125	1
104A1160003	M	68	031985	Neutros(ABS)	2.40	8.10	10.08	11.28	H	125	9
104A1160004	F	44.5	020785	Gluc, random	80.00	160.00	194.00	250.00	H	125	3
104A1160004	F	44.5	021485	GGT	0.00	35.00	51.00	181.00	H	125	9
104A1160004	F	44.5	021485	Platelets	140.00	400.00	174.00	138.00	L	125	2
104A1160004	F	44.5	021485	WBC	4.80	10.80	5.50	4.60	L	125	2
104A1160004	F	44.5	021485	HGB	12.00	16.00	13.10	10.70	L	125	3
104A1160004	F	44.5	021485	HCT	37.00	47.00	39.30	31.60	L	125	3
104A1160004	F	44.5	021485	RBC	4.20	5.40	4.50	3.62	L	125	3
104A1170101	M	46.7	030984	Basos(ABS)	0.00	0.22	0.10	0.22	H	125	2
104A1170101	M	46.7	030984	Gluc, random	80.00	160.00	325.00	382.00	H	125	1

ID	Sex	Age	Date	Test				Flag		
104A1170101	M	46.7	032284	WBC	4.80	10.80	10.30	11.40	H	125	2
104A1170104	M	67.2	022884	Potassium	3.50	5.00	4.90	5.50	H	125	4
104A1170104	M	67.2	022884	Sodium	135.00	145.00	141.00	134.00	L	125	2
104A1170104	M	67.2	022884	Lymphs(ABS)	0.96	4.32	1.86	0.86	L	125	2
104A1170104	M	67.2	031484	Alk.phos	30.00	140.00	135.00	177.00	H	125	9
104A1170104	M	67.2	031484	Gluc, random	80.00	160.00	267.00	364.00	H	125	9
104A1170104	M	67.2	031484	HGB	14.00	18.00	14.00	13.80	L	125	2
104A1170104	M	67.2	031484	HCT	42.00	52.00	42.50	41.30	L	125	2
104A1170104	M	67.2	031484	RBC	4.70	6.10	4.84	4.60	L	125	2
104A1170104	M	67.2	032784	GGT	0.00	65.00	114.00	227.00	H	125	9
104A1170106	F	46.4	041984	Gluc, random	80.00	160.00	417.00	386.00	H	125	1
104A1170106	F	46.4	042684	SGPT	0.00	45.00	49.00	77.00	H	125	9
104A1170106	F	46.4	051084	Sodium	135.00	145.00	135.00	133.00	L	125	2
104A1170106	F	46.4	052484	SGOT	0.00	51.00	22.00	55.00	H	125	2
104A1170106	F	46.4	052484	GGT	0.00	35.00	135.00	165.00	H	125	9
104A1170108	F	63.6	042684	Sglobulin	1.50	3.80	4.20	4.30	H	125	1
104A1170108	F	63.6	051084	GGT	0.00	35.00	76.00	136.00	H	125	9
104A1170108	F	63.6	051084	Sodium	135.00	145.00	136.00	132.00	L	125	2
104A1170108	F	63.6	051084	Chloride	95.00	108.00	95.00	91.00	L	125	2
104A1170108	F	63.6	051084	Gluc, random	80.00	160.00	116.00	195.00	H	125	3

Appendix 7
Patient Laboratory Profile

Patient Number: 13   Female   Age 70 years   Race: Black

Primary diagnoses
  Cellulitis and abscess of foot, except toes

Secondary diagnoses
  Cardiac dysrhythmia, unspecified
  Depressive disorder, not elsewhere classified
  Allergic rhinitis, cause unspecified
  Adult onset diabetes mellitus
  Unspecified essential hypertension
  Osteoarthrosis unspecified: site unspecified

Investigational drugs

	500	250					

Concomitant therapy

Trifluoperazine	X	X	X	X	X	X	
Humulin N insulin	X	X	X	X	X	X	
Lanoxin	X	X	X	X	X	X	
Feldene	X	X	X	X	X	X	
Minizide	X	X	X	X	X	X	
Vistaril	X	X	X	X	X	X	
Tavist-D		X	X	X	X	X	
Vancenase			X	X	X	X	
Tabron						X	
Voltaren							X
Benemid							X

Intercurrent illnesses
  Urinary tract infection   ?? =

Date			03JUL89	07JUL89	12JUL89	19JUL89	01AUG89	Drug lag 36 days		
								Worst Abnormality: 9-PT		
Test	Units	Normal Limits	Week 0	Week 1	Week 1	Week 2	Week 4	B/line	Tmt	Categ
WBC	1000/mm³	4-10.5	7.9	6.7	7.6 *	5.6	6.7	1	1	N
RBC	MILL/mm³	3.5-5.5	4.08	4.19	5.04 *	4.7	4.63	1	1	N
HGB	G/100 ml	12-16	10.6 −	10.5 −	12.5 *	11.8 −	11.6 −	4	4	C1
HCT	%	36-48	32.7 −	31 −	39.3 − *	35.2 −	35 −	2	4	C3
MCV	fl	80-100	80	74 −	78 − *	75 −	76 −			
MCH	pg	26-34	26	25 −	24.8 − *	25 −	25 −			
MCHC	%	31-37	32.4	33.8	31.8 *	33.4	33.1			
NEUTROS	1000/mm³	1.8-7.875	3.871	3.752	4.408 *	2.744	3.484	1	1	N
BANDS	%	0-5	0	0	0 *	0	0			
LYMPHS	1000/mm³	0.8-4.725	3.397	2.077	2.508 *	2.128	2.479	1	1	N
MONOS	1000/mm³	0-1.05	0.237	0.536	0.38 *	0.448	0.402	1	1	N
EOS	1000/mm³	0-0.63	0.395	0.268	0.228 *	0.224	0.268	1	1	N
BASOS	1000/mm³	0-0.21	0	0.067	0.076 *	0.056	0.067	1	1	N
PLATELET	1000/mm³	140-440	298	261	228 *	244	228	1	1	N
ESR	mm/hr	0-20	85 +	23 +	60 + *	22 +	24 +			
PT	sec	0-13	12.6	12.6	12.6 *	13	13.9 +			
APTT	sec	0-50	27	26.7	27.8 *	27.9	28.8			

Test	Units	Reference									
AP	IU/L	20-125	278+	275+	*	238+	211+	120	9	9	C1
GGT	IU/L	0-45	129+	173+	*	142+	114+	105+	9	9	C3
LDH	IU/L	100-250	305+	274+	*	240	207	217	7	3	C1
SGOT	IU/L	0-50	33	62+	*	49	41	43	1	7	C3
SGPT	IU/L	0-50	38	50	*	47	31	38	1	1	N
NA	mEq/L	135-148	131-	141	*	138	141	140	2	1	N
K	mEq/L	3.5-5.5	3.4-	3.7	*	3.8	3.4-	3.4-	2	2	C1
CL	mEq/L	94-109	90-	98	*	101	98	96	2	1	N
CA	mg/dl	8.5-10.6	9.5	9.3	*	9	9.5	8.8	1	1	N
L_PHOS	mg/dl	2.5-4.5	3.4	4.3	*	3.4	3.9	3.7	1	1	N
T_PROT	G/100 ml	6-4.5	6.7	8.2	*	8	8	7.7	1	1	N
S_ALBUM	G/100 ml	3.5-5.5	3.5	4.3	*	4.1	4.2	4.2	1	1	N
T_BILI	mg/dl	0.1-1.2	.4	.2	*	.2	.3	.2	1	1	N
GLUC_F	-		ND	ND	*	ND	ND	ND	?	?	C?
GLUC_RAN	mg/dl	70-115	83	89	*	250+	105	155+	1	9	C9
HAA	Scalar	0-0	0								
TG	mg/dl	10-190	101	159	*	213+	201+	239+			
CHOLEST	mg/dl	115-240	171	179	*	224	238	235			

Appendix 7 (Continued)

Date			03JUL89	07JUL89	12JUL89	19JUL89	01AUG89	Drug lag 36 days		
								Worst Ab-normality: 9-PT		
Test	Units	Normal Limits	Week 0	Week 1	Week 1	Week 2	Week 4	B/line	Tmt	Categ
URIC_ACD	mg/dl	2.2-7.7	11+	11.5+	* 10.9+	11.9+	10.7+	7	9	C1
BUN	mg/dl	7-26	24	33+	* 34+	48+	41+	1	9	C9
CREAT	mg/dl	0.5-1.5	2+	1.6+	* 1.7+	2.3+	2+	7	9	C3
US_GRAV	Scalar	1-1.03	1.01	1.004	* 1.012	1.011	1.01			
U_PH	Scalar	5-7	6	5.5	* 6	5	6			
U_ALBUM	mg/dl	0-0	0	0	*TRACE	TRACE	0			
U_GLUC	mg/dl	0-0	0	0	* 0	0	0			
KETONES	Scalar	0-0	0	0	* 0	0	0			
U_BILI	Scalar	0-0	0	0	* 0	0	0			
U_OCCBLD	Scalar	0-0	0	0	* 0	0	0			
WBC_HPF	/HPF	0-0	0	25-30+	* 6-12+	15-20+	0-4+			
RBC_HPF	/HPF	0-0	0	0	* 0	0	0			
CAST_HPF	/HPF	0-0	0	0	* 0	0	0			
BACT_HPF	/HPF	0-0	0	MANY	*MANY	MOD	MOD			
CRYS_HPF	/HPF	0-0	0	0	* 0	0	0			
EPIT_HPF	/HPF	0-0	0	FEW	* FEW	MOD	FEW			
PREG		-	ND							

Warning : assumption(s) made about SE or intercurrent illnesses

Key to Symbols Used in Patient Profile

!!! : Conflicting Information	Mil : Mild	
X : Dose of Concomitant Therapy	Mod : Moderate	
??? : Unknown Units/Error in Lab Value	Sev : Severe	
+ : Lab Value above NR	Unk : Unknown Severity	
− : Lab Value below NR		

Replace last letter if error:

$\left\{ \begin{array}{l} @ : \text{Missing date of onset} \\ \quad \text{(assume Visit Date)} \\ = : \text{Missing Duration} \\ \quad \text{(assume 1 day)} \\ \& : \text{Both missing} \end{array} \right.$

Worst abnormality classification of lab values (at baseline and during treatment):

1 : Within normal range		
2 : Insignificantly below NR	4 : Minimally below NR	6 : Markedly below NR	8 : Extremely below NR
3 : Insignificantly above NR	5 : Minimally above NR	7 : Markedly above NR	9 : Extremely above NR

* = end of treatment

End of Patient

233

REFERENCES

1. Mitchell JR, Thorgeirsson SS, Potter WZ, Jollow DJ, Keiser H. Acetaminophen induced hepatic injury. *Clin Pharm Ther*. 1974;16:676.
2. Raisfeld IH. Drug induced liver disease. *Gastroenterology*. 1975;69:854.
3. Zimmerman H. The spectrum of hepatotoxicity. *Persp Biol Med*. 1968;12:135.
4. Wallerstein RO, Condit PK, Kasper CK, Brown JW, Morrison FR. Statewise study of chloramphenicol therapy and fatal aplastic anemia. *JAMA*. 1969;208:2045.
5. Yunis AA. *J Clin Lab*. 1980;96:36–46.
6. Zimmerman HJ. *Hepatotoxicity*. New York: Appleton-Century-Crofts; 1978, 428.
7. Zimmerman HJ. *Hepatotoxicity*. New York: Appleton-Century-Crofts; 1978, 428.
8. Zimmerman HJ. Hepatic injury caused by therapeutic agents. In: Becker FF. ed. *The Liver*. Part A. New York: Marcel Dekker; 1974:225–302.
9. Balazs T. Assessment of the value of systemic toxicity studies experimental in animals. In: Mehlman MA, Shapiro RE, Blumenthal H. eds. *Advances in Modern Toxicology*. Vol 1. New York: Wiley; 1976:141–154.
10. Zbinden G. *Progress in Toxicology*, Vols. 1 & 2. New York: Springer-Verlag, 1973, 1976.
11. Zimmerman H. *Hepatotoxicity*. New York: Appelton-Century-Crofts; 1978: 94.
12. Price Evans DA. *Am J Med*. 1963;34:639.
13. 21 C.F.R. §312.32.
14. Pitts NE, Weeks RA, Siegel AM, Zubkoff LA, Hopp DA. A SAS based system for reporting laboratory data from clinical trials. *Drug Inf J*. 1986;20:213–224.

9

A Unified Approach to the Analysis of Safety Data in Clinical Trials

Christy Chuang-Stein and Noel R. Mohberg

The Upjohn Company
Kalamazoo, Michigan

I. INTRODUCTION

Although most of the attention in the statistical analyses of clinical trial data focuses on establishing efficacy of a study treatment relative to a control, a substantial portion of the data in fact pertains to safety concerns. From our experiences, it is not unlikely that 70–80% of the data collected and effort expended concerns safety, but most of these data have little or no relevance in demonstrating efficacy. Because of the surprising lack of analytical tools to handle the broad spectrum of safety data in a unified manner, we direct our attention in this chapter to the organization and analysis of these data using a multivariate approach that encompasses all relevant information. The clinical trials on which we concentrate in this chapter are short-term controlled clinical trials [1] in which the planned treatment period is prespecified and patients are typically followed for the same period of time. We focus on this type of trial because it generally provides the best safety information before a compound's entry into the market and it allows the most meaningful comparisons among treatments with respect to their safety profiles.

Because of the role that efficacy plays in drug development and the fact that most efficacy end points are clearly specified using one or two measurements, statisticians have made substantial advancements in the analysis of efficacy data in clinical trials. In some situations, however, it is impossible to separate efficacy from safety. For example, in many psychopharmacological trials, the same instrument measures efficacy and safety. Thus, statistical procedures that address safety in these situations have efficacy implications as well.

Safety data come from many sources and can be quite different in nature. They may be observations by the clinicians (signs), complaints of untoward events from the patients (symptoms), clinical lab assay reports, and physiological test results such as electrocardiogram (ECG) and computer tomography (CT) scans. Some authors use the phrase *adverse events* to describe all of the above unfavorable results. Because of the possibility of associating adverse events only with adverse clinical symptoms, we choose to use the more general term *safety data* in this chapter to refer to all data that are collected from the safety perspective in a clinical trial. Occasionally, we will use *adverse events* interchangeably with safety data to help with our narration if there is no possibility of confusion. Since there usually are no definite rules governing the collection of these data, their recording is often both amorphous and irregular. Furthermore, since there are so many different medical events that may be reported, especially when patients are instructed to volunteer unfavorable symptoms, statistical methods that concentrate on each individual adverse event are not only cumbersome but are frequently inappropriate.

Most clinical trials are designed to achieve the objectives in efficacy. As a result, very few of them are adequate to evaluate safety. O'Neill [1] points out that the magnitude of rates that can feasibly be studied in most clinical trials is about .01 or higher although large observational cohort studies usually can assess rates on the order of .001 or higher. This translates to low statistical power for comparisons on the incidence rates when the rates themselves are low. In spite of this deficiency, methods are needed to summarize these data and various statistical procedures have been proposed. Peace [2] advocated the use of confidence intervals. He argued that confidence intervals are statistically more appropriate than hypothesis testing in the absence of design considerations for safety. As Rampey and Enas [3] point out, opinion regarding how safety data should be analyzed varies widely. Some individuals believe that only descriptive summary statistics should be used while others believe that p values for adverse events not considered in a formal hypothesis testing framework can also help manage the inferences. Abt [4,5] proposed descriptive data analysis (DDA), which calculates p values for treatment contrast for each adverse event reported during a phase III trial. The p values obtained are descriptive in the sense that they are used for exploratory rather than confirmatory purpose. Using the reasoning that safety information is monitored throughout the efficacy trials and then combined with different studies, Huster [6] felt that formal statistical inference of safety information is invalid. On the other hand, Enas [7] supported the use of inferential statistical methods for both formally and informally helping to characterize the safety profile of a new drug and guide the resulting inference to the broader population. Even though the FDA [8] requires that rigorous statistical methods be applied only to events with substantial differences that are potentially useful to prescribing physicians, the identification of such events is by no means trivial and can result in a safety analysis that is mostly data-driven. When drug exposure duration is an important factor, life table analysis has been suggested by Abt et al. [9] to analyze time to the occurrence of adverse events. A good exposition on methods to analyze safety data in general can be found in O'Neill [1] and the numerous references cited in that paper.

Currently, the most commonly used method for comparing the safety profiles of two treatments is to compare the incidence rates of each individual adverse event. If the sample sizes are adequate, the distributions of the event's severity are compared as well. An example for the former is the comparison of the incidence rates of nausea observed with the test drug and the control. Such a comparison will possess all the desirable statistical properties if planned in advance in the protocol with safety concerns clearly specified. Unfortunately, statisticians often encounter a number of reports from different sources that have safety implications and they are asked to make comparisons based on these reports. Several statistical problems ensue. For example, can one compare an elevated liver enzyme on one drug directly with a report of nausea and jaundice on the other drug? Can one deal with ECG and clinical lab data simultaneously? In addition to the question as to what one can compare, there is an inherent multiple hypotheses testing problem that can erode the p values and reduce all but the most dramatic differences to statistical nonsignificance. Ironically, this problem pervades almost all new drug applications (NDAs) that entail several dozens or even hundreds of comparisons on the reported medical event rates. The validity of the conclusions based on such comparisons is often questionable.

Since laboratory data are routinely collected to ensure that patients are not experiencing any undesirable systemic toxicities while on a study, analysis of lab data has long been part of the safety analysis in a clinical trial. Typical analyses of lab data include the examination of changes from baselines and the comparison of the mean changes among different treatment groups. In addition, the extent to which a laboratory parameter deviates from its associated reference range is frequently tabulated and used to determine the grade of the underlying toxicity. Thompson et al. [10] discussed comprehensive procedures for analyzing lab data. Chuang-Stein [11] proposed a procedure to handle lab data when they come from different laboratories with different ranges as in many multicenter clinical trials.

Despite the fact that most statistical procedures examine safety data in a univariate fashion, some multivariate approaches do exist. For example, competing risk analysis has been suggested by some authors to look at several adverse events simultaneously [1]. Westfall and Young [12] proposed a procedure to adjust p values for multiple tests with the use of a multivariate binomial model. Rampey and Enas [3] applied the vector-based resampling method of Westfall and Young to a cluster of adverse events within a body system. Rampey and Enas treat the adverse events within a body system as having come from multivariate binomial distributions. The purpose of their approach is to adjust the p values generated from multiple comparisons of individual adverse event incidence rates within a body system. Brown et al. [13] proposed a method to compare the safety of two antibiotics based on lab data obtained during and after therapy. They first selected tolerable limits for lab results and ranked abnormalities according to the frequencies of abnormal values detected. They then analyzed pairs of related test results concurrently. Sogliero-Gilbert et al. [14] proposed a way to combine lab results to study the lab abnormality profiles of drugs. They constructed a score, called the Genie Score, for each functional group for each patient as well as an overall score. Gilbert et al. [15] also used Genie Scores to compare drug safety in controlled clinical trials. While the focus of the above authors is mostly with either lab abnormalities or the incidence rates of adverse events, our goal in this chapter is to include *all* safety data as well as their severities in one analysis. Thus, the basis for the comparison of treatment safety proposed in this chapter is much broader than the bases available in the literature. This is an appealing feature considering the diverse nature of safety data.

As with any valid comparison technique, we assume in this chapter that safety data pertaining to the treatments under comparison are obtained in a similar way. This means that for a particular safety end point, identical tests are performed according to the same schedule and the same mechanisms are used to collect the untoward medical events. The latter can be based on elicitation or patient volunteering, which produces structured or unstructured medical event data.

In this chapter, we propose to structure the massive safety data into a more manageable framework by consolidating them into a number, K, adverse event classes, characterized by body systems and determined in conjunction with the underlying disease as well as the treatment(s) involved. Within each class, we propose assignment to each patient of an overall intensity grade based on all relevant safety information. The determination of the intensity grade allows for the combination of data from different sources. The analysis of such organized data concentrates on comparison of the mean intensity grades for different treatments within the K classes simultaneously with use of scores that reflect the acceptability to an individual of the various intensity levels. In addition, we propose a statistic that can also incorporate the relative seriousness of the various adverse event classes to each other. The approach lends itself to conducting a comparison specified a priori and facilitates the understanding of the study outcome insofar as regards drug safety. Furthermore, we demonstrate that the proposed multivariate comparison has much higher power than the existing univariate comparisons to detect differences in certain cases. We provide examples to illustrate the proposed procedures and discuss how the proposed procedure can be generalized.

II. A PROPOSAL TO ORGANIZE AND ANALYZE THE SAFETY DATA

To organize the safety data, we assume that we can summarize the available information regarding patients' safety experience in a study with K adverse event classes characterized by body systems and determined in conjunction with the underlying disease as well as the treatment(s) involved. Examples of such classes are: *cardiovascular*, *hepatic*, *hematological*, *CNS*, *pulmonary*, *gastrointestinal*, *neurological*, *endocrine*, and *metabolic*, etc. (Depending on the circumstances, one might find it desirable to treat *hepatic* as part of *gastrointestinal*.) The determination of the K classes is the first step under our approach and should precede any data analysis. Within each class, we assume that we can determine an overall intensity grade (e.g., none, grade 1, grade 2, . . ., etc.) for each patient, based on clinical observations as well as test results that are considered as physiologically related to the body system representative of the class. The higher the grade, the more severe a condition that the adverse events in an event class collectively imply. For convenience, we will sometimes refer to the various intensity grades as *intensity levels*, or *levels* for short. For example, we might call grade 0, which suggests no adverse reaction, *level 0*; call grade 1 *level 1*, and so forth. For our presentation, we assume the same number of intensity levels for all classes and denote it by J. The process of consolidating safety information in this way requires extensive input from medical personnel as we will illustrate with the example in Section III. Like the determination of the K classes, the decision on intensity grades should be objective and take place before any data scrutiny. Notice that safety data are used to come up with individual indices that suggest the severities of impairment to the body functions represented by the various classes. Thus, the reduced data represent more than just the incidence of adverse events in different classes.

To analyze the consolidated safety data, we assume that within class i ($i = 1$, . . ., K), individuals can assign nonnegative scores $\{w_{ij}, j = 0, . . ., J-1\}$ to the J intensity levels in such a way that $w_{i0} = 0$ ($i = 1, . . ., K$) and that $\{w_{ij}\}$ reflect the acceptability to the individuals of the various intensity grades (we assume in this chapter that high scores suggest low acceptability). The zero score for level 0 corresponds to the most favorable outcome within an adverse event class. One can assign scores separately within each class without taking into account the relative seriousness of the K classes. One can also assign scores that not only reflect the acceptability of the various intensity levels within a class but also the seriousness of the various classes relative to one another. These two choices of scores lead to very different inferential interpretation. Since the assignment of the scores pertains to an individual's perspective, and therefore has a subjective component, results from the statistical comparisons discussed in this section are best interpreted at the individual decision level. We wish to point out here that this subjectiveness is deliberately built into the approach to allow the treatment selection made at the individual level.

We will use x_{ij} to denote the number of individuals whose intensity level within the ith class is j, p_{ij} denote the probability of the jth level within the ith class and N the total number of patients in a treatment group. It is easy to see that $\sum_j x_{ij} = N$ for all i. We want to emphasize that under the proposed method we use all relevant information to arrive at a single intensity grade for a patient within a class. Let $f_{ij} = x_{ij}/N$ denote the observed proportion of the jth intensity level within the ith class, and $s_i = \sum_j w_{ij}f_{ij}$ the observed mean score for the ith class. We can easily show that the expected value of s_i is $m_i = \sum_j w_{ij}p_{ij}$. Furthermore, Let $S' = (s_1, \ldots, s_K)$, then $E(S') = (m_1, \ldots, m_K)$. Denote $\mathrm{Cov}(S) = V = (v_{ij})$. We now show how to compute V.

Define W and F as

$$F_{KJ \times 1} = \begin{pmatrix} f_{10} \\ f_{11} \\ \cdot \\ f_{1,J-1} \\ f_{20} \\ \cdot \\ f_{2,J-1} \\ \cdot \\ \cdot \\ f_{K0} \\ \cdot \\ f_{K,J-1} \end{pmatrix}$$

$$W_{K \times KJ} = \begin{pmatrix} w_{10} \cdot & w_{1,J-1} & 0 & \cdot & 0 & \cdot & \cdot & 0 & \cdot & 0 \\ 0 & \cdot & 0 & w_{20} \cdot & w_{2,J-1} \cdot & \cdot & 0 & \cdot & 0 \\ \cdot & \cdot & \cdot & \cdot & \cdot & \cdot & \cdot & \cdot & \cdot \\ 0 & \cdot & 0 & 0 & \cdot & 0 & \cdot & \cdot & w_{K0} \cdot & w_{K,J-1} \end{pmatrix}$$

We can show that $S = WF$ and $\mathrm{Cov}(S) = W(\mathrm{Cov}(F)) W'$, where $\mathrm{Cov}(F) = (\mathrm{Cov}(f_{ij}, f_{i'j'}))$ is the covariance matrix of F. Thus, our task is to find $\mathrm{Cov}(F)$. Assuming that $(x_{i0}, x_{i1}, \ldots, x_{i,J-1})$ within the ith class has a multinomial distribution with $\{p_{ij}\}$ as the multinomial probabilities, we have

$$\mathrm{Cov}(f_{ij}, f_{ij'}) = \frac{1}{N} (\delta_{jj'}p_{ij} - p_{ij}p_{ij'}) ,$$

where $\delta_{jj} = 1$ if $j = j'$. The above result can be found in most books on categorical data analysis, e.g., Agresti (Ref. 16, p. 424). Next, we compute $\text{Cov}(f_{ij}, f_{i'j'})$ for $i \neq i'$.

To compute $\text{Cov}(f_{ij}, f_{i'j'})$ for $i \neq i'$, we need to consider the joint distribution of the intensity levels in the ith and the i'th classes, for which $\{x_{ij}, j = 0, \ldots, J - 1\}$ and $\{x_{i'j'}, j' = 0, \ldots, J-1\}$ are the observed marginal totals. Let $p_{ij,i'j'}$ denote the probability that the intensity levels in the ith and the i'th classes are at the levels of j and j', respectively, and $x_{ij,i'j'}$, $f_{ij,i'j'}$ *the corresponding observed frequencies and proportions. Then* $\{x_{ij,i'j'}; j, j' = 0, \ldots, J-1\}$ has a multi-nomial distribution with parameters $\{p_{ij,i'j'}; j, j' = 0, \ldots, J-1\}$. We can then compute the covariance between f_{ij} and $f_{i'j'}$ as

$$
\begin{aligned}
\text{Cov}(f_{ij}, f_{i'j'}) &= \text{Cov}\left(\sum_{l'=0}^{J-1} f_{ij,i'l'}, \sum_{l=0}^{J-1} f_{il,i'j'}\right) \\
&= \sum_{l'=0}^{J-1} \sum_{l=0}^{J-1} \text{Cov}(f_{ij,i'l'}, f_{il,i'j'}) \\
&= \text{var}(f_{ij,i'j'}) + \sum_{(l,l')\neq(j,j')} \text{Cov}(f_{ij,i'l'}, f_{il,\,i'j'}) \\
&= \frac{1}{N}\left[p_{ij,i'j'}(1 - p_{ij,i'j'}) - \sum_{(l,l')\neq(j,j')} p_{ij,i'l'}p_{il,i'j'}\right]
\end{aligned}
$$

Substituting the observed proportions $f_{ij,i'j'}$ for the true proportions $p_{ij,i'j'}$ in $\text{Cov}(f_{ij}, f_{ij'})$ and $\text{Cov}(f_{ij}, f_{i'j'})$ we obtain an estimate for V that we denote by $\hat{V}$.

Now suppose that we have two treatments and that we want to compare their safety profiles. We can compute $S^{(i)}$ and $\hat{V}^{(i)}$ ($i = 1, 2$) for the two treatments using the same weights $\{w_{ij}\}$. We can construct a multivariate test based on $S^{(i)}$ as

$$
T_1 = (S^{(1)} - S^{(2)})' (\hat{V}^{(1)} + \hat{V}^{(2)})^{-1} (S^{(1)} - S^{(2)}) \tag{1}
$$

which, if the two treatments have identical safety profiles, has an asymptotic χ^2 distribution with K degrees of freedom (df). We form the statistic T_1 by comparing the two treatments with respect to their mean intensity grades within the K classes simultaneously.

A special case regarding the choice of $\{w_{ij}\}$ deserves mentioning. If $w_{ij} = 1$ for all i and j such that $j \neq 0$, then $s_j^{(1)}$ is the sample proportion of individuals who receive the ith treatment and who have a nonzero grade in the jth event class. Under this choice of scores, the comparison between two treatments reduces to that of the vectors of incidence rates.

What should one do if the statistic T_1 is significant at a prespecified level, say α? How should one interpret the results? Obviously, one can compare the distributions of the intensity level within each event class separately. However, as the example in Section VI will demonstrate, it is possible that all such comparisons are nonsignificant at the (100α)th level even though T_1 is significant. This is because T_1 can accumulate small but consistent differences to come up with a significant result. If this is the case, it will be easy to decide which treatment has a better safety profile. If the individual comparisons within event classes give some significant results [at the (100α)th level] and the significance favors one treatment, the choice is still very clear. However, there will be cases when one treatment has a more favorable safety profile with respect to some body functions while the opposite is true with some other body functions. One question ensues in the latter case; can one say anything about the overall safety advantages when the importance of the various body functions is taken into account?

In the last case discussed above, the ability to judge the importance of the various event classes can be translated to that of assigning scores $\{w_{ij}\}$ that reflect not only the severity of the grade levels within an event class but the seriousness of the event classes among themselves. Under this scenario, we can use a single mean score to summarize the safety profile of a treatment by adding the components $s_j^{(i)}$ in $S^{(i)}$ together. If we let $1' = (1, 1, \ldots, 1)$ be a $K \times 1$ vector of 1's, then we can use $1'(S^{(1)} - S^{(2)})$ $(= \Sigma_j s_j^{(1)} - \Sigma_j s_j^{(2)})$ to quantify the difference in the overall safety profiles between the two treatments. A test statistic can be constructed as

$$T_2 = (S^{(1)} - S^{(2)})' \{1(1'(\hat{V}^{(1)} + \hat{V}^{(2)})1)^{-1} 1'\} (S^{(1)} - S^{(2)}) \tag{2}$$

which, if the two treatments have identical safety profiles, has an asymptotic χ^2 distribution with 1df.

The measure $1'(S^{(1)} - S^{(2)})$, which summarizes the difference between the two treatments under comparison, has only one dimension. If T_2 is significant at a prespecified level and $1'(S^{(1)} - S^{(2)})$ is positive, then T_2 has a better safety outlook. Such a conclusion is based on an overall assessment that weighs the various event classes according to their importance and relevance to the underlying disease and the treatments involved.

We can generalize statistics T_1 and T_2 to compare more than two treatments. Suppose that there are I treatments. We can compute $\{s_j^{(i)}, j = 1, \ldots, K\}$ for each treatment i, $i = 1, \ldots, I$. Let $S^{(i)} = (s_1^{(i)}, \ldots, s_K^{(i)})$, and Ω be an $IK \times 1$ vector of the following form:

$$\Omega = \begin{pmatrix} S^{(1)} \\ S^{(2)} \\ \cdot \\ \cdot \\ \cdot \\ S^{(I)} \end{pmatrix}$$

There are $(I - 1)$ contrasts among $\{s_j^{(i)}, i = 1, \ldots, I\}$ for each $j, j = 1, \ldots, K$. Let H be an $(I - 1)K \times IK$ matrix whose $(I - 1)K$ rows give the coefficients of the $(I - 1)K$ contrasts among $\{s_j^{(i)}, i = 1, \ldots, I\}$ for $j = 1, \ldots, K$. Thus, $H\Omega$ is an $(I - 1)K \times 1$ vector whose components are contrasts in $\{s_j^{(i)}, i = 1, \ldots, I\}$ for different j. The covariance matrix Λ for Ω can be computed as before since we only need to be concerned with the covariance matrix for each individual $S^{(i)}$.

The null hypothesis of identical safety profiles among the I treatments implies that $E(H\Omega) = 0$, i.e., a zero vector of length $(I - 1)K$. A statistic can be constructed as

$$T_3 = (H\Omega)' \, (H\hat{\Lambda}H')^{-1} \, (H\Omega)$$

where $\hat{\Lambda}$ is the estimated covariance matrix obtained by substituting the observed proportions for the true proportions. Under the null hypothesis of identical safety profiles, statistic T_3 has an asymptotic χ^2 distribution with $(I - 1)K$ df.

As for the generalization of T_2 to compare I treatments, denote the single measure that can summarize the safety profile of the ith treatment by $g^{(i)}$. It can be shown easily that $g^{(i)}$ is $\Sigma_l\Sigma_j \, w_{lj}f_{lj}^{(i)}$. Denote by σ_i^2 the variance of $g^{(i)}$. The computation of σ_i^2 can be carried out as before. Furthermore, let $G' = (g^{(1)}, g^{(2)}, \ldots, g^{(I)})$, D a diagonal matrix with σ_i^2 as the ith diagonal element, and C an $(I - 1) \times I$ matrix whose rows give the coefficients of the $(I - 1)$ contrasts among the I treatments. A test statistic can be constructed to test the null hypothesis of identical safety profiles by examining the contrasts in $\{g^{(i)}, i = 1, \ldots, I\}$ as

$$T_4 = (CG)' \, (C\hat{D}C')^{-1} \, (CG)$$

where $\hat{D}$ is an estimate for D obtained by substituting the observed proportions for the true ones. The statistic T_4 has an asymptotic χ^2 distribution with $(I - 1)$ df under the null hypothesis.

If either T_3 or T_4 is significant, one might want to follow it up with a pairwise comparison. Since the number of treatment groups included in a randomized controlled clinical trial is generally not high, the issue of multiplicity arising from pairwise comparison is not a serious one. We recommend using Bonferroni's rule to adjust the significance level when pairwise comparisons are to be conducted.

The theory underlying the proposed procedure is not new. The computation of the covariance matrices, however, requires a bit more attention since it is not a common practice to examine the joint distributions of adverse events. What is unique about the proposed approach is the idea of condensing safety data in a reasonable way, one that allows meaningful comparisons among treatments with regard to their overall safety profiles.

III. AN EXAMPLE

In this section, we use data from two randomized clinical trials to illustrate the proposed procedure. Both trials were double-blind studies that compared two drugs for the treatment of angina pectoris. For convenience, we call the two *drug A* and *drug B*. One study had 19 patients on drug A and 21 on drug B, while the other had 24 on drug A and 22 on drug B. Because these two studies were conducted according to the same protocol, we combined data from the two studies to compare the two drugs with respect to their safety profiles.

A.   Determination of Classes

The data collected included clinical signs and symptoms, ECG examinations, and the regular safety laboratory assays (i.e., hematology, chemistries, and urinalyses). For convenience, we use the term *clinical event* to represent both clinical signs and symptoms. Based on the disease treated and the adverse reactions expected of the two drugs, we used the following 10 classes to consolidate the safety information: *cardiovascular, hematological, gastrointestinal (GI)/ hepatic, genitourinary/renal, neurological/psychiatric, pulmonary, special senses, metabolic/nutritional, dermatological,* and *musculoskeletal.*

B.   Determination of the Intensity Grade Within a Class

Determination of the intensity grade for each patient within a class is the most challenging component of the proposed procedure. With the data collected, we created a set of rules to determine these grades. While we recognize that there is no definitive way to determine the grades, we feel that the rules we chose were both rational and consistent with ordinary medical judgment. Our rules are as follows:

(1)   We considered reports of clinical events as primary and those based on laboratory findings and physiological testing as secondary. (In other situations, it might be desirable to rely more on laboratory findings. In either case, it is important to choose before looking at the data, an order based on certainty of diagnosis and anticipated adverse reactions, which may include clinical impressions, signs, symptoms, lab tests, etc.) Thus, if a patient had a clinical event in a class and also had a laboratory abnormality related to the same class, we determined the grade based on the intensity of the clinical event. In situations where the clinical event was innocuous but the laboratory results suggested a more severe problem, such as nocturia and sharply elevated creatinine, we sought additional medical input. To incorporate lab data into the determination of the intensity grades, we specified the relationships between certain lab parameters and the 10 classes. Table 1 indicates such relationships where the number 1 suggests a primary relationship and the number 2 suggests a secondary one. For example, we considered both ALKP and bilirubin to have a primary relationship to the GI/hepatic class and a secondary relationship to hematology.

(2)   We accepted the treating physician's judgment on whether a clinical event was *unrelated, possibly related,* or *probably related* to the treatment. (A

Table 1 Relationships Between Certain Biochemical Assays and the 10 Identified Classes

	CV	Hem	GI/ hep	GU/ ren	Neur/ psyc	Pulm	SS	Met/ nut	Derm	MS
Albumin			2[a]	1[b]				2		
Alk. phosphatase		2	1							
Amylase			1	2				2		
Bilirubin		2	1							
BUN			2	1				2		
Calcium		2	2	2				1		
Chloride			2	1				2		
Creatinine				1						
CK	1									1
Glucose								1		
LDH	2	2	1							
Inorg. phosphate		2	2	2	1			2		
Potassium				1				2		
Total protein			2	1				2		
SGOT	2		1							
SGPT			1	2						2
Sodium								1		

[a]Suggests a secondary relationship.
[b]Suggests a primary relationship.

cautionary note in using physician's judgment in this context is that one has to be sure that the treating physician is not biased in favor of a particular treatment because of financial relationships with the pharmaceutical sponsor). Table 2 provides an outline of how we graded the intensity based on a single reported clinical event. In Table 2, a "yes" to the question *related to treatment* includes both a possible and a probable relationship. For example, with mild intensity of a clinical event judged as unrelated to treatment, we assigned grade 0. The same event, if judged as treatment-related, would receive grade 1. Generally speaking, the grade increases as the intensity of the clinical event increases. Also, those events related to the treatment have an intensity grade one level higher than the corresponding events not related to the treatment.

(3) We followed the treatment emergent philosophy with regard to temporal relationships for the lab and ECG data and considered observations from both the treatment and the close follow-up periods. We used results reported prior to the treatment to reflect changes in the status. For example, if a pretreatment laboratory or ECG abnormality did not further deteriorate during the course of the treatment, we disregarded the abnormality. On the other hand, if a lab assay

Table 2 Rules from Grading a Single Adverse Clinical Event

Intensity of a clinical event	Related to treatment	Grade assigned
Mild	No	0
Mild	Yes	1
Moderate	No	1
Moderate	Yes	2
Severe	No	2
Severe	Yes	3
Intolerable	No	3
Intolerable	Yes	4

normal prior to the treatment became abnormal during the course of the treatment, we assigned grade 1 to the abnormality. If an abnormality was incompatible with life we would have assigned grade 2, but this situation did not occur in our example. Unlike the lab or ECG results, we graded clinical events according to Table 2 regardless of their documented presence prior to treatment.

(4) When a patient had more than two separate reports of a clinical event, or more than two clinical events that fell in the same class (with classes defined in Section III.A), we raised the intensity grade for that class by 1. For example, if a patient had three reports of mild headache related to treatment, we would assign grade 2 for the corresponding class. Also, if a patient had headache, dizziness, and somnolence, all of which were mild and related to treatment, we would raise the grade from 1 to 2.

The Appendix gives a detailed example of how we determined the intensity grades for one patient. We wish to point out that grade levels are not equally spaced; the increase in intensity from grade 1 to grade 2 is much less than the increase from grade 3 to grade 4.

Using the above rules, we obtained data similar to those displayed in Table 3. We slightly modified the original data to better illustrate the proposed procedure. In Table 3, we use four levels to summarize a study participant's safety experience within each class. The four levels are: none, grades 1, 2, and 3.

To compare the two drugs with respect to their overall safety profiles, we first used the statistic in Eq. (1) with the same equally spaced scores w_{ij} for each of the 10 classes, e.g., $w_{i0} = 0$, $w_{i1} = 1$, $w_{i2} = 2$, and $w_{i3} = 3$, $i = 1, \ldots, 10$. The test statistic T_1 has a value of 21.96, which, upon comparison to a χ^2 distribution with 10 dfs yields a p value of .015 and suggests a significant difference in the safety profiles at the 5% level. The use of the χ^2 distribution in this example serves as an approximation because of the small frequencies for some intensity categories.

Table 3 Results from Consolidating the Safety Data from the First Set of Two Randomized Studies

Class	Drug	None	Grade 1	Grade 2	Grade 3
Cardiovascular	A	29	3	8	3
	B	38	4	1	0
Hematological	A	40	3	0	0
	B	40	3	0	0
Gastrointestinal/hepatic	A	37	3	2	1
	B	36	3	4	0
Genitourinary/renal	A	40	2	1	0
	B	38	2	3	0
Neurological/psychiatric	A	26	4	13	0
	B	15	11	10	7
Pulmonary	A	37	4	2	0
	B	41	1	1	0
Special senses	A	41	1	1	0
	B	41	0	2	0
Metabolic/nutritional	A	40	1	2	0
	B	39	2	2	0
Dermatological	A	41	1	1	0
	B	41	0	2	0
Musculoskeletal	A	39	3	1	0
	B	37	4	2	0

A closer look at the data in Table 3 reveals the possible sources of difference between the two drugs. The two drugs differ most in the cardiovascular and the neurological/psychiatric classes. While drug A has a higher incidence of cardiovascular events, drug B has a higher incidence of neurological/psychiatric events. Applying the Pearson's χ^2 test to the corresponding 2 × 4 subtables in Table 3, we obtain p values of .02 (cardiovascular) and .004 (neurological/psychiatric). If we collapse grades 1, 2, 3 in Table 3 and compare the proportions of nonzero grades for these two drugs, we obtain p values of .02 for both classes. All the above comparisons are significant at the 5% level. Nevertheless, these results need cautious interpretation since the tests concerning the cardiovascular and neurological/psychiatric classes are data-driven. A possible remedy is to adjust the significance level for each test using Bonferroni's criterion, in anticipation of a test to be conducted within each class.

To see how the differences between the two drugs in the various classes affect the overall comparison when we combine the 10 classes with use of the statistic in Eq. (2), we computed the 1 df statistic under various choices of $\{w_{ij}\}$. The $\{w_{ij}\}$ we considered all had the form $w_{ij} = c_i w_j$ where c_i reflects the relative seriousness of the 10 classes to an individual and $w_0 = 0$, $w_1 = 1$, $w_2 = 2$, $w_3 = 3$. We found the computed statistic robust to the choice of c_i for $i \neq 1$ and $i \neq 5$. This is due to the comparable distributions of the intensity level of the two treatments in the corresponding eight classes. Thus, for presentation, we set $c_i = 1$ for $i \neq 1$ and $i \neq 5$. On the other hand, the computed statistic was sensitive to the values of c_1 (cardiovascular) and c_5 (neurological/psychiatric), a result due to the opposite configurations of the intensity level within these two classes. We therefore concentrated on the relative magnitude of c_1 to c_5. In the first half of Table 4, we report the p values obtained under various choices of c_1 and c_5 with c_5 set to 1; using different c_1 and c_5 amounts to weighing the two classes differently in computing the overall test statistic in Eq. (2).

The results in Table 4 are revealing. When an individual regards the cardiovascular and neurological/psychiatric events as equally serious (i.e., $c_1 = 1$), the 1 df analysis fails to show differences in the two drugs' overall safety profiles at the 5% level despite our earlier findings. This is because the observed differences between the two treatment groups in these two key classes occurred in opposite directions and in the combined statistic they balanced one another. With the cardiovascular events regarded as more serious through the use of a higher c_1 in Table 4, however, the associated p value decreased. When $c_1 = 4.7$, the p value is .049, which suggests that drug B has a more favorable safety profile. In other words, if an individual weighs the cardiovascular events at least 4.7 times more serious than the neurological/psychiatric events of the same intensity level, he or she would choose drug B based on the available data.

Table 4 p Values of the Statistic in Eq. (2) Applied to the Data in Table 3 for Various Choices of c_1 and c_5 with $c_i = 1$ for all i, $i \neq 1$ and $i \neq 5$

Statistic	p Value
$c_1 = 1$, $c_5 = 1$	.743
$c_1 = 2$, $c_5 = 1$	.475
$c_1 = 3$, $c_5 = 1$	.171
$c_1 = 4$, $c_5 = 1$	.076
$c_1 = 4.7$, $c_5 = 1$	.049
$c_1 = 5$, $c_5 = 1$	.041
$c_1 = 1$, $c_5 = 2$	.256
$c_1 = 1$, $c_5 = 3$	.123
$c_1 = 1$, $c_5 = 4$	.078
$c_1 = 1$, $c_5 = 5.7$	.050
$c_1 = 1$, $c_5 = 6$	.047

We also reversed the roles of c_1 and c_5 by setting $c_1 = 1$ in the second half of Table 4. Note that as c_5 increases, drug A becomes more appealing. When c_5 increases beyond 5.7, drug A is judged as more favorable. Thus, depending on how an individual weighs one class against the other, he or she will obtain different conclusions on which drug has a more favorable safety profile from his or her own perspective. This dependence, a result of weighing the seriousness of the various classes to one another, demonstrates how the seriousness issue translates to that of treatment selection. For the given data, the ratio of the weights for the two relevant classes has to be relatively high for a treatment to be declared as a clear winner. This is due to the fact that the evidence provided by these two classes, although of the opposite direction, is about the same strength. This comparable strength is demonstrated by the high p value reported in Table 4 (i.e., .743) when the two classes are given the same weight.

In this example, the highest intensity grades assigned were several 3's. There were a few instances where the intensity grades were close to grade 4. Within a class, this draws attention to the latitude within the steps for determination of the intensity grade. It is true that the creation of more intensity grades is likely to increase the sensitivity of the grading system, but it will also lead to insoluble decision problems. Our goal in this chapter was to determine the intensity grades within a class while recognizing the necessity for compromises. It is possible that the choice of intensity grades may vary among different researchers. However, our experience suggests that as long as the choice is unbiased, consistent, reasonable, and made before any data analysis, it is unlikely that the choice will lead to misinterpretation of study results. As a safeguard toward possible bias in determining the intensity grades, we recommend that individuals blind to the treatments determine these grades. The ideal situation is when a group of experts in the target disease area jointly decide the rules that govern the assignment of intensity grades.

IV.   COMBINING RESULTS FROM TWO SETS OF STUDIES

So far we have concentrated on comparing treatments based on results from one clinical trial. Although the data for the example in the previous section came from two studies, we pooled the data and treat them as if they came from a single trial because the two studies are identical for all practical concerns. One can generalize the approach to compare treatments based on results from similar trials, i.e., trials with similar treatments and the same patient population. To do so, one first needs to apply the same set of rules to determine the intensity grades for the same set of medical event classes. This should not be a problem since the determination of the classes and the intensity grades should only depend on the underlying disease and the treatments involved and not on data obtained in any trial. However, it is desirable to ascertain first if the safety data from different trials are poolable. If not, one should use the idea of Mantel–Haenszel to conduct comparisons within trials first and then aggregate the summary statistics across trials.

To illustrate the above point, we will consider the data in Table 5. Data in Table 5 also come from two studies conducted under one protocol (which is slightly different from the one that generated the data in Table 3). However, the drugs under comparison are the same. Since the same drugs and the same patient population were involved in these two sets of studies, we chose to use the same event classes and the same rules to consolidate the safety information. The consolidation led to the results in Table 5. We would like to point out that while consolidating the safety data to produce Table 5, we did encounter some grade 4 events. However, since there are only a few of them, here we will group them with the grade 3 events and treat them as grade 3. The occurrence of grade 4 events is comparable between the two treatment groups.

A quick comparison between data in Table 5 and those in Table 3 suggests that the second set of studies seems to have more genitourinary/renal and gastrointestinal/hepatic events. On the other hand, patients who received drug A in the

Table 5 Results from Consolidating the Safety Data from a Second Set of Two Randomized Studies

Class	Drug	None	Grade 1	Grade 2	Grade 3
Cardiovascular	A	34	1	3	3
	B	41	2	3	1
Hematological	A	37	4	0	0
	B	41	6	0	0
Gastrointestinal/hepatic	A	28	6	5	2
	B	39	3	3	2
Genitourinary/renal	A	31	8	2	0
	B	35	7	5	0
Neurological/psychiatric	A	24	4	7	6
	B	18	6	5	18
Pulmonary	A	35	3	3	0
	B	43	2	2	0
Special senses	A	40	1	0	0
	B	46	0	0	1
Metabolic/nutritional	A	39	2	0	0
	B	45	2	0	0
Dermatological	A	38	1	1	1
	B	43	2	2	0
Musculoskeletal	A	39	1	0	1
	B	44	2	0	1

second set of studies seemed to report fewer cardiovascular events than their counterparts in Table 3. Pearson's χ^2 statistic applied to the incidence of nonzero grade events suggest that patients receiving drug A in Table 5 reported significantly more genitourinary/renal events than those on drug A in Table 3 ($p = .027$). None of the other univariate comparisons between the two tables within the same drugs produce significant results at the 5% significance level.

When applying the multivariate statistic T_1 in Eq. (1) to compare the two drugs using the data in Table 5, we obtained a value of 15.45 with 10 df that yields a p value of .116. Despite this nonsignificant result, one may suspect from Table 5 that patients receiving drug B experienced many more neurological/psychiatric events. The same phenomenon was observed in the previous set of studies. The question is how can we combine data in Tables 3 and 5 knowing that the safety data for the same drug display some subtle differences with respect to some medical event classes in trials leading to Tables 3 and 5.

For convenience, we will use d_i to represent the difference in the summary scores for the ith set of studies. This summary score can be either the vector of scores used to construct the statistic T_1 in Eq. (1) or the overall score used to construct the statistic T_2 in Eq. 2. In other words, d_1 is either $S^{(1)} - S^{(2)}$ or $1'(S^{(1)} - S^{(2)})$ (see the definitions of these terms in Section II) for the first set and d_2 is the corresponding difference in the summary score for the second set. We will use V_i to represent the covariance of d_i. The computation of V_i can also be found in Section II. An idea that is attributed to Mantel and Haenszel is to form a statistic based on $d_1 + d_2$ and its covariance. Since d_1 and d_2 are independent, the covariance for $d_1 + d_2$ is equal to $V_1 + V_2$. Applying the Mantel–Haenszel (M-H) idea to our case, we obtain an M-H modified statistic that takes the following form:

$$(d_1 + d_2)' (V_1 + V_2)^{-1} (d_1 + d_2) \tag{3}$$

where "'" is for the case when d_i is a $K \times 1$ ($K = 10$ in our case) vector. Notice that we use the same formula for the K df statistic and the 1 df statistic. Under the null hypothesis of equal safety profiles, the M-H modified statistic in Eq. (3) will have an asymptotic χ^2 distribution with K df or an asymptotic χ^2 distribution with 1 df depending on whether d_i is a vector or a scalar.

Applying the 10 df M-H modified statistic to the data in Tables 3 and 5, we obtained a value of 31.46 which yields a p value less than .001. An examination of the data suggests that this significant result comes primarily from the difference in the neurological/psychiatric class even though the first set of studies also demonstrates some difference between drug A and drug B with respect to the cardiovascular class. To ascertain the strength of these differences, we include in Table 6 results from applying the 1 df M-H modified statistic to the combined data. Table 6 is laid out similarly to Table 4. With all $c_i = 1$ for i not representing the cardiovascular and the neurological/psychiatric classes, we vary the values of c_1 (for cardiovascular) and c_5 (neurological/psychiatric) and report the

Table 6 p Values of the 1 df Mantel–Haenszel
Modified Statistic in Eq. (3) Applied to the Data
in Tables 3 and 5 Combined for Various Choices of c_1
and c_5 with $c_i = 1$ for all i, $i \neq 1$ and $i \neq 5$

Statistic	p Value
$c_1 = 1, c_5 = 1$	.552
$c_1 = 3, c_5 = 1$	.347
$c_1 = 6, c_5 = 1$	.068
$c_1 = 7, c_5 = 1$	.049
$c_1 = 8, c_5 = 1$	.038
$c_1 = 1, c_5 = 2$	.106
$c_1 = 1, c_5 = 2.6$	.050
$c_1 = 1, c_5 = 3$	.033

p value associated with the 1 df M-H modified statistic. The interpretation of
the results in Table 6 is similar to that based on the results in Table 4. Basically, as
the cardiovascular events become more undesirable compared to the neuro-
logical/psychiatric events, drug B represents a better choice. On the other hand,
if the neurological/psychiatric events become less tolerable, drug A is preferable.
However, the somewhat consistent evidence about the different incidence
of neurological/psychiatric events associated with the two drugs in the two sets of
studies changes the threshold of the ratios c_1/c_5 and c_5/c_1 when one drug will be
declared as a clear winner. With the combined evidence, drug A becomes
preferable when neurological/psychiatric events are judged to be at least 2.6
times as unacceptable as the cardiovascular ones. On the other hand, the cardiovascular events have to be at least 7 times as unacceptable as the neurological/
psychiatric ones for drug B to be more desirable. The lowering of the ratio c_5/c_1
to favor drug A is a result of the added information from the second set of the
studies.

The above procedure can be generalized to more than two clinical trials. If we
use d_i ($i = 1, \ldots, G$) to represent the difference in the summary score in the ith
trial and V_i the covariance associated with d_i, then the M-H modified multivariate
statistic takes the following form:

$$\left(\sum_{i=1}^{G} d_i \right)' \left(\sum_{i=1}^{G} V_i \right)^{-1} \left(\sum_{i=1}^{G} d_i \right)$$

which has an asymptotic χ^2 distribution with either K df or an asymptotic χ^2
distribution with 1 df under the null hypothesis of identical safety profiles among
the G trials.

V. ROBUSTNESS OF THE PROPOSED APPROACH

One question that follows the analyses in the previous two examples concerns how much the results depend on the classification rules used to determine the intensity levels within the chosen medical event classes. To obtain some answer to this question, we investigated the robustness of the M-H modified statistic in Eq. (3) to the classification rules using data in Tables 3 and 5. We assume that different rules lead to the reclassification of certain events. The latter may be either an upgrading or a downgrading of the events' intensities. We made three basic assumptions concerning how different rules will affect the classification: (1) An individual judged to be in the grade 0 category for a class under one set of rules will be judged the same under a different set of rules, (2) The rules affect the classification of events associated with the two treatment groups in a symmetrical way. This assumption implies that if a different set of rules leads to the reclassification of 25% of grade 1 events in one treatment group to grade 2, the rules will also reclassify about 25% of grade 1 events in the other group to grade 2, (3) When reclassification occurs, it only results in an event's moving up or down one category on the intensity scale. Since the rules are usually generic to the medical event classes, we can expect that the percentage of events that get a different grade under a different set of rules stays about the same for different classes. Nevertheless, we did try to vary the percentages of reclassification in different event classes in our investigation.

Selected results from our investigation are reported in Table 7. Since for the data in Tables 3 and 5, cardiovascular and neurological/psychiatric classes are the two classes where differences occur, we concentrated on reclassification percentage within these two classes. In Table 7, we first reported the results from the analyses conducted in Sections III and IV. In particular, we report the c_1 value (with $c_i = 1$ for the rest of the medical event classes and $w_{ij} = c_i w_j$, $w_0 = 0$, $w_1 = 1$, $w_2 = 2$, $w_3 = 3$) that is necessary to declare drug B to be the preferable one at the 5% significance level using the 1 df M-H modified statistic. We also include the c_5 value to declare drug A to be preferable under the same choice of $\{w_{ij}\}$. We next report the results if certain percentages (e.g., 25% or 50%) of events are reclassified into one grade above (i.e., G1 $\rightarrow$ G2, or G2 $\rightarrow$ G3) or below (i.e., G2 $\rightarrow$ G1 or G3 $\rightarrow$ G2) the current one. The selection of which individuals will be affected by the new rules was done by a random number generator. In other words, we randomly selected a designated percentage of individuals and had their grades moved up or down one grade. With the modified results, we report the p value from the 10 df M-H modified statistic as well as the c_1 and c_5 thresholds that permit a clear choice between the two drugs. The second block of the results in Table 7 pertains to situations in which the new rules tend to grade events more severely while the third block pertains to situations when the new rules tend to downgrade events.

Table 7 Results from Studying the Robustness of the Proposed M-H Modified Statistic to the Classification Rules Using the Combined Data in Tables 3 and 5

Cardiovascular	Neurological/psychiatric	p Value of the 10 df M-H modified statistic when $w_{ij} = w_j, i = 1, \ldots, 10,$ $w_j = j, j = 0, \ldots, 3$	c_1 Value ($c_5 = 1$) to declare drug B better ($\alpha = 5\%$) under the 1 df M-H modified statistic	c_5 Value ($c_1 = 1$) to declare drug A better ($\alpha = 5\%$) under the 1 df M-H modified statistic
Original	Original	<0.001	7.0	2.6
25% G1 → G2[a] 50% G2 → G3	25% G1 → G2 50% G2 → G3	0.004	8.0	3.5
50% G1 → G2 25% G2 → G3	25% G1 → G2 50% G2 → G3	0.003	7.5	3.0
25% G1 → G2 25% G2 → G3	25% G1 → G2 25% G2 → G3	0.002	7.5	2.8
50% G1 → G2 50% G2 → G3	50% G1 → G2 50% G2 → G3	0.003	7.6	3.1
50% G2 → G1[b] 25% G3 → G2	50% G2 → G1 25% G3 → G2	0.001	9.2	2.2
50% G2 → G1 25% G3 → G2	25% G2 → G1 50% G3 → G2	<0.001	9.0	2.2
25% G2 → G1 25% G3 → G2	25% G2 → G1 25% G3 → G2	0.002	8.7	2.5
50% G2 → G1 50% G3 → G2	50% G2 → G1 50% G3 → G2	<0.001	8.4	2.4

[a] 25% of the grade 1 events were reclassified as grade 2 events.
[b] 50% of the grade 2 events were reclassified as grade 1 events.

Results in Table 7 are reassuring. While minor differences do exist, the basic conclusions are the same for all the different scenarios reported. Similar findings were obtained with other cases that were investigated but not reported in Table 7. It is interesting to note that when a portion of the events is moved one grade higher, it becomes slightly easier to declare drug B to be the preferable one. The opposite is true when a portion of the events is moved one grade lower.

Even though the conclusions based on the combined data in Tables 3 and 5 do not seem to depend very much on the rules in our investigation, we recommend conducting an investigation similar to the above when applying the approach proposed in this chapter. If the conclusions are found to be relatively robust to the rules, one would have the added confidence in the results. If the contrary is true, one needs to find out what causes the conclusions to be sensitive to the rules and study the medical event patterns more carefully.

VI. OTHER APPLICATIONS

In addition to a multivariate comparison of the safety profiles of two treatments, the proposed analytical procedure has an additional appeal as described by the data in Table 8. Table 8 gives the safety summaries of two treatments in eight

Table 8 Summaries of the Overall Safety Data Within Eight Medical Event Classes in a Clinical Trial Involving Two Treatments

Class	Treatment	None	Grade 1	Grade 2	p Value
Renal	1	129	13	5	.351[a]
	2	134	9	2	.183[b]
Psychiatric	1	123	18	6	.622
	2	127	14	4	.341
Hepatic	1	122	20	5	.247
	2	129	11	5	.142
Cardiovascular	1	134	8	5	.297
	2	138	3	4	.174
CNS	1	104	32	11	.250
	2	114	25	6	.122
Hematological	1	132	11	4	.291
	2	137	5	3	.137
GI	1	124	17	6	.362
	2	130	10	5	.178
Metabolic	1	127	13	7	.293
	2	133	9	3	.145

[a]The p value from the Pearson's χ^2 test applied to the original 2×3 table.
[b]The p value from the Pearson's χ^2 test applied to the collapsed 2×2 table.

classes. Within each class, there are three intensity levels (none, grade 1, and grade 2). One hundred and forty-seven patients received treatment 1 and 145 patients received treatment 2. The number in the table represents the number of patients in each treatment group whose overall safety experience within a particular class was at the level described by the column heading. For each class, there are two p values in the table. The first is from Pearson's χ^2 test applied to the original 2 × 3 table and the second is from the same test, but applied to the 2 × 2 table obtained by collapsing grade 1 with grade 2. Although treatment 1 consistently has a higher incidence of nonzero grades in all classes, all the p values are greater than 10%. The univariate test that compares each class separately does not provide much evidence for a statistically significant difference between the two treatments at the 5% level.

Combining grade 1 with grade 2, treatment group 1 totaled 181 cases of nonzero grades in the eight classes. The corresponding number for treatment group 2 is 118. Various joint distributions of the eight classes can lead to the marginal distributions in Table 8. We considered three such distributions; the first two represent two extreme situations while the third is somewhere between the two extremes.

Case 1: Each patient in treatment group 1 experienced at least one treatment-related event. The 32 patients who experienced grade 1 CNS events and 2 (of 11) patients who experienced grade 2 CNS events are also responsible for the 11 grade 1 hematological events and the 23 GI events. As for patients who received treatment 2, 118 experienced exactly one treatment-related event. With this scenario, the total number of patients who experienced any treatment-related events is the highest.

Case 2: Forty-three patients in treatment group 1 and 31 in treatment group 2 are responsible for all the cases documented. Specifically, in treatment group 1, patients 1–18 (1 through 18) experienced adverse renal events, patients 1–24 experienced adverse psychiatric events, patients 1–25 experienced adverse hepatic events, patients 1–13 experienced adverse cardiovascular events, and so on. Similarly, in treatment group 2, patients 1–11 experienced adverse renal events, patients 1–18 experienced adverse psychiatric events, patients 1–16 experienced adverse hepatic events, and so on. With this scenario, the total number of patients who reported any treatment-related events is the lowest.

Case 3: The decision on who, in each of the two treatment groups, experienced what adverse reaction(s) was made separately within each class with the use of random numbers. In this case, the total number of patients who experienced any treatment-related events is between those of case 1 and case 2.

We made several choices of $\{w_{ij}\}$. In Table 9, we give the p values for the 8 df statistics T_1 obtained under four different choices of $\{w_{ij}\}$ that satisfy $w_{ij} = w_j$. The p values were obtained by comparing T_1 to a χ^2 distribution with 8 df.

Table 9 p Values of the 8 df Statistic in Eq. (1) Applied to the Data in Table 8

Choice of weights (w_0, w_1, w_2)	Case 1	Case 2	Case 3
(0, 1, 1)	<.001	.619	<.001
(0, 1, 2)	<.001	.879	<.001
(0, 1, 3)	<.001	.872	.011
(0, 1, 4)	.005	.863	.046

The results in Table 9 are revealing. Except for case 2, all the comparisons are significant at the 5% level. It does so by pooling together nonsignificant differences that nevertheless demonstrate consistency. For case 1 and case 3, the level of significance varies as the weights assigned to grade 2 vary. Generally speaking, the level decreases with more weight placed on the grade 2 category. This latter result is not unexpected since the frequencies for this category are usually lower than those for the other categories; therefore a comparison based mostly on the incidence of this category will have less power. Another interesting finding from the results in Table 9 is the nonsignificance observed for all choices of weights for case 2. Recall that case 2 corresponds to the situation where a small portion of the patients are responsible for all the reported events. Even though treatment 1 has more reported medical events than treatment 2 (i.e., 181 vs. 118), as in the other two cases, this same difference in terms of the total number of reported events is not enough to establish the superiority of treatment 2 in this case. Thus, the number of patients experiencing the events is also important when comparing two treatments. From our experience, the pattern of medical events in a clinical trial usually falls between those described by case 1 and case 3. Several datasets fitting this description were also constructed. The comparisons were generally found to be significant at the 5% level except for a few cases when $w_3 = 3$ or 4.

We also compared the two treatments using the 1 df statistic. For this statistic, we considered seven choices of $\{w_{ij}\}$. The first four used the same set of scores reported in Table 9. In other words, we treated the eight classes symmetrically. The fifth to seventh choices involved ranking the eight classes to reflect their relative seriousness to an individual and setting w_{ij} as the product of c_i and w_j with w_j as one of the first three choices in Table 9. The ranking led us to set the class-specific scores $\{c_i\}$ as follows: *cardiovascular* = 6, *renal* and *hepatic* = 5, *hematological* = 4, *metabolic* = 3, *GI* = 2, *CNS* and *psychiatric* = 1, where a higher c_i suggests a more serious and less tolerable class. The test statistics involve a χ^2 distribution with 1 df. The p values for the comparisons under all seven choices and for case 1 and case 3 are all smaller than .01 (and much smaller than .001 on many occasions), again suggesting a highly significant difference between the overall safety outcome of the two treatments. Comparisons for case 2 using the 1 df statistic are still nonsignificant for all the weights considered.

This example demonstrates how the proposed procedure can combine consistent, yet nonsignificant, differences into an overall significant difference on many occasions. The ability to do so is particularly important when two treatments have efficacy judged as equivalent and it is important for a patient to choose a treatment that, from his or her perspective, has a more favorable safety outcome.

VII. FURTHER REFINEMENT AND EXTENSION

For notational convenience, we assumed in Section II the same number of intensity levels J for all classes. We can remove this assumption without affecting the results. Allowing different classes to have different numbers of intensity levels makes the proposed approach more flexible in handling classes that might differ substantially in nature. However, even though the levels of intensity grade in the various medical event classes does not affect the degrees of freedom of the test statistics, we discourage the use of unnecessarily large number of categories because not only might this cause difficulty in consolidating the safety information, it can also make the estimates for the covariance matrices unstable because of the extremely sparse tables.

A possible refinement of the analytical procedure is to include individuals' prognostic factors when estimating the probabilities of the various intensity levels within different classes. That is, instead of using the population-based probability estimates in computing the statistics, one can use individualized probability estimates. One can easily include individuals' prognostic factors or pretreatment information for this purpose with the use of logistic regression models such as those suggested in McCullagh [17], among others.

Since the safety information is expected to be summarized from studies in a combined fashion, one question is whether one can apply the approach to summarize the safety profile of a treatment across all studies that might have very different target populations. It is possible that at the early stage of drug development, a potential drug candidate was tested for various indications, resulting in many studies with diversely different patient populations. If the purpose is to summarize the safety data, we can use the usual body system classification to define the classes to consolidate the safety information with no reference to any disease presentation. When combining data from different studies for this purpose, it is highly desirable to summarize the difference within each study first and combine the differences in a way similar to that illustrated in Section IV. The advantage of summarizing differences within studies is to allow the comparisons to be adjusted for studies.

Although we concentrate on short-term randomized controlled clinical trials in this chapter, the idea of comparing treatments based on consolidated safety data can be applied to other studies as long as treatment exposure is comparable between treatments under comparison. Generally speaking, the approach is applicable if the treatment duration is not an important factor in the evaluation of adverse event profiles. Even though the proposed approach can be further extended so that time to the occurrence of an adverse event is also accounted for by the grading system, such an extension can lead to unjustifiably complicated decision that can reduce the attractiveness of the procedure.

VIII. COMMENTS

In this chapter, we advocated combining the diverse safety data to provide a more informative picture for the safety profile of a treatment. We also proposed a method for treatment selection that incorporates an individual's evaluation regarding the acceptability of the various intensity levels within a functional class as well as among different classes. The procedure extends easily to compare the safety profiles of more than two treatments. The crucial steps in consolidating the safety data are determination of the relevant classes and the overall intensity grade for each patient within a class. With few clinical events reported and with the lab data dominating the decision on intensity grades, one can use procedures like those proposed by Sogliero-Gilbert et al. [14] to determine the extent of the abnormality. As for the statistical comparison of the safety profiles, the proposed method relies on an individual's ability to quantify the degree of acceptability of the various intensity levels. Because different individuals will likely choose different scores that can lead to different conclusions, the interpretation of the comparison results is best done at the individual level.

In this chapter, we concentrate on short-term clinical trials. Because of the relatively uniform follow-up time, we are not concerned with the duration of drug exposure nor are we concerned with the time of the occurrence of a reported adverse event. Instead, we base our comparison entirely on the occurrence of adverse events. We feel that our choice on what is to be compared is appropriate for the type of clinical trials considered in this chapter.

The statistic in Eq. (1) compares the safety profiles of two treatments at the individual class level. If a specific sign, symptom, or lab abnormality is considered detrimental to the target population, it will have a great influence on the determination of the intensity grade within the corresponding class. As a result, a substantial difference in the incidence of the sign, symptom, or lab abnormality will translate to that in the mean intensity grades for the corresponding class. The latter is likely to show up in the statistic in Eq. (1). On the other hand, if one is interested in differences in the incidence of any sign, symptom, or lab abnormality, one should perform an exploratory analysis instead of that proposed in this chapter.

The proposed methodology does not adjust for dropout due to lack of efficacy. On the other hand, if an individual drops out because of adverse event(s), this individual will score high in the class(es) to which the event(s) leading to dropout belongs. However, such a dropout does prevent other event classes from registering more events. Therefore, in order for the comparison proposed in this chapter to be unbiased, the dropout rates for lack of efficacy as well as those for adverse events need to be comparable between the treatment groups. This same assumption applies to any statistical procedure that attempts to compare treatments with regard to their safety.

We recommended determining the classes based on body systems and the anticipated adverse experience. Since under the hypothesis of equal safety profiles the statistic in Eq. (1) has an asymptotic χ^2 distribution with K df, the power of the comparison is affected by choices of the number of classes. Nevertheless, one can always specify a priori examination of only a subset of classes that have primary importance to the target patient population. Thus, the degrees of freedom for the resulting statistics will be the number of classes in the subset. On the other hand, the 1 df statistic in Eq. (2) is less affected by the choice of K. One can handle the less important classes by assigning them near-0 scores when computing the 1 df statistic.

The procedure proposed in this chapter compares the overall safety profiles between two treatments with a set of scores $\{w_{ij}\}$. It is likely that two treatments, although with different safety outlooks in regard to some classes, fail to demonstrate any significant difference in their overall profiles with the statistic in Eq. (2). This phenomenon was illustrated in the example in Section III. This is a direct consequence of the statistic's weighing the various classes and producing one single average difference between the two treatments. On the other hand, if one is interested in comparing the differences at the individual class level, one should use the statistic described in Eq. (1).

The proposed approach does have its shortcoming. It is possible that two treatments that despite different safety outlooks with regard to one medical event class are found not to be significantly different with the statistic in Eq. (1). When the difference in one medical event class is marginally significant at the 5% level under a univariate χ^2 test, the difference can become diffuse under a multivariate test procedure because of the increase in the degrees of freedom of the associated multivariate statistics. This is the case in the example in Section IV if we try to apply the approach to compare the overall safety profiles of drug A in the two sets of trials. Even though drug A has a significantly higher incidence of genitourinary/renal events in the new set (Table 5) of studies at the 5% level, the 10 df statistic comparing the overall safety outlook of drug A in these two sets of studies has a value of 10.21, producing a p value of .264. As a result, we recommend supplementing the multivariate tests with unvariate tests when one has reason to speculate that the treatments under comparison are expected to have similar safety outlook in most medical event classes.

Aggregating experience to decide the safety profile of a treatment is not unknown to practicing physicians, who must routinely evaluate each patient's need to arrive at an individualized treatment strategy. The process of information aggregation and treatment selection, although existing for many decades, is not a precise one. On the other hand, if done properly, it provides a reasonable solution in a field which by nature is inexact. We propose in this chapter to formalize this process. The primary advantage of the proposed procedure results from quantifying the relative seriousness of the intensity levels within different classes and ascertaining how this quantification translates to treatment selection.

Rampey and Enas [3] point out the results in a recent article by Boissel [18] stating that physicians are often unaware of clinical trial findings and do not rely on clinical trials data for decision making regarding patient care. Rampey and Enas speculated that one reason might be that clinical trial data have not been analyzed and presented in a way that is helpful to the medical community. Certainly, the current way of summarizing safety data does not provide a succinct and clear picture on the safety profiles of treatments because the analyses are diverse and multifaceted. By comparison, the approach proposed in this chapter mimics a physician's summarizing the safety information to come up with a general impression regarding the safety of a treatment.

The process of sorting out relevant safety data to arrive at appropriate intensity grades can be tedious. Nevertheless, once a logical plan is in place, one can write computer programs to automate this process. The programs can systematically sift through various numerical results, key words, and clinical event description. With modern computing facilities, the implementation of such programs is quite feasible. In our opinion, with safety data in clinical trials, the effort to implement their analysis is minute compared to that of collecting them.

Our approach, through the choice of $\{w_{ij}\}$, has a subjective component. While it is crucial to have the classes and the overall intensity grades determined in an objective manner, the assignment of the scores is left to be made at the individual level. In other words, subjectiveness is deliberately built into the procedure so that treatment selection can reflect an individual's evaluation of the various intensity levels and possibly the acceptability of the various classes. This subjectiveness does create some ambivalence when one attempts to use this approach to make a population-oriented treatment comparison as in a new drug application. One possible solution for the latter is to use $w_{ij} = j$ for each class and use the statistic in Eq.(1). Many researchers (e.g., Ref. 19) have opted for the equally spaced scores when analyzing ordinal data. This somewhat conventional choice of scores for ordered categories can eliminate the subjective nature of the scores.

In an attempt to delineate a classification of adverse event data, Alexander [20] advocated a system that would take into account the source of the reported data, the potential clinical importance to the clinical trial participants, and the role of adverse event report in the safety profile of the drug under evaluation. Alexander felt that such a classification is desirable because he found it disturbing that 20 cases of nausea might attract more attention than a single case of cardiac arrhythmia under the current system of paying most attention to the incidence rates of adverse events. Our method compensates the deficiency of looking only at the incidence rates of adverse events by allowing the assignment of not only a severity level but also a score that reflects the seriousness of the event class to which an adverse event belongs. In addition, because our approach consolidates safety data with respect to body systems, clustered events within a body system can be easily recognized. The ability to identify patterns is what Abt [4,5] advocated for descriptive data analysis.

Appendix

Determination of the Grades for a Patient

This is an example to illustrate how the data of a patient would be used to grade his or her safety experience in the study. The patient under consideration had the following abnormalities: (1) On the electrocardiogram at baseline, he had an interventricular conduction defect, inverted T waves and abnormal ST waves suggestive of an old myocardial infarct or myocardial ischemia, but no changes were observed while on medication. (2) On the hematology report, he had a normal number of leukocytes at screen and baseline, but the number was elevated after 4 weeks of medication. (3) Urinalysis revealed an elevated protein content and an elevated number of red blood cells after 4 weeks of medication. (4) On the safety forms, he reported perianal pain, headache, tiredness, and arthritis.

CVD:
   No clinical events, score = 0
   ECG:
   QRS—IVCD, T—Inverted, ST—abnormal, old infarct, myocardial ischemia
      at baseline. No changes at follow-up, score = 0
   Overall CVD score = 0
Hematology:
   No clinical events, score = 0
   Leukocytes normal at screen, normal at wk 0, high at wk 4, score = 1
   Overall hematology score = 1

GI/hepatic:
    Perianal pain, wk 7/8, severe, not related, score = 2
    No abnormal labs, score = 0
    Overall GI/hepatic score = 2
GU/renal:
    No clinical events, score = 0
    Urine protein high wk 4; RBCHPF high wk 4, score = 1
    Overall GU/renal score = 1
Neuro/psych:
    Headache, wk 5, mild, related, score = 1; headache, wk 7/8, mild, not
        related, score = 0
    Tiredness, wk 1.5, 2, 2.5, 3, 4, 5, 7/8, mild, related, score = 2. (Raised 1
        grade because of frequency of report >2)
    No abnormal neuro/psych labs, score = 0
    Overall neuro/psych score = 2
Pulmonary:
    No abnormalities, overall pulm score = 0
Special senses:
    No abnormalities, overall SS score = 0
Metab/nutrit:
    No abnormalities, overall M/N score = 0
Dermatology:
    No abnormalities, overall derm score = 0
Musculoskeletal:
    Arthritis, wk 1.5, wk 4, severe, not related, score = 2
    No lab abnormalities, score = 0
    Overall MS score = 2

REFERENCES

1. O'Neill RT. Assessment of safety. In *Biopharmaceutical Statistics for Drug Development*. Peace KE. ed. New York: Marcel Dekker; 1988.
2. Peace KE. Design, monitoring, and analysis issues relative to adverse events. *Drug Inf J*. 1987; 21:21–28.
3. Rampey AH, Enas GG. Current issues and innovative approaches in adverse event data analysis. Presented at the 1991 Drug Information Association meeting, Washington DC.
4. Abt K. Descriptive data analysis: a concept between confirmatory and exploratory data analysis. *Meth Inf Med*. 1987; 26:77–88.
5. Abt K. Statistical aspects of neurophysiologic topography. *J Clin Neurophysiol*. 1990; 7:519–534.

6. Huster WJ. Clinical trial adverse events: the case for descriptive techniques. *Drug Inf J*. 1991; 25:447–456.
7. Enas GG. Making decisions about safety in clinical trials: the case for inferential statistics. *Drug Inf J*. 1991; 25:439–446.
8. *Guidelines for the Format and Content of the Clinical and Statistical Sections of an Application*, Center for Drug Evaluation and Research, Food and Drug Administration, Department of Health and Human Services, 1988; 38.
9. Abt K, Cockburn ITR, Guelich A, Krupp P. Evaluation of adverse drug reactions by means of the life table method. *Drug Inf J*. 1989; 23:143–149.
10. Thompson WL, et al. Routine laboratory tests in clinical trials. In *Clinical Trials and Tribulations*. Cato AE. ed. New York: Marcel Dekker; 1988.
11. Chuang-Stein C. Summarizing laboratory data with different reference ranges in multi-center clinical trials. Drug Inf J. 1992; 26:77–84.
12. Westfall PH, Young SS. P-value adjustments for multiple tests in multivariate binomial models. *J Am Stat Assoc*. 1989; 84:780–786.
13. Brown KR, Getson AJ, Gould AL, Martin CM, Ricci FM. Safety of cefoxitin: an approach to the analysis of laboratory data. *Rev Inf Dis*. 1979; 1:228–231.
14. Sogliero-Gilbert G, Mosher K, Zubkoff L. A procedure for the simplification and assessment of lab parameters in clinical trials. *Drug Inf J*. 1986; 20:279–296.
15. Gilbert GS, Ting N, Zubkoff L. A statistical comparison of drug safety in controlled clinical trials: the Genie score as an objective measure of lab abnormalities. *Drug Inf J*. 1991; 25:81–96.
16. Agresti A. *Categorical Data Analysis*. New York: Wiley, 1990.
17. McCullagh P. Regression models for ordinal data (with discussion). *J Roy Stat Soc*. 1980; B42:109–142.
18. Boissel J. Impact of randomized clinical trials on medical practices. *Controlled Clin Trials*. 1989; 10:120S–134S.
19. Agresti A. *Analysis of Ordinal Categorical Data*. New York: Wiley; 1984.
20. Alexander WJ. Adverse events: a classification system for use in clinical trials. *Drug Inf J*. 1991; 25:457–459.

10

The Use of Hazard Functions in Safety Analysis

David S. Salsburg

Pfizer Inc.
Groton, Connecticut

I. CLINICAL QUESTIONS

Suppose a drug is associated with a potentially serious adverse reaction. The prescribing physician may be told that the incidence is exactly 3.2%. But the most the physician can get from knowing the overall incidence rate is the ability to categorize treatments into rough categories such as

The event is so rare that the possibility can be ignored.
The event is rare but the physician should be alert to the possibility.
The event is so frequent that all patients should be checked on a regular basis.

   The physician needs to know much more about the reaction than the incidence rate. Suppose a patient is put on the drug and does not experience this reaction, or at least not for the first month of therapy. Should the physician continue to be concerned? How long should the patient be observed closely to be sure to catch the event if it occurs?
   Suppose a drug has a particular side effect associated with the initiation of therapy. How many patients do we need to observe and how sure can we be that this side effect only occurs during the first few days of therapy, so the practicing physician can be assured that, if it has not occurred initially, it will most likely not occur at all?
   What emerges from these questions is that chronic therapy is not associated with a count of numbers of patients who have adverse reactions but rather with a

time course of events during which an adverse reaction may occur. This chapter discusses ways to estimate that time course.

II. A LITTLE MATHEMATICS

If we want to look at the time course of treatment in individual patients, we need to model the rough idea that events occur over time, while on therapy. A standard mathematical model deals with the time to the first occurrence of an event. Let T = the time until the first occurrence of a specific adverse reaction for a given patient. In an ideal situation, we can follow this patient for as long as it takes until the event occurs. For some patients we might get T equal to 3 days; for others T might be 120 years. It is obvious that we can never have the ideal situation, primarily because other events will occur that will stop our ability to observe the patient. The study may come to an end. The patient might be hospitalized and taken off the experimental medication. The patient may move from the area and drop out of the study. In statistical jargon, the observed time is censored. We will address the problem of censoring in a later section. For the moment, let us consider the ideal situation where we can observe as long as we need to.

Note that we have introduced the assumption that every patient will eventually suffer this adverse reaction. We can model the event in terms of two types of patients: those who experience the reaction and those who never will. However, the mathematics becomes quite complicated, and we can accomplish the same goal by allowing for values of T that are greater than any human lifespan. Thus, in the standard approach to time-to-event data, we act as if all patients will eventually experience the event and model the probability distribution of the random variable T.

Using theories of mathematical statistics, we can describe the probabilistic characters of T in terms of several different functions:

Cumulative distribution function: $F(s) = \text{Prob}\{T \leq s\}$
Survival function: $S(s) = \text{Prob}\{T > s\} = 1 - F(s)$
Density function: $f(s)$ = derivative of $F(s) = d\,F(s)/ds$
Hazard function: $h(s) = f(s)/S(s)$

Each of these functions was created to allow for easy manipulation of certain mathematical expressions. For instance, the density function provides the basis of maximum likelihood estimation and also a tool for determining the most powerful hypothesis test statistic. Because these functions were created for and are primarily used by mathematical theorists, one seldom finds them in applied statistics books or books on the analysis of clinical data. When they do appear, it is often as something snatched out of the air and applied arbitrarily to a given set of data.

The survival function sometimes appears in the clinical literature, primarily in the form of the nonparametric Kaplan–Meier estimator. In the next section, we will discuss the Kaplan–Meier estimator and where and when it is used. But for the moment let us examine the entire paraphernalia of probabilistic functions and consider why one or another might provide useful information for the practicing physician. Both the distribution and the survival functions describe the cumulative probability as T increases. By definition, the distribution function cannot decrease and the survival function cannot increase over time. Figure 1 displays the distribution and survival functions for the Weibull (a parametric form that has been widely used to model time-to-event data). Consider the figure. There is very little that can be seen about the probabilistic behavior of T from these plots. The longer we watch patients, the lower the survival probability by definition, so that the end points of the curves tell us more about how large is the largest observed value of T than they do about the probability of the reaction. One can compare the shapes of two different curves, but it is difficult to determine what a difference in shape really means, or how great a difference there is, or even if the different shapes have clinical meaning.

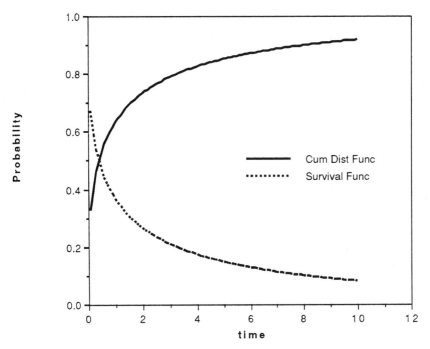

Figure 1 Weibull distribution: cumulative distribution function, and survival function.

Figure 2 shows the hazard function of the same distribution. The hazard function can be thought of as the probability that a patient, who has not yet experienced the event, will have it in the next few days or hours. Thus, a curve with an increasing hazard function describes an event that is more and more likely to occur (if it hasn't yet) the longer patients are treated. A decreasing hazard function implies that the probability of an event occurring decreases with increasing usage, and it can be used to estimate the length of time a patient needs to be watched carefully. A constant hazard function means that the fact that a patient has been on the drug for a long time without experiencing the event is irrelevant. That patient has the same chance of event as one starting on therapy.

Hazard functions need not be all increasing or all decreasing. The hazard function illustrated in Fig. 3 describes the distribution of the first time to increased sweating for a psychotherapeutic agent. The hazard function rises slightly in the first 2 weeks, levels off for a while, and then decreases slowly. This means that most of the patients who will suffer from increased sweating will start doing so within the first 60 days. Thereafter, the longer a patient has gone without the effect the greater is the chance that he or she will not have the reaction.

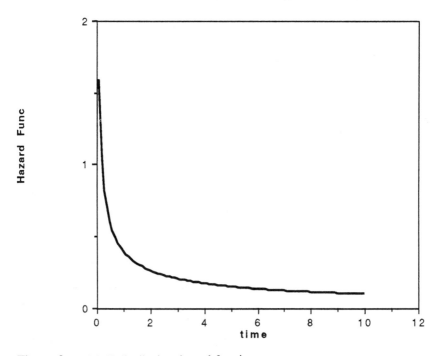

Figure 2 Wiebull distribution: hazard function.

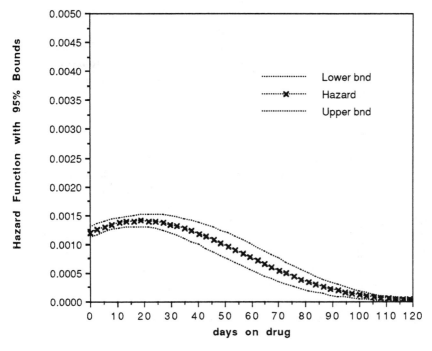

Figure 3 Hazard function (with 95% confidence bounds): first occurrence of in-creased sweating.

Thus, if we could characterize the hazard function associated with a given adverse reaction, we could tell the practicing physician.

1. How soon after initiating therapy the patients will begin experiencing the reaction, if it is going to occur;
2. Over what interval of time the bulk of events will occur; and
3. Whether the probability of the event's occurring diminishes or increases with increasing time on therapy.

Furthermore, we can compare two treatments, and the shapes of the two hazard functions would give use relative information similar to the three items mentioned above.

III. ESTIMATING THE HAZARD FUNCTION

"Aiy, there's the rub!" Once we have a well-defined mathematical concept, we need to be able to estimate its values from data in order to use it in the analysis of clinical trials. Because it is defined as the ratio of two related functions, the hazard function is difficult to estimate. For estimation in general, there are two paths we can take: parametric and nonparametric.

For parametric estimation, we assume that the time to event T has a distribution function taken from a family of distributions, which differ from one another by values of a small set of parameters. For instance, the three-parameter Weibull family defines

$$F(s) = 0 \qquad \text{if } s < \mu$$
$$\exp\{\beta\ (s\ -\ \mu)\gamma\} \qquad \text{if } s \geq \mu$$

The three parameters describe different aspects of the probabilistic functions, but there is no need to worry about the mathematical meaning they have in this context. It is sufficient to think of a large collection of hazard functions, such that the data can be used to estimate the values of the three parameters and allow us to pick one curve as the "best fitting." There are no simple algebraic expressions that can be used to compute these estimates, but they can be calculated on a computer as the solution to the maximum likelihood equations. Furthermore, statistical theory can be used to compute confidence bounds on these parameters and, from those confidence bounds, to compute upper and lower bounds on the hazard function.

Thus, no matter how complicated the data, and no matter how complicated the parametric form being used, the modern computer can supply useful estimates of the hazard function. Also, we can provide the practicing physician with information about the time course of events she or he might expect.

Experience with time-to-event data from a wide range of applications has convinced many statisticians that the three-parameter Weibull (or the two-parameter version when the truncation is set at zero) provides a rich enough set of distributions to fit any situation. SAS, version 6.06, provides the maximum likelihood estimates in PROC LIFETEST [1] for a two-parameter Weibull. Unfortunately, the hazard function produced by PROC LIFETEST is a nonparametric estimate that does not have good probabilistic properties (it is not consistent or unbiased, and there is no good way of estimating its variance). However, the Tanner–Wong nonparametric estimator proposed below provides a curve that is uniformly consistent and for which confidence intervals can be calculated [2].

This brings us to nonparametric estimation of the hazard function. A naive estimate (which can sometimes be quite effective) is to divide the data into groups of values lying between fixed points. For instance, suppose the times to event were 1, 1, 4, 6, 7, 12, 12, 15, 25, 60, 65, 95, 100, 130, 148. We could combine the values between 0 and 10, 11 and 50, 50 and 100, and greater than 100. If we approximate the hazard function by assuming a constant hazard within each of the three intervals, we can estimate the hazard as in the following table:

Time	Density	Survival	Hazard
0–10	0.3333	0.8333	0.4000
11–50	0.2267	0.5333	0.4250
51–100	0.2667	0.4333	0.6160
>100	0.1333	0.1000	1.3333

and produce a plot like Fig. 4. Estimation based on grouped data is reasonably accurate, provided there are a relatively large number of observations in each short interval of time. Otherwise, either the intervals are too long and the fine shape of the curve is missed or the number of observations per interval is so small that the point estimates have high variance and uncertainty.

SAS PROC LIFETEST estimates the hazard function from short intervals containing only one or two observations. If we want to characterize the fine

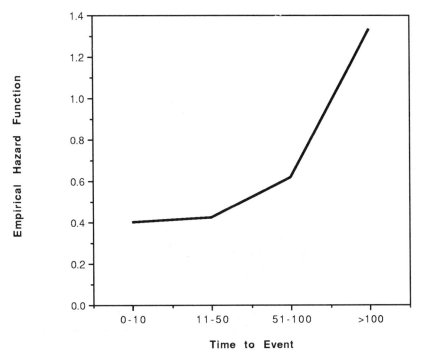

Figure 4 Empirical estimate of a hazard function.

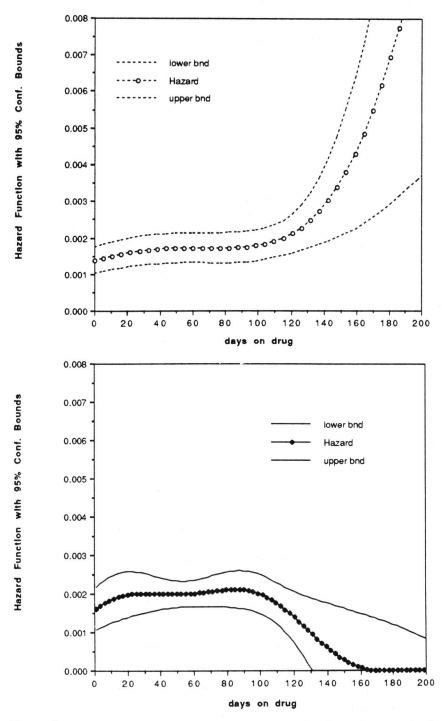

Figure 5 (top) Drug A: hazard function (with 95% bounds), first occurrence of palpitations. (bottom) Drug B: hazard function (with 95% bounds), first occurrence of palpitations.

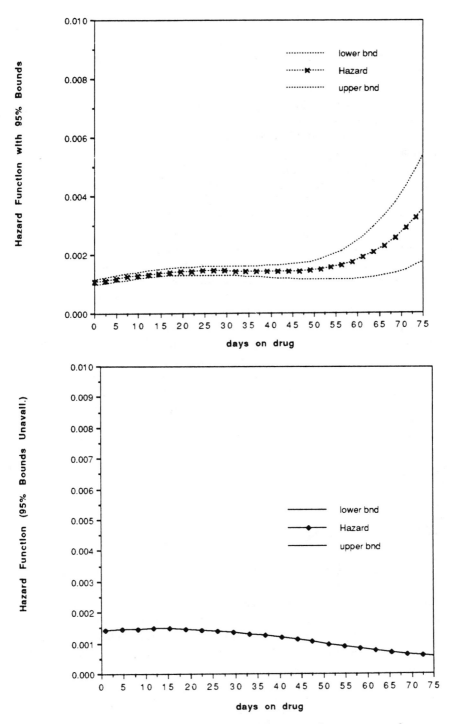

Figure 6 (top) Drug A: hazard function (with 95% bounds), first occurrence of tremor. (bottom) Drug B: hazard function (with 95% bounds), first occurrence of tremor.

shape of the curve by using individual points, we can do much better with a Tanner–Wong nonparametric estimator.

Tanner and Wong [2] showed that a hazard function based on the principles of kernel-type nonparametric density estimation is uniformly consistent, asymptotically normally distributed, and has a known variance. Thus, we can construct a nonparametric estimate of the hazard function and also put confidence bounds around it. The opposite page gives the FORTRAN code for a FORTRAN-callable subroutine that computes the Tanner–Wong estimate and its variance. Tanner and Wong ran a Monte Carlo simulation study to see how well their estimator fits the known hazard function for several different families of curves.

One problem with the Tanner–Wong estimator is that the variance gets quite high when only a few patients are left in the study (the rest having had the adverse event or dropped out). We have run the estimator on data from several programs, and it appears that the confidence intervals are too wide to be useful when the number of patients left is too few. Thus, the FORTRAN program produces values only until the point where 50% of the patients are left.

Figures 5 and 6 display Tanner–Wong estimates of hazard functions for two active drugs from randomized controlled trials. Over a 200-day interval drug A shows a gradually increasing hazard for palpitations, increasing more rapidly as time goes on. Palpitations also occur with drug B, but here the hazard is relatively constant for the first 100 days and then decreases. Tremor, followed for 75 days, shows a similar pattern. For drug A, the hazard is constant out to 55 days and then begins to increase. For drug B, the hazard slowly decreases.

Thus, the prescribing physician could be told that for both drugs there is a very low probability of tremor or palpitations, but that patients on drug A will be at increasing risk as time goes on, whereas patients on drug B who have not yet experienced these adverse reactions have a diminishing chance as time goes on.

IV. CONCLUSIONS

From the rich collection of mathematical functions that have been derived to describe probabilities associated with time to event, we have suggested that the hazard function may be one of the most useful. We have shown how the practicing physician might use a plot of the hazard function or plots of comparative hazard functions to determine what might be expected. We have described how these functions can be estimated in both a parametric and a nonparametric setting.

```
C   KHAZARD.FOR COMPUTES AN ESTIMATE OF THE HAZARD FUNCTION FOR
C   RANDOMLY CENSORED DATA, USING KERNEL DENSITY ESTIMATORS
C
C   SEE: TANNER AND WONG, (1983) THE ESTIMATION OF THE HAZARD FUNCTION FROM
C        RANDOMLY CENSORED DATA BY THE KERNEL METHOD
C        ANNALS OF STATISTICS, VOL 11, NO. 3 PP 989-993
C
C   INPUT, N= NUMBER OF UNCENSORED OBSERVATIONS
C          M= TOTAL NUMBER OF OBSERVATIONS (CENSORED AND UNCENSORED)
C          R(I) = RANK ORDER (WITHIN THE TOTAL SET) OF ITH UNCENSORED OBSERVATION
C          X(I) = TIME VALUE OF THE ITH UNCENSORED OBSERVATION
C          IT ASSUMED THAT THE X'S AND R'S ARE ORDERED FROM SMALLEST TO LARGEST
C
C   OUTPUT, ALAMB(J,1) = HAZARD FUNCTION ESTIMATE AT TIME ALAMB(J,2)
          SUBROUTINE KHAZARD(M,N,R,X,ALAMB)
          DIMENSION R(N),X(N),  ALAMB(100,2)
          FM=M
          U0=X(1)
          FN=N
          T=3.*(M+.05)/4.
          DO 200 I=1,N
          IF (R(I).LE.T) U1=X(I)
200       CONTINUE
          FN=N
          H=(U1-U0)/(10.)
          DELT=(U1-U0)/100.
          T=U0
          CONST=H*2.5066
          DO 250 J=1,100
          ALAMB(J,1)=0.
          ALAMB(J,2)=T
          DO 230 I=1,N
          T1=-0.5*((X(I)-T)/H)**2
          IF (T1.LT.-10.) GO TO 230
          ALAMB(J,1)=ALAMB(J,1)+EXP(T1)/(FM-R(I)+1.)
230       CONTINUE
250       T=T+DELT
          DO 280 J=1,100
280       ALAMB(J,1)=ALAMB(J,1)/CONST
          RETURN
          END
```

REFERENCES

1. SAS Institute. *SAS/STAT User's Guide* version 6, 4th ed. vol 2. 1990.
2. Tanner MA, Wong WH. The estimation of the hazard function from randomly censored data by the kernel method. *Ann Stat.* 1983; 989–993.

11

Meta-Analysis of Drug Safety Data

Gary G. Koch

University of North Carolina
Chapel Hill, North Carolina

Judith E. Schmid, Janet M. Begun, and William C. Maier

Pharmaceutical Product Development, Inc.
Morrisville, North Carolina

I. INTRODUCTION

In analyzing the safety data from phase I–IV clinical trials, a number of difficulties arise. Foremost among these is the matter of sample size. In many cases, an adverse drug experience of interest occurs rarely enough that it is not possible to test the association between the adverse event (AE) and the treatment drug within an individual study. One strategy to alleviate this is to use meta-analysis. In addition to the issue of sample size, the data structure may be complex, with time at risk and duration and frequency of adverse events varying among patients and across studies. Several methods of meta-analysis will be presented that deal with some of the complexities of safety data.

II. META-ANALYSIS OF SAFETY DATA

A. Issues and Advantages of Meta-Analysis

Meta-analysis refers to a statistical analysis that combines the results of some collection of related studies to arrive at a single conclusion to the question at hand [1]. There are several advantages in using meta-analysis [2,3]. The increased sample size gained by including the data from several studies increases the power of the analysis to investigate questions that could not be adequately addressed in the individual studies. There may also be sufficient sample size for analysis of subpopulations. Qualitatively, by juxtaposing different studies, differences in quality and design can be evaluated, and questions of generalizability of the result can be addressed.

There are several issues to be addressed before performing a meta-analysis. The most immediate of these is the decision as to which studies to include in the analysis [4-6]. Should studies be included that differ in scientific quality or in other factors such as design, population studied, type of data collected, or outcome measurement? The question of quality has to do with the believability of the results. Some authors will only include studies with certain characteristics such as randomized double-blind studies, while others include all studies regardless of quality. Differences in the other study factors raise questions regarding whether and how to combine studies that may measure slightly different outcomes. If only very similar studies are combined, the analysis is simpler and the result is clearer than if very diverse studies are combined [7]. When diverse studies are combined, the generalizability of the result is more evident; however, an effect that is present only under specific conditions may be obscured.

Most methods of meta-analysis assume that the individual studies are independent. This may not be the case, e.g., if investigators or patients are involved in more than one study [8]. The effect of variables such as investigator, center, and year of study should be examined and adjusted for as necessary.

In deciding how to combine the studies, it must first be decided how to weight the studies. In most cases, if quality of the studies is not an issue, studies are weighted in a way that reflects sample size. Larger studies are assumed to give a better estimate of the result under study and so are given more weight in the analysis. Another approach is to assume that each study gives an equally valid estimate and to weight all studies equally [7].

There has been much discussion of the merits of combining the results, rather than the data of the individual studies, and so adjusting for individual study differences [9]. For instance, one study may have a higher rate of occurrence of an adverse event but still show the same difference in occurrence rates across treatment groups as another study. In the analysis of rare events, however, the individual study results may be negligible, and analysis of the pooled data may be necessary.

B. Application to Drug Safety Data

Meta-analysis has been used in many fields, in each for slightly different reasons and with slightly different methods. In clinical trials, as analysis of safety data and efficacy data require different approaches, so meta-analysis differs in each case. Efficacy data can often be analyzed using a straightforward and traditional meta-analysis, while safety data often present additional difficulties. In both safety and efficacy meta-analyses, determining the presence of an association between a treatment and an outcome is generally the main focus of the analysis;

however, in the efficacy analysis, evaluation of the consistency of the individual studies in this association is also of major concern. In a safety analysis, the occurrence of the event in question may be infrequent enough that an evaluation of this type is not possible. If the event occurs more frequently, this analysis of homogeneity may be of interest [10-13].

A situation that is ideal for meta-analysis occurs when the studies to be combined are all very similar. If the studies all have similar design, treatment regimens, indications, populations, methods and times for collecting data, duration, and early withdrawal rates, then the more traditional methods of meta-analysis, described in Section III.A, may be used. For many of these factors, the studies can be categorized into a few groups, or the factor can be considered a numerical variable (such as dose) to be determined for each patient or within each study. Then, either by using stratification or by adding factors to a model, the methods of Section III.A can still be used when the studies differ in one or more characteristics. The total sample size and the rate of occurrence of the adverse event may still limit the number of factors that the analyses can take into account.

For instance, if the studies vary in design, stratification or model factors can often be used to adjust for differences in outcome that are associated with the design. When some studies are multicenter studies, stratification by center or adding center as a predictor to the model will adjust for differences in outcome related to center. If it can be shown that center is not associated with outcome or if the sample size is too small to allow stratification by center, then the data may be pooled for the centers in each study. If some studies are unblinded and others blinded, then stratification for this factor should take place unless it can be shown that there is no association between blindedness of the study and the outcome.

If some studies are crossover studies, however, it is difficult to combine them with parallel studies. In any case, the data of crossover studies can be added to the analysis up to the point of the first crossover, but beyond this point it becomes more difficult to know which treatment the event should be classified under and how the time of exposure should be evaluated.

There are two situations that commonly occur in collections of safety studies that may require very different analysis strategies. First, the studies may vary in factors related to time [14]. If the studies have different treatment or follow-up times, or the patients of different studies have different withdrawal rates, or reports of safety problems are collected at different intervals, then an analysis that takes time into account is appropriate. Some methods which account for time are presented in Section III.B.

Second, the data structure may be complicated [15,16]. In many cases the occurrence of an adverse event or an abnormal laboratory finding can be thought of as dichotomous, i.e., for each patient it is either present or not. In some cases severity or duration of the event is of interest. The methods of Section III.A are useful in analyzing dichotomous and ordinal outcomes (where an outcome, such as severity, can be classified into one of several discrete, ordered categories, such as absent, mild, moderate, or severe). Analysis of outcomes that are continuous numerical values are not discussed in this chapter, but methods can be found in the Refs. 9, 12, and 17. If a patient can experience an event more than once in a study, then the outcome can still be considered ordinal (the number of events per patient), and the methods of Section III.A can be used. If, however, the total number of events across all patients is the outcome of interest, then the events for each patient must be considered as correlated and the analysis adjusted accordingly. Severity or duration as well as multiple events for each patient may also be of interest. One analysis strategy for these two cases is discussed in Section III.C and other methods can be found in Refs. 18 and 19.

The methods of this chapter deal only with the univariate analysis of single adverse drug reactions. In reality, many adverse experiences are analyzed in each study and may be of interest in the meta-analysis. In many cases, an analysis is considered exploratory, and separate tests are performed for several different event outcomes, without adjusting for multiplicity of tests or considering possible correlations between events. Outcomes that show significant results are then subjected to further testing and examined in future studies. References that deal with multiple testing issues and multivariate analysis methods include Refs. 14–16, 20–22.

III. STATISTICAL METHODS FOR META-ANALYSIS

A. Basic Methods

The methods in this section are appropriate when the studies are similar in all aspects of design that can affect the outcome. If the studies differ in a factor that has only a few categories, the factor may be used as a stratification variable in addition to study. A categorical or numerical factor may be added as a predictor in a model.

1. Analysis of Data with a Dichotomous Outcome

In the simplest case, there are two treatment groups (test and reference) and the outcome of occurrence or nonoccurrence of the adverse event (AE) can be considered to be dichotomous. The data for each study can then be arranged in a 2×2 table (Table 1). In the table, $a + b + c + d = N$, the total number of patients in the study. The row and column totals of the 2×2 table ($a + b, c + d, a + c, b + d$) are considered to be fixed, the row totals by assignment to treatment group, and the column totals by occurrence of the event in the study population, under the hypothesis of no association with treatment.

If the occurrence of the adverse drug experience is rare, so that stratification by study is not practical, then the data from the individual studies may be

Table 1   2 × 2 Table

Drug	AE occurs	AE does not occur
Test	a	b
Reference	c	d

combined into one 2 × 2 table. (It may be of interest to combine the data in any case to obtain a first approximation to a result.) Fisher's exact test can be used to test for an association between the treatment and the occurrence of the adverse event. In Fisher's test, the exact probability is calculated for each table with the same row and column totals as exhibited by the data. The p value is calculated by summing the probabilities of all tables as likely or less likely to occur, under the null hypothesis of no association between treatment and AE occurrence. The probability of each table under the null hypothesis is:

$$\text{pr}\,(a|H_0) = [(a + b)\,!\,(c + d)\,!\,(a + c)\,!\,(b + d)\,!\,]\,/\,[N\,!\,a!b!c!d!]$$

Fisher's exact test is easily available from software products such as the SAS procedure FREQ [23] and StatXact [24].

If the occurrence rate and sample size are sufficiently large that within-study estimates of the association between the AE and the treatment groups can be calculated, the individual study results can be combined as in classical meta-analysis. The sign test or the signed rank test may be used to determine if the AE occurs more frequently in one treatment group, while weighting all studies equally [7].

The Mantel–Haenszel procedure also tests the AE treatment association and weights larger studies more heavily than smaller studies [3,25]. In the Mantel–Haenszel (M-H) test, the data from each study is arranged in a 2 × 2 table (as above). For each study the expected value of a, $E(a) = (a + b)(a + c)/N$, and the variance of a, $V(a) = (a + b)(c + d)(a + c)(b + d)/N^2(N - 1)$, are calculated. The M-H statistic, using the subscript h to indicate the hth study, is:

$$Q = \frac{\{\Sigma_h[a_h - E\,(a_h)]\}^2}{\Sigma_h V(a_h)}$$

which has a χ^2 distribution, with 1 df. This statistic may be calculated using the SAS procedure FREQ. The M-H test is more powerful when the direction of association between treatment and outcome is the same for most of the studies. For adverse events with moderately large occurrence rates, the homogeneity of the association of treatment with outcome should be examined.

A logistic regression model can also be used to determine if there is an association between the occurrence of the AE and the test drug group, while taking into account study and any other variables that may be important. The model is specified by:

$$\pi_{hik} = \frac{1}{1 + e^{-x'_{hik}\beta}} \qquad \text{or} \qquad \log \frac{\pi_{hik}}{1 - \pi_{hik}} = x'_{hik}\beta$$

where π_{hik} is the probability of occurrence of the AE for the kth patient in the ith treatment group in the hth study or group within a study, x_{hik} is the vector of predictor values for the patient, and β is the vector of parameters to be estimated for the model. Many software packages are available for logistic regression, including the SAS procedures CATMOD and LOGISTIC.

2. Analysis of Data with an Ordinal Outcome

If the outcome is not dichotomous but ordinal, e.g., if the AE is classified according to severity, then extensions of the M-H test and the logistic regression model may be used [26]. The data from each study can be arranged in a $2 \times r$ table as shown in Table 2. In the table, if a set of scores (a_1, a_2, a_3, a_4) is assigned to the outcome possibilities [e.g., the integer scores $(1, 2, 3, 4)$; for other types of scoring, see Ref. 26], then the extended M-H test would look at the difference in mean scores between treatment groups. Using the subscript g to indicate the gth level of severity, the mean score for the individual study for the test treatment group is:

$$m_t = \frac{\Sigma_g a_g n_{tg}}{n_{t+}}$$

and for the reference group is:

$$m_r = \frac{\Sigma_g a_g n_{rg}}{n_{r+}}$$

Under the hypothesis of no association between treatment and AE severity,

$$E(m_t) = \frac{\Sigma_g a_g n_{+g}}{N}$$

Table 2 $2 \times r$ Table: Adverse Event Severity

Drug	Severe	Moderate	Mild	None	Totals
Test	n_{t1}	n_{t2}	n_{t3}	n_{t4}	n_{t+}
Reference	n_{r1}	n_{r2}	n_{r3}	n_{r4}	n_{r+}
Totals	n_{+1}	n_{+2}	n_{+3}	n_{+4}	N

and

$$V(m_t) = \frac{n_{r+}}{n_{t+} (N - 1)} \Sigma_s \frac{n_{+g}}{N} [a_g - E(m_t)]^2$$

$$= \frac{n_{r+}}{n_{t+} (N - 1)} V_a$$

If the data are to be pooled across centers without adjustment, then

$$Q = \frac{[m_t - E(m_t)]^2}{V(m_t)}$$

has a χ^2 distribution, with 1 df. The extended M-H χ^2,

$$Q = \frac{\{\Sigma_h n_{ht+}[m_{ht} - E(m_{ht})]\}^2}{\Sigma_h[n_{ht+}n_{hr+}/ (N_h - 1)] V_{ha}}$$

also with 1 df, tests the association between treatment and AE severity while adjusting for individual study differences.

Similar tests can be performed in the case where there are several ordinal treatment categories, such as levels of dose, as well as an ordinal outcome variable. Scores are assigned to the levels of treatment and to the levels of outcome and trends in the mean scores across treatment levels are examined. If the data are pooled into one contingency table, a correlation χ^2 statistic can be calculated. There is also an extended M-H test that incorporates stratification by study into the analysis.

An extension of logistic regression that can take into account an ordinal outcome variable is the proportional odds model [16,26]. This looks at the successive logits of more vs. less severe outcomes; in this case, within one study or group within a study, the logit for severe vs. less than severe AE $\{\log[\pi_1/(\pi_2 + \pi_3 + \pi_4)]\}$, the logit for moderate or severe vs. less than moderate AE $\{\log [(\pi_1 + \pi_2)/(\pi_3 + \pi_4)]\}$, and the logit for any AE vs. no AE $\{\log [(\pi_1 + \pi_2 + \pi_3)/\pi_4]\}$. The model assumes that each successive logit has a different intercept but the same vector of regression parameters, i.e., logit (ψ_{hk}) $= \alpha_k + x'_h\beta$, for the kth of the successive logits within the hth study or group within study. With β_t as the coefficient estimated by the model for test drug, $\exp(\beta_t)$ is the ratio of test drug to reference drug for the odds of each more severe to less severe AE occurrence category, as predicted by the model. The proportional odds model can be applied with the SAS procedure LOGISTIC.

In the analysis of safety data, it is usually assumed that there is a true rate of occurrence for an adverse event and that each study (or each subgroup within each study) provides an estimate of this rate. Analyses with this assumption use a fixed effects approach to analysis. Alternatively, a random effects approach assumes that different populations may have different rates of occurrence and that there is not one true rate. In this case a mean rate is estimated. When the occurrence rate is fairly large, this may be of interest. If the studies to be combined demonstrate similar trends in the association between the treatments and the occurrence of the AE, then a fixed effects approach is adequate. If, however, the studies are not homogeneous in this way, a random effects approach may be more appropriate. One type of analysis that incorporates a random effects strategy is the use of survey regression methods that consider each study as a cluster of patients and adjust the estimate and its variance accordingly. Sources for the random effects approach include Refs. 10, 12, and 17.

B. Methods That Account for Time at Risk

If the studies have different durations, or if there is considerable variation between patients in the length of time on treatment or time of follow-up, then several strategies can be considered. The strategies discussed earlier did not take time into account, although time could be included as a stratification variable or a model factor. One approach that does account for time at risk is consideration of the incidence density as the rate of interest, rather than the proportion of patients experiencing the adverse event.

1. Incidence Density

The incidence density is the ratio of the total number of events to the total number of time units of risk (both sums across all patients) [27]. If the patients are considered in the analysis only to the time where the first occurrence of the AE takes place, then the observations can be considered independent. If the number of events occurring during each time interval is considered under the null hypothesis of no association with treatment to have a Poisson distribution with a rate of λ per unit of time, then within each study the expected number of AEs in the test drug treatment group is $E(n_t) = \lambda N_t = nN_t / N$, where n is the number of AEs for all treatments in the study, N the sum of time at risk for all patients in the study, and n_t and N_t are the number of AEs and amount of time at risk for the test drug group. The variance of $(n_t - E(n_t))$ is $nN_t N_r / N^2$, where N_r is the amount of time at risk for the reference group. The M-H statistic adjusting for study, with h indexing the hth study, is:

$$\frac{\{\Sigma_h[n_{ht} - E(n_{ht})]\}^2}{\Sigma_h V[n_{ht} - E(n_{ht})]}$$

and has a χ^2 distribution with 1 df.

Use of the incidence density assumes that the risk of an AE occurring remains constant over time. This may not be true [14]. Adverse events associated with drug use occur in many different patterns, which may not be accurately accounted for by an incidence density. For instance, the incidence density underestimates the risk of occurrence of an AE that appears only after a long exposure to a drug. Life table rates can be used to calculate a cumulative incidence rate, while accounting for the changing number of patients at risk over time and estimating the risk of AE occurrence separately in each time interval.

2.   Life Table Analysis

For each treatment group in each study, the data can be arranged in a life table (Table 3). The censored patients, those lost to follow-up or withdrawn from the study during the interval, are assumed to have left the study uniformly throughout the interval, and so are assigned a time at risk of $t/2$. It is also assumed that censoring is not associated with the effects of the drug and that the rate of AE occurrence for the censored patients for the remainder of the study would not have been different from the occurrence rate of those remaining in the study. Patients who experience an AE during the interval are sometimes assigned a time at risk of $t/2$, which assumes that the events occurred uniformly throughout the interval. Often, however, they are assigned a time of t, since the outcome for the interval is known.

The cumulative probability of completing the study throughout the sth time interval without experiencing the AE is the product of the probabilities of completing each of the intervals without the AE: $(1 - P) = \Pi_s (1 - p_s)$, where p_s is the probability of experiencing the event in the sth interval. The cumulative probability of experiencing the event is $P = 1 - \Pi_s (1 - p_s)$. If the number of patients is large throughout the study, Greenwood's formula for estimating the standard error can be applied [28]:

$$SE = (1 - P) \left(\Sigma_s \frac{n_{sa}}{T_s (T_s - n_{sa})} \right)^{1/2}$$

If the data from the individual studies have been collected at similar time intervals, one strategy would be to combine the data for each treatment within

Table 3 Life Table

Interval	Time in interval	No. patients at beginning of interval	No. with AE	No. lost or withdrawn	Person-time at risk	Probability of event
1	t_1	N_1	n_{1a}	n_{1b}	$T_1 = (N_1 - n_{1b}/2)t_1$	$p_1 = n_{1a}/T_1$
2	t_2	N_2	n_{2a}	n_{2b}	$T_2 = (N_2 - n_{2b}/2)t_2$	$p_2 = n_{2a}/T_2$
3	—	—	—	—	—	—
4	—	—	—	—	—	—

each time interval and compare the treatment-specific cumulative rates directly. A weighted average of the within-study difference scores could also be evaluated.

When the actual time of each adverse event is known the cumulative rate can be estimated by the Kaplan–Meier product limit method. In this case, a new time interval begins with the occurrence of each AE, so that each interval usually contains one occurrence. Intervals containing more than one event are possible when two or more AEs have the same actual time of occurrence.

The Mantel–Cox test (also called the Mantel–Haenszel test and the log-rank test) can be used to compare the cumulative AE rates of the treatments across all studies [16,28]. The data are rearranged as shown in Table 4. Each row can be viewed as a 2×2 table, and the M-H χ^2 statistic,

$$ Q = \frac{\{\Sigma_s[n_{st1} - E(n_{st1})]\}^2}{\Sigma_s V(n_{st1})} \qquad \text{(with 1 df)} $$

can be used to test the difference between treatment groups in AE occurrence. Where the data from the individual studies are combined within each time interval, the sum in the M-H statistic is over all intervals. When the data are stratified by study, the sum is over all study by interval combinations. The Mantel–Cox test is most effective where there is a consistent trend in the difference between treatment groups throughout the time intervals. The SAS procedure LIFETEST will calculate the cumulative incidence rate and its standard error and the log-rank test.

3. Piecewise Exponential Model

A model that can be used which takes time at risk into account is the piecewise exponential model [16,26]. The model assumes a separate independent exponential distribution of AE occurrences within each time interval. Within each time interval, the incidence density within each subpopulation for AE occurrence is described with the structure $\lambda_{his} = \exp(x'_{his}\beta)$, where x'_{his} is a vector of predictor variables encompassing study, treatment, and time interval and β is a

Table 4 Arrangement of Data for Mantel–Cox Test

	Test		Reference	
Interval	No. with AE	No. without AE	No. with AE	No. without AE
1	n_{1t1}	n_{1t2}	n_{1r1}	n_{1r2}
2	n_{2t1}	n_{2t2}	n_{2r1}	n_{2r2}
3	—	—	—	—
4	—	—	—	—

vector of parameters to be estimated for the model. Since the likelihood function for the piecewise exponential model is proportional to the likelihood function from a Poisson regression, Poisson regression software such as procedure NLIN of SAS can be used to estimate the regression parameters. (The SAS procedure LOGISTIC can also be used.)

4. Analysis of Data with Multiple Occurrences of the Outcome

When each patient can experience the AE more than once, a ratio can be formed that is analogous to an incidence density. Let y_{hik} be the number of events for the kth patient in the ith treatment group in the hth study, N_{hik} the time of exposure of the patient, and n_{hi} the number of patients in the hth study and ith group. The weight given to the hth study is $w_h = [(n_{ht} n_{hr} /n_h)/\Sigma_h(n_{ht} n_{hr} /n_h)]$.

For each treatment group, the ratio can be formed:

$$R_i = \frac{f_i}{g_i} = \frac{\Sigma_h \Sigma_k (w_h y_{hik} /n_{hi})}{\Sigma_h \Sigma_k (w_h N_{hik} /n_{hi})}$$

where f_i is a weighted sum of adverse event occurrences and g_i is a weighted sum of time at risk. The variance of R_i is estimated by

$$V(R_i) = R_i^2 \left[\frac{V(f_i)}{f_i^2} - \frac{2 \operatorname{Cov} (f_i, g_i)}{f_i g_i} + \frac{V(g_i)}{g_i^2} \right]$$

where $V(f_i) = \Sigma_h w_h^2 (1/n_{hi}(n_{hi} - 1)) \Sigma_k (y_{hik} - \bar{y}_{hi})^2$ with $\bar{y}_{hi} = \Sigma_k (y_{hik} /n_{hi})$;

$V(g_i) = \Sigma_h w_h^2 (1/n_{hi}(n_{hi} - 1)) \Sigma_k (N_{hik} - \bar{N}_{hi})^2$ with $\bar{N}_{hi} = \Sigma_k (N_{hik} /n_{hi})$;

and $\operatorname{Cov} (f_i, g_i) = \Sigma_h w_h^2 (1/n_{hi} (n_{hi} - 1)) \Sigma_k (y_{hik} - \bar{y}_{hi}) (N_{hik} - \bar{N}_{hi})$.

In a similar way, the ratio can be formed where y is a measure that incorporates number of times the event occurred, duration, and/or severity. For instance, y could be the number of events multiplied by their average severity or the sums of durations over which the events took place.

IV. EXAMPLES

The methods of this chapter will be illustrated with artificial data from five studies, each with approximately 500 patients. A summary of the data is shown in Tables 5–8. The studies had durations between 4 and 16 weeks, with information on the adverse event collected at between 2 and 4 time points. A total of 129 of the 2417 patients experienced the AE at least once, and 31 of these had two or more occurrences of the event. The patients were also categorized by sex and age category (<40 and ≥ 40 years).

Table 5 Number of Adverse Events Reported by Time of Exposure

Study	Treatment	2	4	6	8	12	16	Total patients
		\multicolumn{6}{c}{Weeks on study drug}		
A	Reference	4	2	0	—	—	—	249
A	Test drug	2	1	0	—	—	—	237
B	Reference	4	4	0	—	—	—	256
B	Test drug	4	4	1	—	—	—	235
C	Reference	7	1	—	—	—	—	217
C	Test drug	10	1	—	—	—	—	228
D	Reference	—	6	—	6	14	6	232
D	Test drug	—	8	—	6	7	4	261
E	Reference	—	16	—	10	3	3	269
E	Test drug	—	10	—	12	5	2	233

Table 6 Frequencies for Patients Experiencing Adverse Events (AE) by Sex

Study	Treatment	Sex	Patients with AE	Total patients
A	Reference	F	2	122
A	Reference	M	2	127
A	Test drug	F	2	126
A	Test drug	M	0	111
B	Reference	F	4	135
B	Reference	M	1	121
B	Test drug	F	3	119
B	Test drug	M	2	116
C	Reference	F	8	111
C	Reference	M	0	106
C	Test drug	F	6	109
C	Test drug	M	5	119
D	Reference	F	13	117
D	Reference	M	13	115
D	Test drug	F	11	126
D	Test drug	M	10	135
E	Reference	F	13	131
E	Reference	M	14	138
E	Test drug	F	11	116
E	Test drug	M	9	117

Table 7 Frequencies for Patients Experiencing Adverse Events by Age Category

Study	Treatment	Age category	Patients with AE	Total patients
A	Reference	<40	3	165
A	Reference	≥40	1	84
A	Test drug	<40	2	152
A	Test drug	≥40	0	85
B	Reference	<40	3	159
B	Reference	≥40	2	97
B	Test drug	<40	4	161
B	Test drug	≥40	1	74
C	Reference	<40	1	140
C	Reference	≥40	7	77
C	Test drug	<40	4	153
C	Test drug	≥40	7	75
D	Reference	<40	11	146
D	Reference	≥40	15	86
D	Test drug	<40	9	169
D	Test drug	≥40	12	92
E	Reference	<40	13	173
E	Reference	≥40	14	96
E	Test drug	<40	11	148
E	Test drug	≥40	9	85

Table 8 Frequencies for Patients Experiencing One or More Adverse Events

Study	Treatment	Patients with AE 0 AE	1 AE	≥2 AE	Total patients
A	Reference	245	2	2	249
A	Test drug	235	1	1	237
B	Reference	251	2	3	256
B	Test drug	230	1	4	235
C	Reference	209	8	0	217
C	Test drug	217	11	0	228
D	Reference	206	21	5	232
D	Test drug	240	17	4	261
E	Reference	242	22	5	269
E	Test drug	213	13	7	233

A. Example 1: Illustration of Basic Methods

1. Dichotomous Adverse Event Outcome with Dichotomous Treatment
    Categories

For the first illustrative analysis, the outcome was considered as dichotomous (occurrence or nonoccurrence of the event), and the duration of the studies was not taken into account. To examine the effect of treatment on the outcome, the data were arranged in a 2 × 2 table, and Fisher's exact test was applied (Table 9). For Fisher's exact test, the p value of .416 was compatible with no association between the treatment and the occurrence of the AE. Similarly, Fisher's exact test was performed to examine the association of sex and age category with the outcome when AE frequencies were pooled across studies. AE frequencies relative to age category are shown in Table 7; frequencies relative to sex are shown in Table 6. For sex, the p value was .148, and for age category $p < .001$. Although more females than males reported the adverse event, there was not a significant association between sex and the outcome, whereas older patients did experience the event significantly more often than younger patients.

An M-H test was performed to examine the association between treatment and the outcome while controlling for study (see Table 8). For instance, for study A the 2 × 2 table is presented in Table 10. Under the hypothesis of no association between treatment and AE occurrence, $E(a) = (249 \times 6)/486 = 3.07$ and $V(a) = (249 \times 237 \times 6 \times 480)/(486^2 \times 485) = 1.48$. The M-H statistic, $Q = \{\Sigma_h[a_h - E(a_h)]\}^2/\Sigma V(a_h)$ (where the sum is taken across all five studies) was 0.890, with a p value of .345, which supports the nonassociation between the treatment drug and occurrence of the AE. The Breslow–Day test for homogeneity of the odds ratios was also given by the SAS procedure FREQ ($Q = 1.797$, with 4 df and $p = .773$), indicating that the studies were similar in the association between the treatment and the outcome.

An M-H test was additionally performed to examine the association of sex with AE occurrence while controlling for study. Here, $Q = 2.776$, with 1 df and $p = .096$, suggesting some association between sex and the outcome. For the M-H test for association of age category with AE while controlling for study, Q

Table 9   2 × 2 Table for Treatment vs. Adverse Event Occurrence

	AE occurrence		
Treatment	Yes	No	Total
Reference	70	1153	1223
Test	59	1135	1194
Total	129	2288	2417

Table 10 2 × 2 Table for Study A for Treatment vs. Adverse Event Occurrence

Treatment	AE occurrence		Total
	Yes	No	
Reference	4	245	249
Test	2	235	237
Total	6	480	486

$= 17.740$ and $p < .001$. There is a strong association between age category and AE occurrence. For age, the Breslow–Day statistic was 10.004, with 4 df and $p = .040$, which indicates some heterogeneity in the age effect across the different studies.

A logistic regression model was applied to describe the relationship between AE occurrence and explanatory variables for study, treatment, sex, and age category. The parameter estimates given by the SAS procedure CATMOD are shown in Table 11. The difference in adverse event occurrence between older and younger patients is evident; the odds of occurrence to nonoccurrence is $\exp(0.7430) = 2.10$ times higher for the patients over 40 years old. The nonsignificant likelihood ratio test is consistent with a reasonably good fit of the model to the data and thereby supports the assumption of homogeneity of the effects for each of the explanatory variables in the model relative to the others.

Table 11 Parameter Estimates from SAS Procedure CATMOD for Logistic Regression Model

Effect	Estimate	Standard error	χ^2	Prob.
Intercept	−5.5095	0.5136	115.09	.0000
Study B	0.5030	0.5211	0.93	.3345
Study C	1.2860	0.4738	7.37	.0066
Study D	2.1453	0.4394	23.84	.0000
Study E	2.1153	0.4393	23.19	.0000
Treatment	−0.1656	0.1853	0.80	.3714
Sex	0.2545	0.1862	1.87	.1718
Age group	0.7430	0.1849	16.14	.0001
Goodness-of-fit:	df	χ^2	p value	
Likelihood ratio statistic	32	35.30	.3151	

2. Ordinal Adverse Event Outcome with Dichotomous Treatment Categories

To illustrate methods for an ordinal outcome, the patients were categorized based on the number of occurrences of the adverse event: 0, 1, and 2 or more (see Table 12). The mean score for the reference group is $m_r = [0(1153) + 1(55) + 2(15)]/1223 = 0.0695$. Under the hypothesis of no association, $E(m_r) = [0(2288) + 1(98) + 2(31)]/2417 = 0.0662$ and $V(m_r) = (1194/1223 \times 2416)[(2288/2417)(0 - .0662)^2 + (98/2417)(1 - 0.0662)^2 + (31/2417)(2 - 0.0662)^2] = 3.53 \times 10^{-5}$. The χ^2 statistic for comparing the mean scores of the two treatment groups (from the SAS procedure FREQ) is $Q = (m_r - E(m_r))^2/V(m_r) = 0.309$, with 1 df and $p = .578$. The distribution of the number of AE occurrences within each study is shown in Table 8. The analogous M-H statistic for testing if the row mean scores differ for the treatments, while controlling for study, is $Q = 0.356$, with 1 df and a p value of .551.

The proportional odds model extension of logistic regression analysis was used to describe the relationship between the number of AE occurrences (0, 1, and ≥ 2) and the explanatory variables for study, sex, age category, and treatment. In this model, the odds of at least one AE vs. none and the odds of at least two AEs vs. at most one AE have parallel relationships to the explanatory variables through a single set of corresponding regression parameters, but they have distinct intercepts. The parameter estimates and χ^2 tests from the SAS procedure LOGISTIC are shown in Table 13.

As noted for other analyses, age category is significant, with older patients having $\exp(0.7436) = 2.10$ times the odds of more prevalent occurrence of AE than younger patients. The individual studies are also seen to differ from each other in the odds of AE occurrence. One possible reason for the difference between studies is the variation in the length of study. The studies varied from 4 to 16 weeks in length, with patients in the longer studies having greater opportunity to experience and report AEs. For purposes of completeness, one can note that the LOGISTIC procedure provides a score statistic for evaluating the appropriateness of the proportional odds assumption. However, its result of $Q = 45.87$ with 7 df and $p < .001$ should be viewed skeptically because of the

Table 12   2 × 3 Table for Treatment vs. Adverse Event Occurrence

Treatment	AE occurrences			Total
	0	1	≥ 2	
Reference	1153	55	15	1223
Test drug	1135	43	16	1194
Total	2288	98	31	2417

Table 13   Parameter Estimates from SAS Procedure LOGISTIC for Proportional
Odds Model

Variable	Parameter estimate	Standard error	Wald χ^2	Pr $> \chi^2$	Standardized estimate
Intercept 1	-7.0118	0.5387	169.4152	0.0001	—
Intercept 2	-5.5129	0.5131	115.4574	0.0001	—
Study B	0.5091	0.5196	0.9600	0.3272	0.112951
Study C	1.2678	0.4739	7.1569	0.0075	0.270961
Study D	2.1385	0.4387	23.7640	0.0001	0.475180
Study E	2.1133	0.4385	23.2276	0.0001	0.472732
Sex	0.2619	0.1863	1.9768	0.1597	0.072214
Treatment	-0.1613	0.1852	0.7587	0.3837	-0.044479
Age group	0.7436	0.1849	16.1739	0.0001	0.195840

potentially spurious influence of 0 frequencies for ≥ 2 AE in study C and the small frequencies (≤ 4) of both 1 AE and ≥ 2 AEs in studies A and B. If the model is simplified by pooling study B with study C and study D with study E, the score statistic for the proportional odds assumption is $Q = 6.66$ with 5 df and $p = .247$. This result is interpreted as providing reasonable support for the use of the proportional odds model.

3.   Ordinal Adverse Event Outcome with Ordinal Treatment Categories

In Tables 14 and 15, frequencies of 0, 1, and ≥ 2 adverse events are shown for a modification of the studies under consideration to compare four treatment groups: a placebo and three doses of a test drug. The frequencies within each study are shown in Table 14. After pooling the data across studies, the numbers of patients experiencing 0, 1, or ≥ 2 adverse events are shown in Table 15. The correlation χ^2 statistic using integer scores is 3.29, with 1 df and $p = .070$; there is a nearly significant tendency for AE occurrences to be more prevalent at higher doses. The extended M-H statistic, testing for correlation between dosage and AE occurrence with adjustment for study, is $Q = 3.359$, with 1 df and $p = .067$.

B.   Example 2: Illustration of Methods Accounting for Time at Risk

A restructuring of the data from Example 1 that considers the first occurrence of the AE and takes time into account is provided in Table 16. The previous discussion considered only patients who had either completed the study without an AE or had experienced at least one AE. Patients who withdrew from the study before its completion without having an AE are now also included in the analysis.

Table 14 Adverse Event Occurrences for Patients from a Four-Dose Study

Study	Treatment	Patients with AE			Total patients
		0 AE's	1 AE	≥2 AE	
A	Placebo	121	1	1	123
A	Dose 1	122	1	0	123
A	Dose 2	132	0	0	132
A	Dose 3	105	1	2	108
B	Placebo	128	0	2	130
B	Dose 1	113	2	3	118
B	Dose 2	129	1	0	130
B	Dose 3	111	0	2	113
C	Placebo	112	3	0	115
C	Dose 1	111	4	0	115
C	Dose 2	108	2	0	110
C	Dose 3	95	10	0	105
D	Placebo	118	10	1	129
D	Dose 1	112	7	4	123
D	Dose 2	106	14	2	122
D	Dose 3	110	7	2	119
E	Placebo	128	6	3	137
E	Dose 1	106	8	2	116
E	Dose 2	123	10	2	135
E	Dose 3	98	11	5	114

1. Incidence Density

Since the exact times of withdrawal from the study or occurrence of the adverse event were not known, those events were regarded as happening (on average) halfway through the appropriate time interval. Time at risk was then calculated over all patients by summing the weeks of the completed intervals and half the weeks from intervals where an AE occurred or a patient withdrew from the

Table 15 4 × 3 Table of Treatment vs. Adverse Event Occurrence

Treatment	AE occurrences			Total
	0	1	≥2	
Placebo	607	20	7	634
Low dose	564	22	9	595
Middle dose	598	27	4	629
High dose	519	29	11	559
Total	2288	98	31	2417

Table 16   Patient Outcome and Incidence Density Calculations

Study	Treatment outcome	Interval ending at week						Completed study	Weeks of study	Time at risk	Incidence density
		2	4	6	8	12	16				
A	Reference										
	AE	4	0	0	—	—	—				
	Withdrawn	29	6	1	—	—	—	245	6	1526	.0026
	Test drug										
	AE	2	0	0	—	—	—				
	Withdrawn	33	0	3	—	—	—	235	6	1460	.0014
B	Reference										
	AE	4	1	0	—	—	—				
	Withdrawn	32	1	3	—	—	—	251	6	1563	.0032
	Test drug										
	AE	4	0	1	—	—	—				
	Withdrawn	24	4	3	—	—	—	230	6	1440	.0035
C	Reference										
	AE	7	1	—	—	—	—				
	Withdrawn	50	3	—	—	—	—	209	4	905	.0088
	Test drug										
	AE	10	1	—	—	—	—				
	Withdrawn	52	0	—	—	—	—	217	4	933	.0118
D	Reference										
	AE	—	6	—	6	11	3				
	Withdrawn	—	25	—	3	5	0	206	16	3614	.0066
	Test drug										
	AE	—	8	—	6	7	0				
	Withdrawn	—	23	—	0	7	0	240	16	4078	.0049
E	Reference										
	AE	—	16	—	6	2	3				
	Withdrawn	—	19	—	4	4	0	242	16	4104	.0065
	Test drug										
	AE	—	10	—	5	3	2				
	Withdrawn	—	24	—	1	2	0	213	16	3590	.0056

study. The incidence density was calculated for each of the two treatment groups for each study as (number of events/time at risk). Relative to the hypothesis of no association between treatment and event occurrence, and using the Poisson distribution for AE frequency, for study A, $E(n_t) = ((4 + 2) \times 1526)/(1526 + 1460) = 2.93$, and $V(n_t) = ((4 + 2) \times 1526 \times 1460)/(1526 + 1460)^2 = 1.50$. The M-H statistic was calculated using this method for the Poisson distribution, as discussed earlier (Section III.B). M-H χ^2 (with 1 df) was 0.679, with p value of .410.

2. Life Table Methods

The SAS procedure LIFETEST was used to calculate life table statistics. In determining time at risk, LIFETEST uses an estimated number of patients at risk for each of the respective time intervals. This quantity is the sum of all patients completing the interval, patients experiencing the event in the interval, and one half the patients withdrawing during the interval. Patients who completed a study were viewed as having withdrawn from the study during the day after the end of the study (within 0.14 week). To standardize the end points of the intervals for all studies, the events occurring between weeks 4 and 8 in studies D and E were

Table 17   Life Table Survival Estimates from SAS Procedure LIFETEST

Study	Interval (weeks)	Number failed (with AE)	Number withdrawn	Effective sample size	Conditional probability of AE	No AE to beginning of interval
A	0–4	6	68	524.0	.0115	1.0000
	4–4.14	0	0	484.0		0.9885
	4.14–6	0	4	482.0		0.9885
	6–6.14	0	480	240.0		0.9885
B	0–4	9	61	527.5	.0171	1.0000
	4–4.14	0	0	488.0		0.9829
	4.14–6	1	6	485.0	.00206	0.9829
	6–6.14	0	481	240.5		0.9809
C	0–4	19	105	497.5	.0382	1.0000
	4–4.14	0	426	213.0		0.9618
D	0–4	14	48	532.0	.0263	1.0000
	4–4.14	0	0	494.0		0.9737
	4.14–6	6	2	493.0	.0122	0.9737
	6–6.14	0	0	486.0		0.9618
	6.14–8	6	1	485.5	.0124	0.9618
	8–8.14	0	0	479.0		0.9499
	8.14–12	18	12	473.0	.0381	0.9499
	12–16	3	0	449.0	.00668	0.9138
	16–16.14	0	446	223.0		0.9077
E	0–4	26	43	534.5	.0486	1.0000
	4–4.14	0	0	487.0		0.9514
	4.14–6	5	2	486.0	.0103	0.9514
	6–6.14	0	0	480.0		0.9416
	6.14–8	6	3	478.5	.0125	0.9416
	8–8.14	0	0	471.0		0.9298
	8.14–12	5	6	468.0	.0107	0.9298
	12–16	5	0	460.0	.0109	0.9198
	16–16.14	0	455	227.5		0.9098

equally divided between weeks 4–6 and weeks 6–8, and 4, 6, 8, 12, and 16 weeks were used as the applicable end points of the interval. The life table results for the pooled treatment groups are shown in Table 17. The results for the log-rank (Mantel–Haenszel) tests from the procedure LIFETEST are shown in Table 18.

3. Piecewise Exponential Model

A Poisson regression analysis was used to estimate parameters in a piecewise exponential model for incidence densities like those in Table 16. For each patient, the time at risk was defined as the length (in weeks) of each completed interval or one half the length of an interval in which the patient withdrew from the study or experienced the adverse event for the first time. For each interval, the number of events and sums of time at risk were then determined for the patients in each subpopulation with respect to the study by treatment by sex by age category cross-classification. After multiplication of the times at risk by 100 to simulate Poisson distributions (see Ref. 29), these quantities were then analyzed in a (numerator/denominator) model with the SAS procedure LOGIS-TIC. The model included explanatory variables for study, treatment, sex, age category, and time interval. The results are shown in Table 19. (The estimate for the intercept was obtained by adding $\log_e$ (100) to the value of -11.8663 obtained from the LOGISTIC procedure in order to remove the influence of the multiplication of the times at risk by 100.)

As in previously described analyses, age category is significant, with the rate of AE occurrence for older patients being $\exp(0.7082) = 2.03$ times higher than that for younger patients. There were significantly lower rates of occurrence in the later time intervals than in the first; for instance, in the 4- to 8-week interval, the rate of AE occurrence is 0.47 times lower than in the 0- to 4-week interval.

C. Example 3: Illustration Using Multiple Occurrence Data

Finally, to take into account multiple occurrences of the event experienced by individual patients, a ratio of a weighted mean of AE occurrences to a weighted mean of time at risk was formed, where the mean was calculated over all patients within each study, and then over all studies. The time at risk was calculated as

Table 18 Univariate Log-Rank Tests from SAS Procedure LIFETEST

Variable	Test statistic	Standard deviation	χ^2	$Pr > \chi^2$
Treatment	5.1354	5.6704	0.8202	0.3651
Sex	−9.0996	5.6777	2.5686	0.1090
Age category	−23.3704	5.4027	18.7119	0.0001

Table 19 Analysis of Maximum Likelihood Estimates for Piecewise Exponential Model from SAS Procedure LOGISTIC

Variable	Parameter estimate	Standard error	Wald χ^2	Pr $> \chi^2$	Standardized estimate
Intercept	−7.2611	0.5083	544.8830	0.0001	
Study B	0.5909	0.5076	1.3552	0.2444	0.118881
Study C	1.6646	0.4746	12.3032	0.0005	0.235131
Study D	1.6470	0.4395	14.0442	0.0002	0.418740
Study E	1.6398	0.4397	13.9110	0.0002	0.417227
Treatment	−0.1383	0.1762	0.6163	0.4324	−0.038122
Sex	0.2639	0.1776	2.2074	0.1374	0.072746
Age category	0.7082	0.1761	16.1767	0.0001	0.185779
4–8 weeks	−0.7479	0.2412	9.6117	0.0019	−0.191023
8–12 weeks	−0.5426	0.2550	4.5302	0.0333	−0.106618
12–16 weeks	−1.5817	0.3828	17.0750	0.0001	−0.308605

the sum of completed intervals and one half the sum of intervals in which a patient withdrew from the study. (No patients with AEs withdrew before the completion of the study; had they withdrawn, their time at risk would have been determined in the same way as for those who withdrew and had no adverse events.) Table 20 shows the calculations for total events and total time at risk in each study.

The weight for study A was (285 × 273)/(285 + 273) divided by (285 × 273)/(285 + 273) + (292 × 266)/(292 + 266) + (270 × 280)/(270 + 280) + (265 × 291)/(265 + 291) + (296 × 260)/(296 + 260) or 139.435/693.200 = 0.20015. The weighted values for the portion of f and g (ratio numerator and denominator) due to study A for the reference group were 0.00423 and 1.09114, respectively, and the ratio across all studies for the reference group was R_r = 0.061359/8.72658 = 0.0070. For the patients on the test drug, R_t = 0.056255/8.73963 = 0.0064. The weights and numerator and denominator values for each study are displayed in Table 21.

For the reference group, the variance of the numerator was $V(f_r)$ = 5.739 × 10^{-5}, the variance of the denominator was $V(g_r)$ = 5.378 × 10^{-3}, and the covariance between them was Cov(f_r, g_r) = 5.096 × 10^{-5}. For the test drug group, $V(f_t)$ = 6.049 × 10^{-5}, $V(g_t)$ = 5.550 × 10^{-3}, and Cov(f_t, g_t) = 4.4787 × 10^{-5}. The variances of the two ratios, then, were $V(R_r)$ = 7.477 × 10^{-7} and $V(R_t)$ = 7.874 × 10^{-7}. Because of the large sample size, $Z = (R_t - R_r)/[V(R_t) + V(R_r)]^{1/2}$ is approximately normally distributed and is equal to −0.489, with a two-sided p value of .631. Thus, for the combined studies, the weighted rates of

Table 20 Total Event and Time at Risk Calculations for Ratio Estimate

Study	Treatment	No. patients	Outcome	Total events	End of interval	Time at risk	Total time
					Time (weeks)		
A	Reference	29	Withdrawn	0	2	1	29
		6	Withdrawn	0	4	3	18
		1	Withdrawn	0	6	5	5
		245	No AE	0	6	6	1470
		2	1 AE	2	6	6	12
		2	2 AE	4	6	6	12
Totals		285		6			1546
A	Test drug	33	Withdrawn	0	2	1	33
		3	Withdrawn	0	6	5	15
		235	No AE	0	6	6	1410
		1	1 AE	1	6	6	6
		1	2 AE	2	6	6	6
Totals		273		3			1470
B	Reference	32	Withdrawn	0	2	1	32
		1	Withdrawn	0	4	3	3
		3	Withdrawn	0	6	5	15
		251	No AE	0	6	6	1506
		2	1 AE	2	6	6	12
		3	2 AE	6	6	6	18
Totals		292		8			1586
B	Test drug	24	Withdrawn	0	2	1	24
		4	Withdrawn	0	4	3	12
		3	Withdrawn	0	6	5	15
		230	No AE	0	6	6	1380
		1	1 AE	1	6	6	6
		4	2 AE	8	6	6	24
Totals		266		9			1461
C	Reference	50	Withdrawn	0	2	1	50
		3	Withdrawn	0	4	3	9
		209	No AE	0	4	4	836
		8	1 AE	8	4	4	32
Totals		270		8			927
C	Test drug	52	Withdrawn	0	2	1	52
		217	No AE	0	4	4	868
		11	1 AE	11	4	4	44
Totals		280		11			964

Table 20 (*Continued*)

Study	Treatment	No. patients	Outcome	Total events	Time (weeks) End of interval	Time (weeks) Time at risk	Time (weeks) Total time
D	Reference	25	Withdrawn	0	4	2	50
		3	Withdrawn	0	8	6	18
		5	Withdrawn	0	12	10	50
		206	No AE	0	16	16	3296
		21	1 AE	21	16	16	336
		4	2 AE	8	16	16	64
		1	3 AE	3	16	16	16
Totals		265		32			3830
D	Test drug	23	Withdrawn	0	4	2	46
		7	Withdrawn	0	12	10	70
		240	No AE	0	16	16	3840
		17	1 AE	17	16	16	272
		4	2 AE	8	16	16	64
Totals		291		25			4292
E	Reference	19	Withdrawn	0	4	2	38
		4	Withdrawn	0	8	6	24
		4	Withdrawn	0	12	10	40
		242	No AE	0	16	16	3872
		22	1 AE	22	16	16	352
		5	2 AE	10	16	16	80
Totals		296		32			4406
E	Test drug	24	Withdrawn	0	4	2	48
		1	Withdrawn	0	8	6	6
		2	Withdrawn	0	12	10	20
		213	No AE	0	16	16	3408
		13	1 AE	13	16	16	208
		5	2 AE	10	16	16	80
		2	3 AE	6	16	16	32
Totals		260		29			3802

events per week at risk are similar for the two treatments. Additionally, one can note that $\log_e(R_t/R_r) = 0.0883$ and $\mathrm{Var}\{\log_e(R_t/R_r)\} = \mathrm{Var}(R_t)/R_t^2 + \mathrm{Var}(R_r)/R_r^2 = 0.0341$; and so a .95 confidence interval for the ratio of weighted rates of events per week at risk for the two treatments is $\exp\{(-0.088) \pm 1.96\sqrt{0.0341}\}$ or (0.64, 1.31). The advantage of this confidence interval is that it quantifies the degree of similarity of the weighted rates of events per week at risk for the two treatments.

Table 21 Weights and Contributions to the Ratio Numerator and Denominator for each Study

Study	Weight	Reference group contribution to		Test group contribution to	
		Numerator	Denominator	Numerator	Denominator
A	0.20115	0.00423	1.091	0.00221	1.083
B	0.20080	0.00550	1.091	0.00679	1.103
C	0.19829	0.00588	0.681	0.00780	0.683
D	0.20008	0.02416	2.892	0.01719	2.951
E	0.19968	0.02159	2.972	0.02227	2.920

V. DISCUSSION

Meta-analysis is a useful strategy in the analysis of drug safety data, particularly when the sample size in individual studies is insufficient to allow a meaningful interpretation. There are several issues to keep in mind while performing a meta-analysis, such as which studies to include and how much weight to give to each one, but the statistical methods for the most part are very straightforward. In many cases, methods that are used in multicenter clinical trials can be adapted for use in meta-analysis. The methods presented in this chapter take into account some of the difficulties common in drug safety data such as varying time at risk and multiple occurrences of an adverse event in individual patients.

REFERENCES

1. Glass GV. Primary, secondary, and meta-analysis of research. *Educ Res.* 1976;5: 3–8.
2. Peto R. Why do we need systematic overviews of randomized trials? *Stat Med.* 1987;6:233–240.
3. Chalmers TC, Buyse ME. Meta-analysis. In: Chalmers T. ed. *Data Analysis for Clinical Medicine: The Quantitative Approach to Patient Care in Gastoenterology.* Rome: International University Press; 1988:75–84.
4. Light RJ. Accumulating evidence from independent studies: What we can win and what we can lose. *Stat Med.* 1987;6:221–228.
5. Bulpitt CJ. Medical statistics: meta-analysis. *Lancet.* 1988;2:93–94.
6. Einarson TR. Meta-analysis of the pharmacotherapy literature. In: Hartzema AB, Porta M, Tilson HH. eds. *Pharmacoepidemiology: An Introduction.* 2nd ed. Cincinnati: Harvey Whitney; 1991:236–268.
7. Elashoff JD, Koch GG. Statistical methods in trials of anti-ulcer drugs. In: Swabb E, Szabo S. eds. *Ulcer Disease: Investigation and Basis for Therapy.* New York: Marcel Dekker; 1990:375–406.
8. Wachter KW. Disturbed by meta-analysis? *Science.* 1988;241:1407–1408.

9. Hedges L, Olkin I. *Statistical Method for Meta-analysis*. New York: Academic Press; 1985.
10. DerSimonian R, Laird N. Meta-analysis in clinical trials. *Controlled Clin Trials*. 1986;7:177–188.
11. Bailey KR. Interstudy differences: how should they influence the interpretation and analysis of results? *Stat Med*. 1987;6:351–358.
12. Schmid JE, Koch GG, LaVange LM. An overview of statistical issues and methods of meta-analysis. *J Biopharm Stat*. 1991;1(1):103–120.
13. Gail M, Simon R. Testing for qualitative interaction between treatment effects and patient subsets. *Biometrics*. 1985;6:341–348.
14. O'Neill RT. Assessment of safety. In: Peace KE. ed. *Biopharmaceutical Statistics for Drug Development*. New York: Marcel Dekker; 1988:543–604.
15. Koch GG. Discussion: statistical perspective. *Drug Inf J*. 1991;25(3):461–464.
16. Edwards S, Koch GG, Sollecito WA, Peace KE. Summarization, analysis, and monitoring of adverse events. In: Peace KE. ed. *Statistical Issues in Drug Research and Development*. New York: Marcel Dekker; 1990:19–170.
17. Whitehead A, Whitehead J. A general parametric approach to the meta-analysis of randomized clinical trials. *Stat Med*. 1991;10:1665–1677.
18. Chevart B. A nonparametric model for multiple recurrences. *Appl Stat*. 1988;37(2):157–168.
19. Thall PF, Lachin JM. Analysis of recurrent events: Non-parametric methods for random-interval count data. *J Am Stat Assoc*. 1988;83(402):339–347.
20. Enas GG. Making decisions about safety in clinical trials; the case for inferential statistics. *Drug Inf J*. 1991;25(3):439–446.
21. Huster WJ. Clinical trial adverse events: the case for descriptive statistics. *Drug Inf J*. 1991;25(3):447–456.
22. D'Agostino RB, Heeren TC. Multiple comparisons in over-the-counter drug clinical trials with both positive and placebo controls. *Stat Med*. 1991;10(1):1–6.
23. SAS/STAT Users Guide. version 6. 4th ed. vols 1 and 2. Cary, NC: SAS Institute; 1990.
24. StatXact. Statistical software for exact nonparametric inference. User Manual. version 2. Cambridge, MA: Cytel Software Corporation; 1991.
25. Fleiss JL. *The Design and Analysis of Clinical Experiments*. New York: Wiley; 1986.
26. Koch GG, Edwards SE. Clinical efficacy trials with categorical data. In: Peace KE. ed. *Biopharmaceutical Statistics for Drug Development*. New York: Marcel Dekker; 1988:403–457.
27. Kleinbaum DG, Kupper LL, Morgenstern H. *Epidemiologic Research: Principles and Quantitative Methods*. New York: Van Nostrand Reinhold; 1982:98–115.
28. Harris EK, Albert A. *Survivorship Analysis and Clinical Studies*. New York: Marcel Dekker; 1991:1–54.
29. Vine MF, Schoenbach VJ, Hulka BS, Koch GG, Samsa G. A typical metaplasia and incidence of bronchogenic carcinoma. *Am J Epidemiol*. 1990;131:781–793.

12

Design and Analysis Considerations for Safety Data, Particularly Adverse Events

Karl E. Peace

Biopharmaceutical Research Consultants, Inc.
Ann Arbor, Michigan

I.   INTRODUCTION

In the clinical development of drugs for which it is possible to design trials to provide definitive information on aspects of safety, there are few, if any, issues. One would develop the protocol. The protocol would include a background section, an objective section, a plan of study section, a data analysis section, an administrative section, and a bibliography (see the Appendix). The plan of study would include description of the study population, description of the study design, and criteria regarding dealing with problem management. The data analysis section would include criteria for defining safety end points, would address statistical design considerations, would address early termination considerations, if any, and would specify their statistical methods and their appropriateness for use in summarizing and/or analyzing the end points [1]. The administration section of the protocol would include the review and consent requirements, record keeping, and details regarding monitoring.

In my experience, there have been a number of occasions when it has been possible to design trials to provide definitive information about safety objectives. As a first example, in the clinical development of a new antibiotic, a skin rash was observed among several patients at the top dose of a phase II dose comparison trial. Since the top dose appeared to be more efficacious, a trial was subsequently designed and executed to confirm the rash experience before deciding to terminate the top dose from further clinical development. In designing the follow-up trial, the phase II dose comparison trial was considered as a pilot study for the purpose of sample size estimation. The safety trial consisted of a single arm of the top dose, incorporated sequential procedures as discussed by Armitage [2], and required 47 patients for confirmation of the skin rash. The decision was subsequently made to terminate the top dose from clinical development.

A second example was a clinical trial designed and conducted to assess the hypokalemia potential of two doses, 25 mg (B) and 50 mg (C) of hydrochlorothiazide, and 25 mg of hydrochlorothiazide plus 50 mg of triamterene (A). The definition of hypokalemia was serum potassium concentration less than or equal to 3.5 mEq/L. The protocol required patients with mild to moderate hypertension to be treated for 6 months. Analyses of the data were to be performed starting at 6 weeks of treatment. Approximately 171 patients per group were needed to detect a 10% difference in the incidences of hypokalemia among any two regimens with a type 1 error rate of 5% and a power of 80%. The outcome of the trial after 6 weeks of treatment is reflected by the ordering $A < B < C$. That is, the combination exhibited a lower incidence of hypokalemia than 25 mg of hydrochlorothiazide alone, which in turn exhibited a lower incidence than the 50-mg dose of hydrochlorothiazide alone.

As a third example, the phase III clinical development plan for a new antihypertensive compound included a forced-titration, placebo-controlled dose comparison trial, a trial comparing once vs. twice a day administration of the target dose, and a positive control trial against the target dose. Although the latter trial would furnish antihypertensive efficacy information on the target dose of the new drug relative to the positive control, the aim of the positive control trial was to provide a marketing hook. It was thought that patients on the new drug were less likely than patients on the positive control to experience "hypertensive rebound" or "blood pressure overshoot" when therapy was withdrawn. Briefly, design considerations consisted of an initial phase representing 6 months of treatment to control blood pressure, followed by a phase where the antihypertensive compound was withdrawn and blood pressure subsequently monitored for up to 7 days for overshoot. The number of patients required qualitatively was the number necessary to discriminate between the two regimens in terms of overshoot inflated to account for the proportions expected to be controlled over the first phase.

II. EFFICACY TRIALS PRIOR TO MARKET APPROVAL

The previous three examples illustrate areas where it was possible to design clinical trials to provide definitive information on aspects of safety. However, for most drugs, particularly premarket approval ones, it is not possible to do so. Some reasons are (a) inadequate information to formulate the safety objective or question, (b) inadequate information to specify the primary safety end points, and (c) inadequate information to characterize the target population. Even if the end points are specified, the question formulated, and the target population identified, there is usually inadequate information on estimates of end points for sample size determination. In addition, even if the end points are specified, the question formulated, the target population identified, and sufficient information exists to determine adequate sample sizes, logistical and/or financial difficulties usually preclude conducting a trial that large.

Therefore, a rational position to take in the development of new drugs is to design trials to provide definitive information about efficacy, to monitor safety and describe the safety profile in each trial, and to accumulate and describe the safety profile across trials [3]. This position is consistent with the statutory requirement for new drug, regulatory approval in the United States by the Food and Drug Administration (FDA), which is to provide both clinical and statistical evidence of efficacy and to adequately describe the safety profile. It is thus reasonable to expect that a new drug application (NDA), which contains clinical and statistical evidence of the claimed efficacy effects and an adequate description of the safety profile, which in itself represents no unacceptable safety concerns, would be given regulatory approval to be marketed in the United States.

U.S. regulatory requirements for new drug development allow the sponsor to proceed along the lines indicated by two axioms of drug development: (a) drugs in development are considered nonefficacious until proven otherwise; (b) drugs in development are considered safe until proven otherwise. From the statistician's viewpoint, axiom 1 identifies the null hypothesis (HOE) to be "the drug is nonefficacious" and identifies the alternative hypothesis (HAE) to be "the drug is efficacious." Axiom 2 identifies the null hypothesis (HOS) to be "the drug is safe" and identifies the alternative hypothesis (HAS) to be "the drug is not safe."

For a sponsor's drug to be approved as being efficacious, enough information must be accumulated to contradict the null hypothesis (HOE). This implies that the type #1 error is synonymous with the regulatory decision risk regarding approval for efficacy and that the type 2 error is synonymous with the sponsor's risk of failing to detect a truly efficacious drug [4,5]. For the drug to be approved with a decision as to safety, the null hypothesis (HOS) must not be contradicted by the available safety information. This implies that the type #2 error is synonymous with regulatory decision risk regarding approval whereas the type #1 error is synonymous with the sponsor's risk.

III. NATURE OF SAFETY INFORMATION FROM EFFICACY TRIALS

If trials in the clinical development of new drugs are designed to provide definitive information about efficacy rather than safety, it is imperative to consider the quality of safety information from such trials. As a definition, a trial will be regarded as being designed to provide definitive evidence of efficacy if it has a power of 95% to detect a clinically important difference between the target and reference regimens with a false-positive rate of 5% in terms of the primary response measure. For discussion purposes, the clinically important difference is taken as 20% and the response variable is assumed to be dichotomous. A dichotomous response variable for efficacy assessment allows a natural connection between the efficacy end point and safety end points such as the proportion of patients who experience adverse events.

The number of patients required per regimen for a trial defined in terms of these characteristics will range anywhere from 125 to 164 patients, depending on whether one takes the viewpoint that the alternative hypothesis is one- or two-sided [6] and also whether one adopts the worst case of the variance or adopts a position less conservative. It is important to note that a trial designed in the manner described above to detect a δ% difference between two regimens will permit the statistical detection (at the .05 nominal level) of a difference as small as one half δ% at the analysis stage.

However, a trial designed definitively in this manner is very unlikely to be able to furnish any information about an extremely rare event. For example, if the fraction of a population who would develop an adverse experience upon treatment with a drug at a given dose were 0.1%, one would require 4604 (Table 1) patients to be treated with the drug at the given dose in order to be 99% confident of observing at least one patient with a particular adverse experience. If one required a greater degree of certainty, say 99.99%, about 10,000 patients would require treatment. In fact, the definitively designed efficacy trial would not enable one to detect any adverse experiences with certainty that would occur less frequently than in 6% of the treated population.

Taking a trial with 150 patients per arm as representative of the definitively designed efficacy trial, one is not likely to observe in such a trial any patient experiencing a rare adverse event. For example, the probability of observing no patient with an adverse experience among 150 treated patients given that the true incidence in the population is 0.1% is .681. It is therefore highly likely that the outcome of such a trial will be 0 divided by 150, i.e., an incidence of 0% among those patients treated. A corresponding exact 95% confidence interval based on this outcome ranges from 0% to 2.4%. If what was known about the mechanism of action, the pharmacology, and/or the toxicology of the drug suggested certain untoward adverse events were possible, and one monitored specifically for such events in a definitively designed efficacy trial, the fact that no such events were observed among 150 treated patients would probably be insufficient for regulatory approval in view of the upper limit of the 95% confidence interval being 2.4%.

For adverse events that would happen in 6% or greater of the population, the typical definitively designed trial for efficacy would permit discrimination be-

Table 1 Number of Patients Required to be Treated with a Dose of a Drug in Order to be $100(1 - \alpha)\%$ Confident of Observing at Least One Adverse Experience (AE) Given That the True Fraction (P) Who Would Develop AEs in the Population is P

P	$(1 - \alpha)$: 0.90	0.95	0.99	0.999	0.9999
.001	2302	2995	4604	6906	9208
.005	460	599	920	1380	1840
.01	230	300	460	690	920
.015	153	200	306	459	612
.02	114	149	228	342	456
.03	76	99	152	218	304
.04	57	75	114	171	228
.05	45	59	90	135	180
.06	38	50	76	114	152
.07	32	42	64	96	128
.08	28	37	56	84	112
.09	25	33	50	75	100
.10	22	29	44	66	88
.15	15	20	30	45	60
.20	11	15	22	33	44
.30	7	10	14	21	28
.40	5	7	10	15	20
.50	4	6	8	12	16

tween two arms of approximately a 20% difference in the incidences of adverse experiences with a power of 95% and a nominal false-positive rate of 5% or, alternatively, discrimination between two arms of approximately a 10% difference with a power of 50% and a nominal false-positive rate of 5%. The latter quantifies the smallest observed difference at the analysis stage, which would be indicative of a real difference.

IV. MONITORING THE CLINICAL DEVELOPMENT PROGRAM FOR SAFETY

Since a trial designed to provide definitive efficacy information is not likely to provide much information about safety, it therefore becomes highly important to monitor all trials of new drugs for safety. Some reasons are the following: (a) It is in the patient's best interest, i.e., ideally one would want to know the earliest possible moment when anything untoward began to happen to the patient so that appropriate medical procedures could be initiated. (b) It is also in the primary investigator's best interest. (c) It is certainly in the sponsor's best interest in terms of credibility and to prompt reporting to the regulatory agency, and also to minimize legal consequences. However, there are logistical difficulties in monitoring trials for safety (or efficacy) information. These may depend on (a) the frequency of follow-up patient visits, (b) the rate of patient accession, (c) the data collection instrument, (d) the quality of the collection of data, (e) the staff of field monitors, (f) the ability to rapidly generate a quantity-assured database in an ongoing manner, (g) the ability to rapidly generate appropriate displays, summaries, or analyses, (h) the identification of who will make decisions based on such reviews, and (i) possibly other committees as well. Kamm et al. [7] provide an excellent reference on organizational structure reflecting the logistics of being able to rapidly monitor a trial (ticlopidine aspirin stroke study, or TASS) for safety. Briefly, the TASS trial was parallel, was stratified by sex, cardiovascular history, previous stroke, and was quadruply blinded. Organizational structure consisted of an operations committee, a randomization center, a drug distribution center, clinical centers, a central laboratory, an end-point review committee, an interim statistical analysis group, a safety committee that interacted with the FDA and the investigational review board, and a policy committee.

V. STATISTICAL METHODOLOGY

Given that the logistics for monitoring a trial for safety can be put in place, what should be the appropriate analysis or summarization methodology for generating information to be reviewed? First of all, one should distinguish between methodology that might be used for rare events vs. methodology that might be used for common events. For rare events, each event is important, especially if untoward. Procedures aimed at comparing treatment regimens may not be revealing, particularly from individual trials designed for efficacy. Therefore a simple descriptor such as the ratio of the number of patients experiencing the event to the number of patients exposed to treatment may be more appropriate. As more information accumulates, time-to-event methods may be applied as well as some type of meta-analytical techniques that would combine information across trials.

For common events, statistical methodology should be based on confidence intervals. Confidence intervals are statistically more appropriate than hypothesis testing in the absence of design considerations for safety. They also utilize the observed incidence as well as the estimate of the variability of the observed incidence. Confidence intervals should also better facilitate a decision by an informed reviewer. For a two-sided confidence interval with a large confidence coefficient, the lower limit being greater than 0 might represent the drug not being safe, whereas the upper limit, if small enough, might permit a conclusion of proof of safety. This would be particularly true if one were able to set an acceptable safety limit [8]. If the upper limit of the confidence interval with a large confidence coefficient were in fact less than the acceptable safety limit, then proof of safety would be indicated; whereas the lower confidence limit exceeding the acceptable safety limit would be indicative of proof of being not safe. In the utilization of confidence intervals, the confidence level (the compliment of the type-1 error) must be chosen. In addition, statistical rigor would require that the confidence level be preserved or adjusted if multiple or interim analyses are performed. However, it may not be so important to preserve the confidence level or the type-1 error, particularly if "absolute safety" of the sponsor's compound alone is of interest. Presumably, one would want to know the first moment when the accumulated information on an untoward event was different from that of untreated patients at *some* level of confidence. If, however, it is important to preserve the type-1 error, then there are procedures to do so. Most incorporate group sequential methods. Jennison and Turnbull [9] provide an excellent reference.

A. Direct Comparison

In using confidence intervals to display and to help monitor adverse experience information in clinical trials of new drugs, the more traditional approach would be to directly compare two regimens. The aim of the comparison would be to provide estimates of the *difference* between regimen incidences. To construct a two-sided $100(1 - 2\alpha)\%$ confidence interval on the true difference on incidences of adverse experiences between two regimens, one would proceed as follows: Let P_i and P_j denote the true incidences of some adverse event in the populations to be treated with the i and j regimens, respectively; let $\hat{P}_i$ and $\hat{P}_j$ denote the corresponding observed incidences among N_i and N_j treated patients, respectively; then the difference, $\hat{\delta}_{ij} = \hat{P}_i - \hat{P}_j$, in observed incidences would represent the estimate of the difference in true incidences; the estimate of the variance of the observed difference is given by $\hat{V}_i + \hat{V}_j$, where $\hat{V}_i$ is the estimate of the variance of the observed incidence in the i regimen given by $\hat{P}_i(1 - \hat{P}_i)/N_i$. The confidence interval can be represented as

$$\hat{L}_{ij} \leq P_i - P_j \leq \hat{U}_{ij} \tag{1}$$

where $\hat{L}_{ij}$ is the lower limit and $\hat{U}_{ij}$ is the upper limit. The limits may be specified as

$$\hat{L}_{ij} = \hat{P}_i - \hat{P}_j - Z\alpha(\hat{V}_i + \hat{V}_j)^{1/2} \tag{2}$$

$$\hat{U}_{ij} = \hat{P}_i - \hat{P}_j + Z\alpha(\hat{V}_i + \hat{V}_j)^{1/2} \tag{3}$$

where $Z\alpha$ is the upper $100 1(1 - \alpha)$ percentile of the distribution (assumed symmetrical) of $\hat{P}_i - \hat{P}_j$ under the assumption of no difference in true incidences.

The direct comparison of two regimens via $100(1 - 2\alpha)\%$ confidence intervals also permits concluding that two regimens are different. If the lower limit L_{ij} were positive (presuming that the observed incidence in the ith regimen exceeded the observed incidence in the jth regimen), one would conclude that the two regimens were different at the nominal significance level α.

B.   Indirect Comparison Methodology

Another approach may be thought of as an indirect comparison of two regimens. The primary or initial aim of the approach is to provide estimates of the true incidences of each regimen. Let P_i, P_j, $\hat{P}_i$, $\hat{P}_j$, N_i, N_j, and $\hat{V}_i$ and $\hat{V}_j$ be identified as before. A two-sided $100(1 - 2\alpha_1)\%$ confidence interval on the true incidence P_i in the i regimen is

$$\hat{L}_i \leq P_i \leq \hat{U}_i \tag{4}$$

where $\hat{L}_i$ is the lower limit and $\hat{U}_i$ the upper limit. The limits are given by

$$\hat{L}_i = \hat{P}_i - Z\alpha_1(\hat{V}_i)^{1/2} \tag{5}$$

$$\hat{U}_i = \hat{P}_i + Z\,\alpha_1(\hat{V}_i)^{1/2} \tag{6}$$

where $Z\alpha_1$ is the $100(1 - \alpha_1)$ percentile of the distribution of $\hat{P}_i - \hat{P}_j$ under the assumption that $P_i = P_j$.

In addition to such confidence intervals furnishing information on the true incidence in each regimen, they also permit two regimens to be indirectly compared. One would be able to say that regimens i and j were statistically different at the nominal significance level α_1 if the lower limit of the $100(1 - 2\alpha_1)\%$ confidence interval on the true incidence of regimen i was greater than the upper limit of regimen j, i.e., if $\hat{L}_i > \hat{U}_j$ where again the observed incidence in the ith regimen was greater than the observed incidence in the jth regimen.

The direct comparison and the indirect comparison methods connect. To illustrate, think of the null hypothesis as no difference in true incidences (H_0: $P_i = P_j$) among the regimens, and the alternative hypothesis as there is a difference (H_a: $P_i > P_j$). The rejection rule for the direct comparison method is: the incidence of regimen i statistically exceeds that of regimen j at the significance level α if $L_{ij} > 0$. The rejection rule for the indirect comparison method is: the incidence of regimen i statistically exceeds that of regimen j at the significance level α_1 if $L_i > U_j$, presuming that $P_i > P_j$. The equivalence of the rejection rules is expressed as

$$Z\alpha_1 = \left(\frac{(\hat{V}_i)^{1/2} + (\hat{V}_j)^{1/2}}{(\hat{V}_i + \hat{V}_j)^{1/2}} \right)^{-1} Z\alpha \tag{7}$$

That is, they are equivalent if the relationship between the critical point for the indirect comparison is proportional to the critical point for the direct comparison, where the proportionality constant is that ratio of the variances given in Eq. (7). As an example, under the null hypothesis of no difference and equal sample sizes, the critical point corresponding to the indirect comparison would be 1, divided by the square root of 2, times the critical point for the direct comparison. For the specified case where α equals 5%, α_1 would be 12.24%. That is, if one were using a nominal 90% two-sided confidence interval to directly compare two regimens and the lower limit of that confidence interval exceeded 0, one would say with a confidence level of 95% or a type 1 error rate of 5% that the two regimens were in fact different. To reach the same decision using the indirect comparison, one would construct two-sided 75.53% confidence intervals on the true incidence in each regimen and require that the lower limit of one be greater than the upper limit of the other.

VI. SUMMARY

To summarize, it has been recognized that it may be possible to design some trials to provide definitive safety information. Three examples were presented where indeed that was the case. However, for most new drugs in clinical development it is not possible. Therefore, a rational approach is to design definitively for efficacy and monitor and *describe* safety. Parenthetically, if statistical inferential analyses are performed, Ref. 10 may be consulted. This position is in fact consistent with the statutory requirement for approval to market new drugs in the United States. Statistical procedures involving confidence intervals were also suggested for monitoring trials for safety.

In addition, the following suggestions and observations are made. (a) Since open trials do not permit unbiased comparisons of groups and positive controlled trials may reflect an upward bias, the primary assessment of safety should come from double-blind, placebo-controlled trials. (b) Ideally, the clinical development plan for a new compound should address plans for assessing efficacy *and* safety as characteristics of the drug. This should include developing how the null hypothesis that the drug is not efficacious (HOE) and the drug is safe (HOS) would be contradicted. The ideal development plan would also include procedures for monitoring each trial for safety as well as for monitoring the development plan as data accumulate across trials. (c) If rare adverse events are of interest, development plans should be designed to have a high probability of observing one or more events in each dose regimen; this may include postmarketing surveillance studies as well. (d) The preferred statistical methodology for monitoring and analyzing adverse experience data is per-regimen confidence intervals with large coefficients. This approach allows one to provide interval estimates on the true incidence of each regimen; permits sequential procedures such as those of Jennison and Turnbull to be incorporated; also permits sequential procedures such as those of Schultz et al. [11] or Fleming [12] to be incorporated regarding a decision to terminate any arm independent of other arms; and would minimize breaking the blind of studies. (e) The impact on ideal clinical development plans if a Hauck and Anderson [13] approach were taken to reverse the null and alternative hypotheses regarding safety should be investigated. That is, consider the null hypothesis to be "the drug is not safe" and the alternative hypothesis to be "the drug is safe." Such an approach would provide consistency between the regulatory risks for approval based on efficacy as well as on safety. (f) The impact on ideal clinical development plans, if we viewed efficacy and safety as compound hypotheses, should be investigated. That is, view the null hypotheses as "the drug is not efficacious and the drug is not safe" and the alternative hypothesis as "the drug is efficacious and the drug is safe." Other alternative hypotheses less stringent may also be proposed. (g) If we continue to design only for efficacy, what the total sample size provides in the way of safety information per trial and across trials in a particular clinical development plan should be explored. If this is sufficiently uninformative, then larger sample sizes may be called for. (h) Perhaps a safety review committee of impartial observers should be formulated. (i) Finally, since comparisons of groups are usually based on averages, two groups may have similar averages yet differ in the proportions of patients with higher/lower values [14]. Therefore ideally, each patient in each clinical trial conducted in the development of new drugs should be monitored for safety. When changes are noted that would give the physician concern, one should care for the patient and then assess whether such changes are different from those among untreated comparable patients. This in itself argues for accumulating large experimental databases on placebo-treated patients from placebo-controlled trials.

Appendix

Protocol Outline

I.   Background
II. Objective
III. Plan of Study
    3.1   Study population
        3.1.1   Demography
        3.1.2   Criteria for patient inclusion
        3.1.3   Criteria for patient exclusion
    3.2   Study design
        3.2.1   Type of study
        3.2.2   Assignment of treatment
        3.2.3   Blinding, dosage, and administration of study drugs
        3.2.4   Concomitant medications
        3.2.5   Procedures
            1.   Treatment period
            2.   Pretherapy
            3.   During treatment period
            4.   Posttherapy
            5.   Observers
            6.   Data recording
            7.   Dropouts
    3.3   Problem management
        3.3.1   Adverse reactions
        3.3.2   Criteria for discontinuing study drug

REFERENCES

1. Peace KE. Shortening the time for clinical drug development. *Reg Affairs*. 1991;3:3–22.
2. Armitage P. Sequential tests in prophylactic and therapeutic trials. *Quart J Med*. 1954;91:255–274.
3. Peace KE. Design, monitoring, and analysis issues relative to adverse events. *Drug Inf J*. 1987;21:21–28.
4. Peace KE. The alternative hypothesis: one-sided or two-sided? *J Clin Epidemiol*. 1989;42(5),473–476.
5. Peace KE. The alternative hypothesis: one-sided or two sided? A rejoinder. *J Clin Epidemiol*. 1991.
6. Peace KE. One-sided or two-sided P-values: which most appropriately address the question of drug efficacy? *J Biopharm Stat*. 1991;(1):133–138.
7. Kamm B, Maloney B, Cranston B, Roe R, Hassy W. Ticlopidine Aspirin Stroke Study organizational structure. Presented at Society for Controlled Clinical Trials May 13–16, 1984, Miami.
8. Bross ID. Why proof of safety is much more difficult than proof of hazard. *Biometrics*. 1985;41(3):785–793.
9. Jennison C, Turnbull BW. Repeated confidence intervals for group sequential trials. *Controlled Clin Trials*. 1984;5:33–45.
10. Edwards SE, Koch GG, Sollecito WA. Summarization of adverse experiences. In: Peace KE. ed., *Statistical Issues in Drug Research and Development*. 1989;19–150.
11. Schultz TR, Nichol FR, Elfring GL, Weed SD. Multiple stage procedures for drug screening. *Biometrics*. 1973;29:293–300.
12. Fleming TR. One-sample multiple testing procedure for phase II clinical trials. *Biometrics*. 1982;38:143–151.
13. Hauck WW, Anderson S. A new procedure for testing equivalence in comparative bioavailability and other clinical trials. *Commun Stat Theor Meth*. 1983;12:2663–2692.
14. Peace KE: Some comments on the Biopharmaceutical Section and Statistics. *ASA Proceedings Sesquicentennial Invited Paper Sessions*; 1989 and 1988;98–105.

13

Clinical Trial Adverse Drug Experience Reporting Requirements in the Major Countries: One Manufacturer's Approach

Max W. Talbott and Ellen D. Kelso

Eli Lilly and Company
Indianapolis, Indiana

I. INTRODUCTION

The requirements for collecting and reporting adverse drug experience (ADE) information from clinical trials are in a very dynamic state in the world's major countries. Stimulated in part by the increasingly complex nature of clinical trials and in part by political evolution (especially in Europe), some long-established requirements are even now still evolving, becoming generally more detailed and stringent as they develop.

Numerous researchers, among them Huster [1] and O'Neil [2], have described procedures and approaches for analyzing and reporting safety data from clinical trials. Most often these methods relate to the acquisition of clinical trial (CT) safety data for the ultimate registration dossier submissions. Little has been written on the subject of requirements and approaches for the collection and reporting (to regulatory agencies and participating investigators) of significant or serious adverse drug experiences occurring in premarket, clinical trials.

Though regulations covering the collection and reporting of clinical trial adverse events have been in place in the United States, the United Kingdom, and Europe for a number of years, only within the last 5 years have most of these rules attained some significant definition and substance. For example, in the United States, specific definition (and associated time frames) for reportable clinical trial adverse events date primarily from the so-called IND Rewrite of 1987. U.K. requirements were also updated in 1987, Canadian requirements in

1989, and Germany, at least in so far as the explanatory guidelines are concerned, in 1991.

Just as most of the major countries are now seeing increasing harmonization of the registration requirements for new products, so too are the various national requirements for the reporting of clinical trial adverse drug experiences becoming more similar. This form of harmonization most likely is the result of the increasing professional interaction of the staffs of the world's regulatory agencies as well as the ever more global nature of major pharmaceutical companies.

As Eli Lilly and Company has broadened its use of worldwide clinical trials, it has become abundantly clear that despite heroic efforts toward the harmonization of ADE reporting requirements (most notably the CIOMS Working Group I initiative [3]), there is still some divergence of requirements throughout the world for the reporting of adverse drug experiences from clinical trials. Thompson [4] commented on the advantage of harmonization, both in clinical trial and marketing authorization contexts:

> Regulatory harmonization is not meant to homogenize medical practice among all medical cultures. Cultures differ in their definition of health, diagnosis of disease, intensity of therapy, assessments of benefits, risk preferences, patient assertiveness and adherence to prescribed treatments, and physician surveillance of patient responses. Regulatory harmonization can minimize risks of clinical investigation and marketed use of new therapies, facilitate introduction of significant therapeutic advances, and lead to shared responsibility for scientific analysis of increasingly complex and voluminous clinical data.

In the following chapter, Eli Lilly's experience and understanding of trial event reporting rules, gleaned through a survey of the CT ADE reporting requirements in the major countries, will be presented. In addition, an approach will be described that the company has utilized to ensure that each affiliate (to include the U.S. headquarters affiliate) is made aware of significant CT events and complies with the national laws of the various host countries.

A. ADE Survey

Table 1 presents the CT ADE reporting requirements for Japan, Australia, United States, Canada, United Kingdom, France, Germany, Italy, Spain, and the Nordic countries. By way of a disclaimer, the reader is cautioned to verify the requirement representations made by this table. The consequences of failure to comply with ADE reporting rules are too serious for one to uncritically rely on anything other than specific government documents that detail the formal requirements for ADE reporting. To develop a global approach to CT ADE reporting, ''determiner requirements'' have been chosen by the authors from each of the categories of ADE requirements and have been graphically designated in Table 2 by heavy outlines. Once identified, these determiners described a "worse case" requirement for one to employ for standards as ADEs are collected from clinical trials around the world.

It is important to note that certain national reporting requirements make a distinction between ADEs originating from trials conducted within the country and those ADEs from trials outside the country. Invariably, when such distinctions are made, more stringent rules (i.e., more inclusive criteria and/or more rapid reporting time frames) pertain to the adverse events occurring within the specific country. Accordingly, Lilly has established general corporate ADE reporting policies that will enable each affiliate to meet its specific national requirements though Tables 1 and 2 are directed more toward transnational requirements. Additionally, Lilly has developed an interconnected ADE reporting system that provides, in a timely manner, ADE information from all trial locations to all affiliates.

B. The Lilly Research Laboratories Drug Experience Network

The Lilly Research Laboratories Drug Experience Network (DEN) has previously been described in a number of venues, most specifically in a 1987 publication [5]. Currently we have in preparation an update of that publication which describes the second generation of DEN, implemented during 1991.

DEN is a global system for collection, storage, summarization, and reporting of adverse events. Adverse events, with the exception of minor events in clinical trials, are entered into the DEN database. Events are described by FDA CO-START classification terms. A centralized group of physicians facilitates data entry and makes determinations of expectedness and suitability for alert reporting.

Summaries of adverse events are prepared from the DEN central database at intervals that range from daily to annually. Statistical tests of report incidence, corrected for marketing exposure, are made quarterly, annually, or as otherwise required. Reports of individual events are made weekly for events that require expedited reporting. Other events are reported quarterly or annually.

Transnational reporting has been initiated utilizing the CIOMS approach. This system utilizes one form, common submission rules, and the English language for reporting events occurring in one country to other countries. Such reports are provided weekly to Lilly affiliates for submission, as required, to their regulatory authorities.

Our experience with DEN has shown that ADEs may occur immediately, such as an anaphylactic reaction to injection of penicillin. Other events may be delayed, such as a birth defect or cancer arising months or years after drug exposure. Events may be common occurrences, such as automobile accidents, that might be related to use of a sedative drug. Most events during or after drug therapy, whether in CTs or in postmarket use, are identical with events in

Table 1 CT ADE Reporting Requirements in the Major Countries

	US	CAN	JPN	AUS	GBR	FRA	GER	ITA	SPA	NORD
Serious	Fatal, life threatening, hospitalization, congenital, cancer or overdose	Not defined per se for CT ADE	Fatal, permanent significant disability, hospitalization	Not defined per se for CT ADE	Fatal, life threatening, disabling, hospitalization	Not defined per se for CT ADE	Not defined per se for CT ADE	Fatal, life threatening, disabling	Fatal, hospitalization, additional Rx, congenital, disabling	Not defined per se for CT ADE
Expected	Unexpected by nature, severity; or frequency	Not defined per se for CT ADE	Not defined per se for CT ADE	Not defined per se for CT ADE	Not defined per se for CT ADE	Not defined per se for CT ADE	No distinction between expected and unexpected	Unexpected	Not defined per se for CT ADE	No distinction between expected and unexpected

Causal	Reasonably, possibly, causally related	Not defined per se for CT ADE	"Judged by a physician"	"All suspected"	"Suspected"	"French imputation method"	"All causal"	Only causal	Not defined per se for CT ADE	"Associated with the use of the drug"
Timing	3-day telephone alert; 10-day safety alert	"Immediately"	"Within 30 days"	3-day alert; 15-day report	"For-with"	"Immediately"	"Without delay"	"Within 15 days"	"Quickly"	3-day telephone alert, 10-day safety alert
Reference	IND rewrite, 1987	"Conduct of Clinical Investigations," 1989	Derived from Article 62-2, Ministry of Health and Welfare	GCRP Guidelines; CTX Guidelines, 7Jul91	Annex VIII Medicines Control Agency	Derived from Ministry of Health Decree, 1984	Derived from Fourth Drug Law Amendment, 1991	Ministry of Health Regulations	Derived from Ministry of Health pharmacosurveillance policy	Nordic Guidelines; Good Clinical Trial Practice, 1989

Table 2 CT ADE Reporting Requirements in the Major Countries: Determiner Requirements

	US	CAN	JPN	AUS	GBR	FRA	GER	ITA	SPA	NORD
Serious	Fatal, life threatening, hospitalization, congenital, cancer or overdose	Not defined per se for CT ADE	Fatal, permanent significant disability, hospitalization	Not defined per se for CT ADE	Fatal, life threatening, disabling, hospitalization	Not defined per se for CT ADE	Not defined per se for CT ADE	Fatal, life threatening, disabling	Fatal, hospitalization, additional Rx, congenital, disabling	Not defined per se for CT ADE
Expected	Unexpected by nature, severity; or frequency	Not defined per se for CT ADE	Not defined per se for CT ADE	Not defined per se for CT ADE	Not defined per se for CT ADE	Not defined per se for CT ADE	No distinction between expected and unexpected	Unexpected	Not defined per se for CT ADE	No distinction between expected and unexpected

Causal	Reasonably, possibly, causally related	Not defined per se for CT ADE	"Judged by a physician"	"All suspected"	"Suspected"	"French imputation method"	"All causal"	Only causal	Not defined per se for CT ADE	"Associated with the use of the drug"
Timing	3-day telephone alert; 10-day safety alert	"Immediately"	"Within 30 days"	3-day alert; 15-day report	"Forwith"	"Immediately"	"Without delay"	"Within 15 days"	"Quickly"	3-day telephone alert, 10-day safety alert
Reference	IND rewrite, 1987	"Conduct of Clinical Investigations," 1989	Derived from Article 62-2, Ministry of Health and Welfare	GCRP Guidelines; CTX Guidelines, 7Jul91	Annex VIII Medicines Control Agency	Derived from Ministry of Health Decree, 1984	Derived from Fourth Drug Law Amendment, 1991	Ministry of Health Regulations	Derived from Ministry of Health pharmacosurveillance policy	Nordic Guidelines; Good Clinical Trial Practice, 1989

patients who have never taken drugs. Even with complete information, it is rare that a causal relationship between drug and event can be defined, and many reports are fragmentary or incorrect, or both. Nevertheless, by collecting all events in a comprehensive database, it may be possible to recognize patterns of events by comparing groups of patients. Such patterns are important elements in ensuring the safety of clinical trials and the optimal use of drugs.

Five unifying principles have guided development of DEN.

1. *Centralization:* Events worldwide are collected into a central comprehensive database.
2. *Objectivity:* Assessment of severity is made as objectively as possible.
3. *Expertise:* Event investigation and analysis are performed by physicians and experienced staff.
4. *Automation:* Summarization, analysis, and reporting are assisted by highly automated systems.
5. *Globalization:* Timely and complete ADE information is shared with Lilly affiliates around the world.

Adverse event information in a CT is collected systematically at each visit of a patient with an investigator. There are many, generally minor, events in most trials. In one recent yearlong trial in patients with hypertension, 3460 patients attended 39,485 visits at which 37,142 adverse event reports were recorded in the clinical trial database. Almost all of these events were nonserious. Only a few hundred events were of sufficient significance to be entered also in the DEN database.

In sum, all adverse events on Lilly marketed products, and all serious events on Lilly trial products, are collected, analyzed, and subsequently distributed to Lilly affiliates throughout the world. Lilly has established and enforced a corporate policy of reporting serious CT and all spontaneous ADEs to corporate headquarters within 48 hr of the affiliates first becoming aware of the event. Since affiliate personnel do not witness trial events per se, clinical investigators are directed to notify Lilly personnel immediately upon the occurrence of any serious event. As indicated in Table 2, the U.S. IND definition of a serious event is the most rigorous such definition among the major countries' requirements and thus it has been adopted as the standard for interpretation of our "48-hr rule."

Once the serious trial event is entered into DEN, a cascade of actions ensues. These activities are depicted in Figs. 1 and 2. A Lilly headquarters physician, in conjunction with the drug epidemiology unit (DEU*) staff, first determines the "expectedness" of the serious CT ADE. For trial events, expectedness is based on the adverse events listed in the corporate clinical investigation brochure for

---

*The DEU is made up of pharmacists, nurses, and other health care practitioners who collect data on ADEs and perform extensive surveillance and analysis activities.

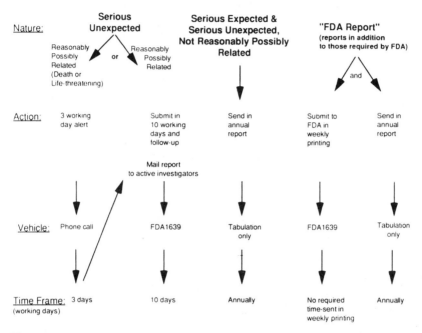

Figure 1 Drug experience network CT ADE activities.

the particular study. This brochure, which is updated frequently, is used throughout the world for any studies of specific investigational drug products. Once a trial event has been determined to be serious and unexpected, the physician monitor and DEU staff evaluate the event to determine whether there is a "reasonable possibility that the experience may have been caused by the drug." This definition originates from the 1987 U.S. IND Rewrite. This causality determination is based on the combined clinical judgment of the physician and DEU staffs and does not rely on any causality algorithms.

A significant challenge is to classify reports so that the essential ones are submitted but the extraneous reports are not. This can be done in part by focusing on explicit outcomes such as death, hospitalization, disability, or discontinuation from trials because of adverse events. Problems still arise. For example, what should be done with the death years after an experimental cancer chemotherapy or rash weeks after antibiotic therapy? Judging causality is difficult.

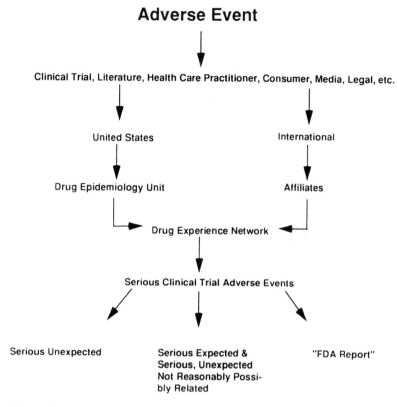

Figure 2   Drug experience network ADE information flow.

A French method utilizes a two-dimensional scoring system in which one dimension relates to the onset and offset chronology and the second dimension relates to the presence of alternative causal factors [6]. A second algorithm [7] includes 56 decisions in each of six separate dimensions: history of association of the event with the drug, alternate causes, timing of onset, evidence of drug overdose, dechallenge course, and course of rechallenge. When this latter algorithm was tested with 30 suspect cases, the agreement of causality made by two clinical pharmacologists increased from 47% to 63% (only 16 percentage points) [8].

When Pere et al. [9] compared six causality assessment procedures, only modest agreement was found. The authors concluded that the procedures had "poor predictive values."

All causality algorithms require extensive information. This generally can be obtained in clinical trials, but this goal is rarely realized with spontaneous reports. The most important information comes from rechallenge. This cannot be performed safely in the most serious events and is infrequently attempted in CTs.

An additional problem with causality judgment is the potential impact on product liability legal actions against the manufacturer and treating physician. If the manufacturer makes a determination, based on preliminary fragmentary information, that the event may be caused by the drug product, this initial assessment may be difficult to reverse when more complete information becomes available. The impact of liability considerations on drug development has been extensively reviewed by Swazey [10] and Lasagna [11].

To be ultraconservative, Lilly generally concludes that an event may be causally related unless there is a specific reason to conclude that it is not. We are constantly evaluating causality algorithms and may eventually embed such an algorithm in our computer system to facilitate the event assessment process.

Once a CT ADE has been judged to be serious, unexpected, and reasonably possibly causally related, i.e., an alert report (this assessment is made within 24 hr of the event's arrival at headquarters), the DEN computer program automatically triages the report for submission to regulatory agencies, clinical investigators, and Lilly affiliates. For FDA reporting purposes, fatal and immediately life-threatening events, which are unexpected and possibly causally related, are telephoned to the FDA consistent with the IND requirements for 3-day alert events. Every week the DEN system mails to the FDA, clinical investigators, and affiliates all alert reports obtained by headquarters during the preceding week. In the not-too-distant future we hope to electronically transfer both alert and periodic ADE reports to the FDA and perhaps other regulatory agencies.

The DEN system has listings of investigators and their addresses (for both IND and non-IND studies) for each study conducted throughout the world. The corporate decision to apprise both IND and non-IND investigators of alert CT ADE reports is based primarily on the FDA regulation [12] which reads in part:

The sponsor shall notify FDA and all participating investigators in a written IND safety report of any adverse experience associated with use of the drug that is both serious and unexpected. Such notification shall be made as soon as possible and in no event later than 10 working days after the sponsor's initial receipt of the information.

Lilly believes that all investigators in premarket CTs should be advised of alert ADEs. Such alert reports, as defined by the U.S. requirement, are provided by Lilly to both IND study and non-IND study investigators. Submissions of nondomestic alert reports can thus be accomplished by each affiliate weekly if so required by local regulation or practice. As indicated previously, affiliates may be required to report domestic CT alert reports more quickly than on a weekly basis and thus may rely on local supplementary manual reporting systems to augment DEN; however, the automated, international coordinating aspects of the

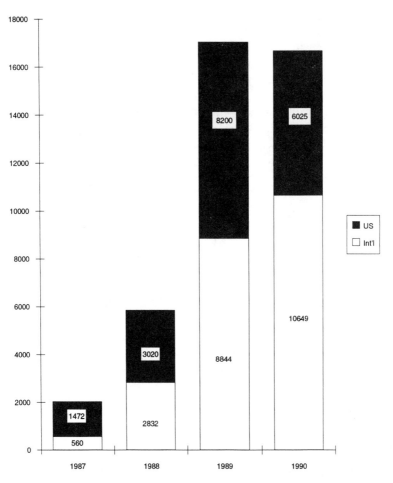

Figure 3 Investigator distribution of IND safety reports. Numbers represent individual mailings to specific investigators. For instance, if a study had 100 investigators, a safety report mailing would represent 100 ''distributions'' in the graphic. The U.S. and international (Int'l) designations indicate the location of the recipient investigators.

DEN system ensure that the affiliates' respective regulatory agencies can be made aware of all alert reports, occurring with an investigational drug anywhere in the world, as frequently as every week. Similarly, all clinical investigators of a particular drug are provided on a weekly basis with all alert reports generated around the world for that drug.

While this system often results in instances of overcompliance with certain countries' clinical trial ADE reporting requirements, we believe that the U.S.

IND Rewrite provisions for alert event reporting within 10 working days (and consequent investigator notification of all alert instances) are appropriate for implementation in all of our studies worldwide. Though demanding in human resource, systems, and administrative contexts, this approach to meeting CT reporting requirements is workable and useful. In order to provide an appreciation of the magnitude of document transmission that accompanies our decision to follow such an exhaustive reporting standard, Fig. 3 illustrates the numbers of alert report investigator mailings (and their follow-ups) that have been processed since 1987.

II. CONCLUSION

Roden [13] succinctly characterized the drug safety responsibility of the world's pharmaceutical companies:

> The pharmaceutical industry has two major roles in drug safety surveillance. First, it must promote the collection and investigation of information relating to adverse reactions for the purpose of advising on drug safety. Second, it must fulfill its obligation to the regulatory authorities by reporting individual ADEs on an expedited basis and/or periodically, according to the regulations in each country in which a drug is licensed for clinical trial or marketing.

Just as there is a clear understanding of the industry's obligation in the monitoring and reporting of ADEs, there is also a growing recognition of the need for harmonization of CT ADE reporting requirements. Certainly, within the last few years the requirements have become more sophisticated. We believe that Lilly has arrived at a reasonable approach to deal with the varying reporting requirements of the countries in which we conduct trials. However, in order to improve the usefulness of the ADE information, we would submit that there is some distance to go. To expedite this process, we suggest that a uniform ADE reporting criteria be considered worldwide. A ready solution exists in the form of the CIOMS Working Group proposal that was previously already referenced. This approach, which focuses on the alert reporting of serious, unexpected, and possibly related CT ADEs (as well as similar spontaneous events), should provide all countries with an assurance of the timely receipt of information about significant clinical trial adverse drug experiences.

REFERENCES

1. Huster WJ. Clinical trial adverse events: the case for descriptive techniques. *Drug Inf J*. 1991;25:447–456.
2. O'Neill R. Assessment of safety. In: Peace K. ed. *Biopharmaceutical Statistics for Drug Development*. vol. 13. New York: Marcel Dekker; 1988:543–604,

3. Bankoswki Z. International Reporting of Adverse Drug Reactions. Final Report on CIOMS Working Group. Geneva; CIOMS: 1990.
4. Thompson WL. Harmonization of clinical trials. Presented at the First International Conference on Harmonization, Brussels, Nov. 5–7, 1991.
5. Talbott MW, Hadley PA, Lister WC, et al. Adverse drug events: global collection, analysis, and reporting. J Clin Res Drug Dev. 1987;1:53–73.
6. Begaud B, Evreux JC, Jouglard J, Lagier G. Unexpected or toxic drug reaction assessment (imputation). *Therapie.* 1985;40:115–118.
7. Kramer MS, Leventhal JM, Hutchinson TA, Feinstein AR. An algorithm for the operational assessment of adverse drug reactions. I. Background, description, and instructions for use. *JAMA.* 1979;242:623–632.
8. Hutchinson TA, Leventhal JM, Kramer MS, Karch FE, Lipman AG, Feinstein AR. An algorithm for the operational assessment of adverse drug reactions II. Demonstration of reproducibility and validity. JAMA. 1979;242:633–638.
9. Pere JC, Begaud B, Haramburu F, Albin H. Computerized comparison of six adverse drug reaction assessment procedures. *Clin Pharm Ther.* 1986;40:451–461.
10. Swazey JP. Prescription drug safety and product liability. In Huber PW, Litan RE. eds. The liability maze: the impact of liability law on safety and innovation. Washington, DC: The Brookings Institution; 1991:291–333.
11. Lasagna L. The chilling effect of product liability on new drug development. In: Huber PW, Litan RE. eds. The liability maze: the impact of liability law on safety and innovation. Washington, DC. The Brookings Institution; 1991:334–359.
12. Code of Federal Regulations: 21 CFR Part 312.32(c)(i); 1990; April 11:70.
13. Roden SM. An introduction to drug safety surveillance. In: Rawlins MD, International Drug Surveillance Department. eds. *Drug Safety: A Shared Responsibility.* London: Churchill Livingstone; 1991:1–11.

14

Safety Surveillance

Norman E. Pitts*

Pfizer Inc.
Groton, Connecticut

Unfortunately there are no therapeutic roses without their thorns.

Sir Derrick Dunlop [1]

I. INTRODUCTION

The research and development (R&D) of new therapeutic agents is a long and complicated process that by the time of regulatory approval represents a very considerable investment in both time and resources. However, notwithstanding the magnitude of this investment, it is unrealistic to expect that the research process will have necessarily defined all significant aspects of a drug's profile prior to marketing. In some instances this may be possible but it is always prudent to proceed on the assumption that this cannot be done consistently with any degree of reliability. While this observation applies to both efficacy and safety issues, it is particularly relevant to questions of safety. Indeed it renders a profound disservice to the concept of a public that is properly informed on health matters to encourage unqualified reliance on a belief that all possible safety risks can be known and defined prior to approval.

The regulatory approval of new drugs is essentially a three-step process. First it must be established that the drug is efficacious and produces a clinically meaningful therapeutic benefit. The second step is to determine the safety profile of the drug when used for the purpose indicated and in the doses recommended. The final step in the decision-making process is a benefit-to-risk assessment. Does the benefit to be achieved justify the potential risk? The precision with which the safety element of this equation can be defined at the time of marketing approval is a function of the interplay of a number of variables. Most impor-

---

*Retired.

tantly, it depends on the nature and frequency of the adverse event and the numbers of patients it is logistically feasible to study in a preapproval research program. Accordingly, approval decisions should always be viewed as being contingent on the results of subsequent postmarketing experience. In many European countries drug regulatory law gives de jure recognition to this fundamental principle by granting a license to market with subsequent periodic license renewal rather than a final and unconditional approval to market as provided for in U.S. food and drug law.

Relative to efficacy, the significant issues relating to a drug's recommended use will have been addressed prior to marketing approval. Nevertheless, there may remain additional therapeutic uses not yet adequately explored, or possibly not even anticipated. Such gaps in existing knowledge may be conveniently and effectively addressed pending further research by suitable labeling with respect to the recommended usage. Of greater moment, however, are those issues relating to safety that are presently unknown. These issues will usually relate as much to the recommended and approved use as they do to any potential, but as yet, unapproved use. They cannot, therefore, be avoided or circumvented by suitable precautionary labeling.

The nature of the potential safety risks may be completely unknown and unanticipated at the time of approval or, if known, their potential severity or frequency may still remain to be defined more precisely. In the preapproval phase the emphasis is almost completely, if not entirely, on the randomized, controlled experimental study as the vehicle for data acquisition and one must recognize certain caveats regarding the ability to extrapolate from this experience to the postmarketing setting. While this may certainly be true for efficacy conclusions, it is much more important with respect to safety assurances.

Once approved for marketing and subject to widespread use in the real-life treatment setting, far larger numbers of patients are exposed to drug than hitherto. In addition, different patient populations, different concomitant pathologies and medications, and different patterns of use and dosage all come into play as factors influencing response to drug and the possible occurrence of hitherto unknown drug effects. It is not uncommon to find that factors contributing to the occurrence of unexpected drug effects have remained undetected during the clinical research program. This is because it is not feasible to explore all the possible permutations of factors that might be responsible for such unexpected effects within the practical constraints of a preapproval research program, at least not unless the study of a certain effect is indicated because good theoretical reasons exist to anticipate the possibility of its presence. As a consequence new and unexpected aspects of the drug's profile may emerge for the first time in the postmarketing period, for reasons completely unrelated to the competence or quality of the clinical research conducted prior to approval.

For these reasons the research and evaluation of a drug should not be regarded as beginning with its discovery and ending with its approval. The acquisition of new knowledge concerning any drug should be viewed as a continuing process that begins with its discovery and extends to approval and beyond to the postmarketing period. Postmarketing drug evaluation, and especially safety monitoring, is as much an integral part of the drug development process as the preapproval clinical research program. The only difference is the progressively narrowing gap between that which is known about the drug and that which remains to be determined. Therefore drug approval does not represent the end of the development process, but merely marks the end of one important phase of that process.

The postmarketing environment with its instant access to large numbers of patients receiving drug in the course of normal medical care provides the necessary statistical power to detect very infrequently occurring safety events. The challenge becomes one of extracting useful data from this uncontrolled setting. In order to achieve this techniques must be perfected that place greater emphasis on data acquisition by observational as opposed to experimental methods.

At this juncture it may be instructive to digress for a moment in order to explore the developmental history of a concern for drug safety.

II. A HISTORICAL PERSPECTIVE

A review of safety monitoring as it has evolved historically possesses more than academic value since it allows an appreciation of the factors influencing and shaping the regulatory philosophy of the various regulatory authorities.

There is a general but nevertheless erroneous perception that a recognition of the problem of drug safety and the need for regulation and safety monitoring is of fairly recent origin dating from the thalidomide experience. This assumption is not unreasonable bearing in mind the magnitude of the thalidomide tragedy and the high level of publicity it attracted. In point of fact, however, a concern for the harm, as well as the benefits, of medical therapies has a much more ancient origin, an origin that even predates the principles embodied in the Corpus Hippocraticum and the articulation of the concept of *Primum Non Nocere*. Its history may be traced back some several thousand years to the dawn of recorded history and the Code of Hammurabi. In Mesopotamia, the practice of medicine involved the administration of a variety of medications that prior experience had shown to be useful. King Hammurabi therefore promulgated the Code in order to control treatment practices with these remedies and protect patients from unnecessary harm. Similar concerns are also evident in the papyri of ancient Egypt that contain information on an enormous number of drugs and set forth a rigid code the purpose of which was also to protect patients from harm by inappropriate treatment [2].

In Europe, the first evidence of a concern for the control of the safety and quality of medicines can be found in Salerno in the 13th century, from whence it extended to France, Germany, and England in the 15th and 16th centuries. As early as 1423, the City of London appointed drug inspectors and in 1540 Henry VIII directed the Royal College of Physicians of London to appoint inspectors for the purpose of monitoring the quality of drugs sold by apothecaries. This action resulted in the compilation of the *London Pharmacopeia* in 1618. Eventually this document was replaced by the *British Pharmacopeia* in 1864 [3]. Contemporaneously with the latter event, a similar compendium of available drugs became available in this country, a document that also owed its origins entirely to the efforts of the medical profession. The *U.S. Pharmacopeia* was first published in 1820 [4].

A. More Recent Safety Concerns

Over the last 100 years the historical record teaches that it was the medical profession rather than government that focused public attention on a need for some formal mechanism to monitor the safety of drugs used in medical practice. For instance, in the latter part of the 19th century, prompted by the experiences with smallpox vaccine, a concern began to develop within the profession regarding adverse drug reactions to drugs. Shortly thereafter, reports began to accumulate of sudden unexpected deaths following the induction of anesthesia with chloroform and a serious question also arose with respect to its potential for liver toxicity. So serious was the concern over these events that in 1877 the British Medical Association (BMA), acting entirely at the instigation of the medical profession, organized a working party to conduct what was probably the very first collaborative study of suspected drug toxicity [5]. It was certainly the first attempt to conduct a formal study of the safety of a drug that was already in wide use as an integral part of established medical practice. Based on the findings of this study, the BMA advocated the establishment of an independent body to monitor and assess drug safety [6].

During the ensuing years (1909–1914) the BMA expanded its interest in drug safety to include investigations into "patent medicines" [7]. Subsequently a Select Committee of the BMA, acting at the instigation of the British Parliament, produced a report that was scheduled for publication in August 1914. As it ultimately transpired, the day on which the report was due to be printed also proved to be the day that the United Kingdom declared war on Germany. Understandably any further progress on the Select Committee's recommendations became lost in the maelstrom of war and sociopolitical upheaval that followed. However, it should be noted that, in what must surely constitute a most remarkable demonstration of prescience, the recommendations of the Select Committee were almost identical to those eventually promulgated in the Medicines Act a full half century later!

In the period following World War I the course of events provided further testimony to the fact that this interest in drug safety had not been an idle concern. A literal epidemic of jaundice and fatal hepatic necrosis developed in soldiers who had received arsenicals as therapy for syphilis during the war. On this occasion the investigation of the untoward events became the subject of a special project conducted in the United Kingdom under the auspices of the Medical Research Committee (predecessor to the present Medical Research Council). A comprehensive study was initiated to investigate and report on this serious adverse reaction and its possible causal relationship to arsenical therapy [8]. In the 1920s this same pattern of events was repeated with the occurrence of a fatal hepatotoxicity that was shown, on this occasion, to be due to the use of cinchophen in the treatment of gout [9].

At three points in time therefore—1877, 1909–1914, and 1922—medical opinion in Europe, supported by similar public sentiment, had been very close to reaching a consensus on the need to establish a system to monitor the safety of drugs. However, the concept was not pursued further and one is legitimately entitled to pose the question of why this should have been so. Why was this idea, which had already been raised by the medical profession, not taken further by governments and developed to provide a system for monitoring and regulating drug safety? Furthermore, in the absence of such government action why did the medical profession itself not press for action in accordance with its expressed views. The reasons are probably not far to seek and have particular relevance for the pattern of regulatory developments both in Western Europe and in the United States.

In this country government concern for the regulation of drugs, as reflected in the Pure Food and Drug Act (1906), had only arisen secondarily as a consequence of a primary concern for the purity of foodstuffs. This act, which was precipitated by an episode concerning contaminated meat, was mainly concerned with ensuring the purity and unadulterated state of foodstuffs. This same focus of attention was then logically extended to include medicines, manifesting as a concern for the adulteration and misbranding of proprietary medicines [10].

Another reason for this regulatory emphasis on drug purity and adulteration, and the universality of this concern, is readily apparent if one considers the status of therapeutics at that time. In the latter part of the 18th century and the early 1900s there was only a handful of drugs available as single entities, e.g., morphine, codeine, digitalis, quinine, aspirin, ether, chloroform, and diptheria antitoxin. For the most part therapy was in the form of multi-ingredient prescriptions prepared by dispensing physicians, with a significant component comprising proprietary nostrums that could be freely purchased by the patient without the participation of a "learned intermediary," i.e., the physician.

Indeed, as one views developments in the United States and the countries of Western Europe, a remarkable parallel is evident between the various countries with respect to the origins, philosophy, and objectives of drug regulation. The concern of most governments, at that time, was not the safety of these remedies per se, in terms of adverse reactions, but rather, in keeping with the primary focus with respect to foodstuffs, a concern for the possibility of adulteration or impurity. The intent of legislation was to ensure that the public was buying what was advertised and that the product was not contaminated or otherwise adulterated. With this purpose in mind the food and drug acts were enacted in England in 1875 [11]. And, on the same time frame, other countries in Europe, such as Germany, the Netherlands, Norway, and Denmark, enacted legislation with these same objectives [12].

B. The Modern Era of Drug Regulation

In the early 1930s a research-based pharmaceutical industry began to emerge and move therapy increasingly in the direction of single-chemical entities, with specific pharmacological activity, as opposed to mixtures and proprietary nostrums. Concomitant with these developments evidence continued to accumulate attesting to the wisdom of a system of safety monitoring, both prior to marketing and subsequently. Reports were beginning to appear in the literature concerning agranulocytosis associated with the analgesic amidopyrine [13] and subsequently the newly discovered sulfonamides were found to possess a variety of toxic effects. Nevertheless, the need for legislation to address safety per se as distinct from questions of purity and adulteration continued to go unrecognized as a statutory need.

Even the large number of deaths associated with the elixir of sulfanilamide incident did not serve to focus legislative attention on the full extent of the safety issue, in the sense that it necessarily involved questions of both preapproval and postapproval safety monitoring. Certainly this tragedy precipitated the enactment of the Federal Food, Drug and Cosmetic Act (1938). And admittedly, in sharp contrast to the 1906 act, the focus of this new legislation now extended beyond issues of purity and adulteration to include safety and adverse reactions per se. However, this new legislation addressed itself only to statutory requirements for evidence of safety prior to marketing approval. Even though these deaths had occurred in the postmarketing period there was no mention whatsoever of a requirement for the continued monitoring of safety after marketing. It appeared to be implicit in the law as enacted that the legislators entertained the completely erroneous view that adequate preapproval safety testing could be relied on to predict and avoid such tragic eventualities in the future. Aside from the sulfanilamide episode, even the past history of other similar safety experiences, which should have been known to the legislators and suggested otherwise, appears to have been ignored in the emotion of the moment.

Nevertheless, this omission need not necessarily have been a fatal flaw in the legislation. Theoretically any substantive deficiencies in the law could be remedied by the regulations subsequently promulgated by the Food and Drug Administration (FDA) to implement the act. Characteristically U.S. food and drug law has been lacking in specifics and detail but has remedied this by delegating broad responsibility and discretion to the agency to establish any system of regulation it saw fit. In effect, the statute empowered the FDA to "legislate by regulation." Unfortunately, the federal regulations, like the legislation, failed to address the issue of postmarketing safety surveillance. In point of fact this is not altogether surprising. There is evidence that this erroneous view of the legislature, regarding the assurances provided by preapproval testing, had wider acceptance and was also shared by the regulatory scientists. For instance, the commissioner of the FDA commented on the value of preclinical animal studies as a means of detecting potential human safety problems and avoiding tragedies such as the elixir of sulfanilamide experience. He noted that such animal studies had not been conducted with sulfanilamide, and his remarks, taken in context, carried the clear implication that proper testing, using state-of-the-art methodology, could be relied on to reveal problems prior to drug approval [14].

Subsequent to the passage of the 1938 act further examples of the scientific invalidity of this legislative and regulatory position continued to occur but, surprisingly, occasioned no desire on the part of the legislature or the agency to make any changes whatsoever in this regulatory philosophy. For instance, serious safety problems in the postmarketing period had arisen with drugs such as phenylbutazone, chlorpromazine, and chloramphenicol, and provided clear and repetitive evidence that a system focused entirely on rigorous approval requirements per se is inadequate to safeguard the public health. The hematological problems attendant on chloramphenicol therapy did, however, evoke a response from the medical profession if not from government. In 1955, prompted by the chloramphenicol experience, the American Medical Association (AMA) Council on Drugs established a Subcommittee on Drug-Induced Dyscrasias. The committee was charged with developing a reporting system to monitor the possible hematological effects of new drugs following their introduction onto the market.

In one sense this apparent legislative inattention to a need for postmarketing surveillance is surprising. But it does nevertheless present a curious parallel to similar events occurring over this same period in Europe. Indeed, no further substantive developments in the direction of drug regulation occurred in any country until thalidomide focused world attention on the issue in such a tragic and dramatic fashion. Given the previous history it is indeed surprising that a tragedy of this magnitude was required to provide the necessary catalyst for the introduction of a more formalized system of statutory drug regulation in the various countries around the world.

It is so surprising that one may legitimately ask why it should have taken so long to address the safety issue in a fully comprehensive manner. The issue was hardly new, since the concept of postmarketing safety monitoring had continued to engage the attention of the medical profession over the years as a consequence of the many prior examples that testified to this need. Perhaps the most reasonable explanation lies in the remarkable nature of the scientific advances that were being achieved in therapeutic research and innovation during this period. It would seem to be axiomatic that significant gains in pharmacological activity, which provided such unprecedented benefits, would also offer the potential risk of significant adverse effects. This was not focused on, however, probably because of the high level of enthusiasm for the remarkable therapeutic gains being achieved. Similarly at the laboratory level there was a preoccupation with the development of animal models bearing on pharmacological efficacy. Indeed it was only after the thalidomide disaster that more attention was paid to preclinical toxicological methodology and interpretation. For instance, prior to thalidomide the science of teratology was entirely analytical in its approach. It was only subsequent to that event that it assumed a more practical orientation seeking to better understand the comparative aspects of placental function between the species and to develop animal screens predictive of teratogenic effects in humans.

This explanation not only has a certain logical appeal but is consistent with the facts. It is also a view that is shared by a representative of at least one regulatory agency. The reason given for the United Kingdom's failure to act in matters of safety until the 1960s has been attributed to the fact that the therapeutic advances led to such amazing improvements in efficacy that adverse reactions, although recognized as a possibility, evinced no great concern [15]. There may also have been an additional element. A preoccupation with research accomplishments in producing drugs for various diseases and the ability to predict such activity from animal screens may have encouraged the erroneous belief that toxicity could similarly be predicted.

Ultimately it was thalidomide that drew attention away from the remarkable therapeutic gains that were being achieved and brought into much sharper focus the potential toxicity risks that may be associated with these newer drugs. Following this event, Sir Derrick Dunlop's aphorism, quoted at the head of this chapter, became the guiding principle underlying the drug legislation now emerging in the different countries. However, there was a subtle but very important pragmatic difference in the manner in which the regulatory implications of this principle were interpreted and implemented in different countries. This difference was the determining factor in shaping the regulatory philosophy and approach that was adopted.

C.   A Divergence in Regulatory Philosophy

These differences in governmental response are evident in the regulatory approach followed in Europe vis-à-vis this country. In all countries there was broad and universal acknowledgment that it was unwise, and entirely without scientific merit, to place complete reliance on preclinical animal studies as a predictor of a drug's safety profile in humans. However, while there was a consensus on this fundamental point, there appeared, at least initially, to be significant differences in regulatory philosophy regarding human studies.

On the one hand, there was the regulatory approach adopted by the United Kingdom. This approach was based on the premise that while animal studies might be potentially flawed as a reliable predictor due to interspecies differences, absolute safety assurance may also be lacking from preapproval human studies. This may occur regardless of the quality of the human studies and arises from logistic and statistical considerations. Since there is a limit as to the extent of the safety guarantees provided by preapproval studies and a detailed review-and-approval process, postmarketing safety surveillance is mandatory. Important knowledge concerning the safety of a drug may be derived from both the preapproval and postmarketing periods. A primary focus on the former can never dispense with a need for the latter. An effective drug regulatory system must therefore give equal emphasis to human safety evaluation in both the preapproval and postmarketing situations.

In essence this legislative approach by the U.K. government reflected the conclusions of a conference of the Royal College of Physicians. This conference was convened to consider the implications of the thalidomide tragedy and advise the government on the form that subsequent legislation concerning drug research and approval should take. In reaching its conclusions the conference acknowledged the sheer logistical impossibility of detecting all potential adverse events prior to approval. It was this view that was instrumental in shaping the direction and emphasis of the subsequent U.K. legislation [16]. For instance, the Medicines Act [17] of the United Kingdom specified the primary objectives of the legislation as follows:

1.   To advise on the safety, quality, and efficacy for human use of any substance or article (not being an instrument, apparatus, or appliance) to which any provision of the act is applicable.
2.   To promote the collection and investigation of information on adverse reactions for the purpose of enabling such advice to be given.

This regulatory approach placed equal statutory emphasis on preapproval requirements and the approval process on the one hand and on postapproval safety surveillance for the emergence of unsuspected toxicity on the other. Even the name of the duly constituted body established to implement the law, the

Committee on Safety of Medicines, clearly emphasized the main focus of concern. The continuing nature of drug safety assessment into the postmarketing period was further emphasized by the fact that permission to market a drug was granted by the issuance of a product license, renewable at fixed intervals, rather than an absolute unqualified approval to market, as in this country.

Undoubtedly this legislative emphasis has been responsible for the well-developed system of government-sponsored postmarketing safety surveillance that has characterized the regulatory approach in the United Kingdom from the very outset. It is an approach that takes due cognizance of the real message of thalidomide and the other equally important, but less publicized, postmarketing drug safety issues that preceded it. Uncertainties will always exist with respect to the reliability of animal studies as a predictor for humans. Because of this fact and for a variety of other reasons, the full safety profile of a drug may only emerge subsequent to marketing.

By contrast, the substantive law that was enacted in this country indicated a significant difference in the manner in which the message of thalidomide had been interpreted. The primary thrust of the 1962 Kefauver–Harris Amendments to the Federal Food, Drug and Cosmetic Act was a requirement that

> there be substantial evidence that the drug will have the effect it purports or is represented to have under the conditions or use prescribed, recommended, or suggested in the proposed labelling thereof [18].

The legislation further stated that

> the term "substantial evidence" means evidence consisting of adequate and well controlled investigations, including clinical investigations, by experts qualified by scientific training and experience to evaluate the effectiveness of the drug involved, on the basis of which it could fairly and responsibly be concluded by such experts that the drug will have the effect it purports or is represented to have under the conditions of use prescribed, recommended, or suggested in the labelling or proposed labelling thereof [18].

The focus was on proof of efficacy as the criterion for approval and all reference to a safety requirement related to the information derived from those investigations conducted prior to approval to establish "substantial evidence" of efficacy. With the exception of a reference to the "imminent hazard" procedure the legislation made no specific reference to any requirement for postapproval safety monitoring. The emphasis of the legislation was on the research phase and the approval process as the safeguard of the public health.

Therefore, as they ultimately emerged, the 1962 Kefauver–Harris amendments to the Federal Food, Drug and Cosmetic Act, enacted in the wake of thalidomide, may be viewed as reflecting a continuation of the same bias that was evident in the legislative response to the sulfanilamide tragedy in the original act. Little seemed to have changed since 1938 and the view was still prevalent that well-executed preapproval drug evaluation constitutes an effective preventive measure for the avoidance of future tragedies of this nature. The extent of the reliance on this approach is supported not only by the omission from the act of all mention of postmarketing surveillance but also by the introduction of a requirement that permission to market be granted by final and unqualified approval of the new drug application (NDA).

This legislative preoccupation with the adequacy of preapproval testing is further exemplified by the fact that the only modification to Senator Kefauver's proposed amendments, which was added as a direct response to the thalidomide episode, was the insertion of a requirement for animal testing prior to clinical use. This constituted a most surprising omission, not only from the 1962 amendments as originally drafted, but also from the federal regulations as they had existed over the previous quarter century. Surprising because, immediately after the sulfanilamide disaster in 1938, the then-commissioner of the FDA, Commissioner Larrick, observed publicly that adequate preclinical animal testing could easily have averted the disaster.

This interpretation of legislative and regulatory philosophy is not entirely speculative since it receives support from other statements made at that time. Immediately following the unfolding of the thalidomide tragedy in the national press, Senator Kefauver sought to use its impact to move forward his proposed amendments to the Food, Drug and Cosmetic Act, which were currently stalled in Congress. He announced to the public at large that his amendments ''would ensure that the American people were safeguarded against such future disasters'' [20]. And, most importantly, no public dissent to this erroneous statement of fact was forthcoming from any other authoritative source, legislative or regulatory. As a consequence this pronouncement, emanating as it did on the authority of one of the two congressional sponsors of the 1962 amendments, served to create unrealistic expectations in the mind of the general public regarding the future performance of the regulatory system in terms of its protecting them from such events.

The regulations subsequently promulgated by the FDA to implement the 1962 amendments to the law displayed a similar focus. They did nothing to dispel the notion that a closely regulated IND process and detailed review and approval of the NDA could be relied on to provide this assurance of safety. Whilst there was some reference to postmarketing safety reporting, such references lacked the same measure of detail and specificity with which the IND and NDA approval process were addressed. A global perspective was also lacking since there was no mention of any reporting requirements with respect to non-U.S. data. For the main part, the regulations were heavily oriented toward regulation of the IND process and NDA approval with the major emphasis on ''substantial evidence'' of efficacy.

The unrealistic expectations engendered in the mind of the general public by Senator Kefauver's statement cannot have been lost on the agency as it set about the task of implementing the regulations. Its attempt to meet these expectations was almost certainly one of the important factors influencing development of the distinctive approach to drug regulation that characterized the activities of the FDA as compared to those of other national agencies.

The result was a slow system that overemphasized detail and focused almost exclusively on the IND research phase and the NDA approval process. It was based on a regulatory philosophy that sought to achieve a level of assurance prior to approval that it is not scientifically reasonable to guarantee. This resulted in the much publicized "drug lag" of the 1970s and with it the dangerous paradox inherent in such an approach. A prolonged and detailed drug approval process may appear superficially to be efficient simply by allowing time for postmarketing experience to accumulate from other countries prior to the approval decision. This opens up the prospect of the regulatory authority appearing to be right, but for the wrong reason. This constitutes at most a political success but never a scientific success. The experience with thalidomide in this country, and later with practolol, could certainly be viewed in this context.

D. A Harmonization of Regulatory Philosophy

Recent years have witnessed a change in which the distinction between these two regulatory philosophies has tended to disappear. In this country there has recently been a shift toward a much greater emphasis not only on the need for postmarketing safety surveillance per se but on its implementation on a global as opposed to a purely national scale. Two events occurring concurrently have been instrumental in refocusing attention on this aspect of drug development.

The first was the emergence of the IND and NDA Rewrite regulations undertaken in response to mounting criticism with respect to delays in drug development and approval relative to other countries. These new regulations now dealt with the issues of postmarketing safety monitoring in great detail and specificity. Of particular importance they now required the collection and submission of safety experiences with a particular drug from all international markets in which the drug is marketed or in clinical trial.

The second was a final recognition by the FDA that all drugs are not created equal and that certain drugs for certain classes of patient merit a very different regulatory approach. As a generic issue the so-called drug lag was certainly the most publicized and debated consequence of the agency's preoccupation with the drug approval process. However, focusing upon this as a general issue tends to divert attention from the serious consequences it created for a specific subset of the patient population. These are the patients with serious, life-threatening diseases for which there are either no effective therapies or for which treatment options are of limited value or have been exhausted. A new oncological agent for instance merits a very different regulatory approach from a drug that is simply "another" sedative.

One can only speculate that if the prevailing regulatory philosophy had been one that placed greater emphasis on postmarketing evaluation to compensate for inevitable deficiencies in the research and approval process, and less on the finality of approval, such differential treatment might have been achieved much earlier. The agency might well have been much more proactive in its willingness to approve drugs earlier for such patient groups supplemented by appropriate postmarketing follow-up. As it was, it required the AIDS crisis and the political impact of its various activist groups to force government bureaucracy to recognize what had long been a medical and ethical need.

There is now a consensus among the different regulatory authorities with regard to the importance of global system of postmarketing safety monitoring for all drugs. It is a process that cannot be replaced by any preapproval research program or drug approval process regardless of its quality or level of detail. In recognition of this fact the various national agencies themselves are now interacting and exchanging information of safety issues in a way that can only be beneficial for the drug evaluation process as a whole.

III. BASIC CONSIDERATIONS

Sound clinical judgment and careful observation of the patient have always been essential to the acquisition of new medical knowledge. Historically, research knowledge was gathered exclusively by applying these skills to the evaluation of the individual patient in the ordinary treatment setting. But, over time, an appreciation developed for the extent to which observer bias and a variety of other variables could operate in this setting to influence, and possibly distort, the conclusions to be drawn from even the most careful clinical observation. As a consequence attention became focused on ways of minimizing the impact of these variables. This resulted in a shift of emphasis from methods based on observation of the individual patient during treatment to those based on the response of patients as a group within the context of a controlled study. Conclusions were now derived from the application of statistical methodology to group response, determined in a study design that sought to minimize bias and control for those variables that would otherwise confound the interpretation of the data. The controlled clinical trial had become established as the fundamental basis of meaningful clinical research and the ability to draw reliable, valid scientific conclusions.

It should be pointed out, however, that while the consensus of scientific opinion holds that this is the only scientifically reliable method for generating valid data, this view has been seriously questioned. These objections have both an ethical and a scientific basis. The former objection would dispute the ethics of a procedure that assigns patients to therapy based entirely on mathematical dictates as opposed to the dictates of what is required for the optimum medical care of the patient. But this ethical objection is also buttressed by a scientific objection that raises issues with respect to the difficulty and validity of generalizing from a controlled study population to the population at large because of informed consent requirements. Issues are also raised with respect to the validity of extrapolating the findings in the contrived artificial environment of a controlled study to the normal treatment setting. As a logical extension of these views it has been suggested that all postmarketing studies of drug efficacy do not necessarily have to be controlled comparative studies [21].

Acceptance of the majority view regarding controlled studies should not, however, blind us to the fact that even though the controlled trial may properly be viewed as indispensable to the development of reliable scientific knowledge, there are limitations to this approach. These limitations are most evident in the evaluation of safety issues, especially when the toxicity to be explored is expressed in the form of isolated, unpredictable events of low incidence. The "gold standard" of clinical research methodology, the double-blind, randomized, controlled trial, faces serious challenges when applied to the evaluation of this type of drug safety issue.

As a general rule the controlled studies in any preapproval clinical research program are designed primarily to provide "substantial evidence" of efficacy and support drug approval. The patient numbers for inclusion in studies are selected so as to provide the desired power to detect predetermined degrees of change in the efficacy parameters selected for the study. Study design is dictated by efficacy considerations rather than safety considerations. However, these efficacy studies, comprising as they do the greater part of the preapproval clinical research program, also serve a secondary purpose. They help to characterize the safety profile of the drug, at least insofar as the more common adverse reactions are concerned. But since they are designed prospectively with the primary objective of addressing efficacy, any information that they may generate with respect to safety is derived secondarily. The study protocol has not been designed to address specific safety issues as it has efficacy issues. Indeed, most commonly safety studies cannot be designed prospectively with any degree of confidence during the preapproval clinical research program. This is because the safety issues that may ultimately give rise to concern are not known or predictable at this stage.

With respect to efficacy issues, the current state of the art with respect to animal pharmacological models is such that it is possible to predict putative drug activity in humans with a reasonable degree of confidence. As a consequence, extensive resources are committed to clinical research programs predicated entirely on the conclusions derived from such animal systems. The clinical evaluation of efficacy is embarked on with prior knowledge of the anticipated effects in humans, the relevant parameters to be monitored, and the degree of change in those parameters which the studies are required to detect. Study design can therefore be specifically tailored to address the relevant efficacy issues.

By contrast, the deficiencies of animal toxicology studies as a reliable predictor of the safety profile in humans preclude the availability of certain knowledge regarding the nature, severity, and frequency of all the safety issues which may exist in humans. It would seem that our capacity to impose additional requirements with respect to animal toxicological studies far exceeds our capacity to interpret them and understand their predictive relevance to humans. Such a view is not so much meaningless hyperbole as it is truth standing on its head to attract attention. While the patient numbers employed in a clinical research program are intended by design to be adequate to establish substantial proof of efficacy, the same cannot be said of safety issues. There can never be a similar assurance regarding the adequacy of these same patient numbers for the detection of adverse reactions whose nature and frequency is presently unknown and unsuspected. Using the efficacy analogy, knowledge concerning the existence, nature, and characteristics of a drug safety issue is an essential prerequisite to being able to design a study prospectively with the desired power to address the problem. This information is not available, and cannot be expected to be available, with respect to all the safety issues that may be present.

Aside from these problems relating to the poor predictability of animal toxicology studies, the evaluation of drug safety during the clinical research program poses other problems. These relate to the ability to detect low-incidence toxicities, to accurately define the true incidence, and to differentiate the investigational drug group from a control group when the toxicity simulates non–drug-induced background noise.

For instance, if an adverse event has a true underlying incidence of 1%, there is a high probability (95%) that at least one event will be observed if 300 patients are exposed to the drug. From the opposite perspective there still remains a 5% probability of not seeing at least one event. If, as is not uncommonly the case, the incidence of a serious toxicity is only a fraction of 1%, then the probability of seeing at least one event in this number of patients is considerably diminished.

Preapproval clinical research programs most commonly contain a total of approximately 2000–5000 patients exposed to the investigational drug in a series of different studies. A representative figure would probably be somewhere in the order of 3000 patients. If a serious toxicity is present with a true underlying incidence of only 1 in 1000 (0.1%), this total number of patients (3000) would provide a 95% probability of seeing at least one such event during the course of the clinical program. Once again, the fact that the toxicity does not manifest does not exclude the possibility (5%) that a toxicity with an incidence of 0.1% actually exists. Clearly, if the incidence is appreciably less than 0.1% the probability increases that a preapproval research program of average size might not uncover it prior to approval. These statistics may be placed in their proper clinical perspective by noting that some serious drug-induced toxicities, sufficient in themselves to place significant constraints on the therapeutic use of the drug, may occur much less frequently than 0.1%. Chloramphenicol-induced aplastic anemia with an incidence in the order of 1 in 40,000–60,000 would be one such example [22]. An incidence of this order would require the exposure of 120,000–180,000 patients in a preapproval research program in order to provide this same level of confidence (95%) of seeing at least one such event. Clearly then, serious toxicities may exist that may not be discoverable in the preapproval clinical research program.

However, there is a very important caveat to this line of reasoning. The above discussion makes the assumption that the adverse event, once detected, is easily identified and characterized as drug toxicity. It assumes that the only problem relates to the probability of the event actually occurring during the course of the preapproval clinical program. Unfortunately, this whole issue of preapproval detection of safety problems can be, and often is, more complicated than these statistics would appear to suggest. This arises because the problem of detecting rare toxic events may be further compounded by the fact that adverse reactions do not necessarily present clinically as unique and distinctive syndromes clearly identifiable as drug-induced toxicity. On the contrary, the clinical manifestation of drug toxicity is often similar, if not identical, to that of other clinical syndromes that can occur spontaneously in the general population for reasons quite unrelated to the drug in question. This has the potential to lead to serious diagnostic difficulties in determining causality and relationship to drug, especially when there is no definitive or conclusive diagnostic test to confirm or refute a drug-induced etiology. Hemopoietic toxicity and hepatotoxicity are two examples of serious, low-incidence drug-induced toxicities that may mimic spontaneous non–drug-induced events in their manner of clinical presentation. This phenomenon was particularly relevant to establishing causality in instances of suspected drug-induced hepatotoxicity before the development of serological testing for certain types of viral hepatitis. Indeed, it is more than likely that this diagnostic deficiency may have been responsible for the widely varying estimates of the incidence of gold-induced hepatotoxicity that characterized the published reports of the early studies.

A more recent example of this phenomenon is provided by the drug practolol. This drug is responsible for serious eye involvement that may cause blindness in a small number of patients who receive the drug. A milder manifestation of this same eye disorder occurs with much greater frequency (20%) and could have provided warning of the possibility of more serious toxicity. However, recognition of this much more frequent and less serious manifestation of drug toxicity was delayed because of the confusion caused by its close resemblance to a clinical syndrome that occurs spontaneously in the general population in which the drug is used.

When there is a need to differentiate between a drug-induced effect and "background noise" of this nature in the general population a whole new dimension is added to the problem presented. The total number of patients studied, as the determining factor for the probability of uncovering an infrequently occurring adverse reaction, is no longer the sole issue. Study size, as opposed to total patients exposed, now becomes an important consideration since in these situations it is often helpful, for purposes of establishing causality, to determine whether or not the incidence of the event in the investigational drug group is significantly different from that in the control group. The focus has now shifted from the total number of patients exposed, which determines the probability of an event of given incidence occurring, to the individual study, which is critical to making comparisons of incidence in the investigational drug and control groups.

Unfortunately, patient numbers that provide a high level of confidence with respect to simply discovering an infrequently occurring adverse event do not provide the same power for making intergroup comparisons to assist in the causality attribution of that event. For instance, it was previously noted that 300 patients exposed to drug in an uncontrolled setting provides a 95% probability that at least one adverse reaction will occur if the underlying incidence of the toxicity is 1%. If, however, this same number of patients (300) is included as the investigational drug group in a controlled study and intergroup comparisons are attempted, the statistical power is considerably diminished. If one event occurs in the drug group and there are no events in the control group, the difference between the two groups will not be significant. It now requires several events to occur in the drug group before intergroup comparisons find significance (Table 1). Furthermore, if there is background noise in the control group closely resembling the adverse reaction the problem is compounded. Suppose, for instance, that only one non–drug-induced event, closely mimicking the suspected toxicity, occurs in the 300-patient control group. The suspected toxicity must now occur with an incidence in excess of 2% in the 300 patient investigational drug group in order to find a significant difference ($\leq .05$) between the two groups and support a conclusion that something more than non–drug-induced background noise is present in the investigational drug group (Table 1).

Even greater problems arise when the incidence of the adverse event is only a fraction of 1%. In such situations (Table 2) very large numbers of patients are required to show significant differences between the investigational drug and control groups. Suppose that the suspected adverse reaction occurs with an incidence of 1 in 500 (0.2%) and that a clinically similar syndrome, unrelated to drug, occurs with the same incidence in the general population as represented by

348   Pitts

Table 1 Comparison of Two Groups of 300 Patients

| Observed incidence (%) | | Number of events | | Statistical significance |
Treated	Controls	Treated	Controls	
1.3	0	4	0	≤.05
1.7	0	5	0	≤.05
2.0	0	6	0	≤.05
2.3	0	7	0	≤.05
2.7	0	8	0	≤.01
2.3	0.3	7	1	≤.05
2.7	0.3	8	1	≤.05
3.0	0.3	9	1	≤.05
3.3	0.3	10	1	≤.05
3.7	0.3	11	1	≤.01
3.7	0.7	11	2	≤.05

the control group. The total number of patients required for a controlled study must reach 18,000 evaluable patients in order to provide 80% power to find a difference (≤.05) between the investigational drug and control groups. The logistics of controlled studies of this magnitude are formidable and present obvious problems of implementation. Events that occur even more infrequently, such as the myelotoxicity of chloramphenicol (0.002%), are for all practical purposes completely beyond the reach of the controlled study approach.

When safety evaluation is considered strictly from the perspective of low-incidence adverse reactions there is clearly a serious limitation with respect to the useful contribution that may be expected from the controlled study. Furthermore,

Table 2 Number of Patients Needed to Detect ($p \leq .05$) a Drug Effect of 1/500 (0.002) with Different Levels of Background Noise in the Placebo Control Group

| Patients needed per study to provide following power: | Incidence of event in the control group | | | | |
	$p = .0001$	$p = .001$	$p = .002$	$p = .05$	$p = .1$
50%	2,106	5,040	7,862	130,956	245,698
75%	4,172	9,982	15,572	259,358	486,600
80%	4,814	11,520	17,972	299,328	561,594
90%	6,670	15,956	24,894	414,610	777,886
95%	8,426	20,160	31,450	523,826	982,794
99%	12,276	29,368	45,818	763,126	1,431,762

controlled studies to definitively establish a certain aspect of the safety profile can only be designed prospectively when knowledge is available regarding the nature and frequency of the safety event to be evaluated. Commonly during the research phase potential safety hazards are as yet unknown, and consequently information is not available with regard to these two variables.

From a pragmatic point of view, an excellent case can be made for dispensing with controlled studies in the evaluation of low-incidence toxicity. If 3000 patients are available and all receive the investigational drug, there is a 95% probability of detecting toxicity with an incidence of 0.1%. But if this same number of patients is allocated equally between investigational drug and control groups in a controlled study, this potential to detect low-incidence toxicity is reduced without any concomitant gains in the ability to make intergroup comparisons. For instance, if an effect occurs with a frequency of 0.2% in the investigational drug group but there is a minimal background noise of 0.01% in the control group, a study of this size will not have the requisite power (80%) to detect a significant difference ($\leq.05$) between the two groups. Overall the interests of safety evaluation, insofar as it concerns infrequent adverse reactions, will not have been advanced.

This argument is not meant to detract from the value of the controlled trial per se but only to emphasize that its value is not absolute but relative to the nature of the problem being explored. From an overall perspective controlled studies are essential in the research phase to provide "substantial proof" of efficacy, and for whatever they may contribute to a knowledge of safety, recognizing their limitations with respect to certain types of safety problem and the caveats that attach to any secondarily derived data. However, one should not hastily reject open uncontrolled data as being insufficient to make a meaningful contribution to safety evaluation. Once the required number of controlled studies is established in a clinical research program the use of further patients for additional controlled studies does not constitute a prudent use of patient material. A better approach, with the greatest potential for uncovering unsuspected toxicity prior to approval, is to increase overall patient exposure to the investigational drug by placing all additional patients in open uncontrolled studies.

Implicit in this conclusion is much of the rationale for the routine application of one or more of the various methods of postmarketing surveillance. Even with the larger preapproval clinical programs there can never be complete assurance that a safety issue has not evaded detection. In summary, the several contributing factors that conspire to bring this about are as follows:

Animal toxicology is currently unable to define and quantify the safety problems to be expected in humans with the same degree of confidence that animal pharmacology is able to function as a reliable predictor for human efficacy.
Safety evaluation is a two-stage process, first the detection of an adverse event

and second the ability to definitively establish a causal relationship of the event to drug.

Detection of an adverse event is entirely a function of the total number of patients exposed to drug and the underlying incidence of the event. It is independent of study design and does not require that the patients participate in a formal controlled clinical study. The greater the number of patients exposed, the greater the degree of confidence that rare safety events do not exist.

Causality attribution follows logically on the detection of the adverse event and requires the application of diagnostic skills and any tests that may be available. For purposes of causality attribution the ability to differentiate drug effect from normal background noise of a similar nature may be critical. While this is wholly dependent on study design it may be impractical for low-incidence toxicities because of the patient numbers required.

The next section will discuss the various methodologies that may be employed to further explore drug safety in the postmarketing period—methodologies that in the main seek to derive the maximum information relative to safety from the large numbers of patients now exposed to drug and at the same time seek to minimize the impact of the uncontrolled treatment setting on the data collected.

IV. OBJECTIVES OF POSTMARKETING SURVEILLANCE

The postmarketing period must always be approached with the understanding that hitherto unknown safety issues may remain to be discovered and knowledge of known safety issues may require further modification. The possibility of subsequent modification of drug labeling in the light of this accumulating experience postapproval can never be excluded and postmarketing safety surveillance (PMS) is a logical and essential extension of the research program. It should therefore be addressed with the same dedication and thoroughness as the preapproval research program itself.

In this scheme the drug labeling itself serves a very useful precautionary purpose as regards protecting the patient from as yet unknown aspects of the drug's effects. This purpose is most effectively served with respect to efficacy issues. By carefully detailing the recommended mode of use and approved indications the risk of possible untoward effects from unapproved use is minimized. The precautionary value of the labeling with respect to safety issues is, however, somewhat more problematic since drug use strictly in accordance with the approved labeling cannot be relied on to avoid the occurrence of hitherto unsuspected toxicities. This problem can only be addressed by an efficient postmarketing safety surveillance system. It should also be noted that while such vigilance should never be relaxed, it is particularly critical in the immediate postmarketing period.

In this context it is relevant to note that some drugs very rapidly gain wide market acceptance and usage. The entry of the drug into the marketplace in such cases can best be described as explosive. This places an added emphasis on the adequacy of the postmarketing surveillance system in place since in the early years after approval, when patient exposure is increasing exponentially, there is the likelihood that new toxicities may emerge suddenly and dramatically. It has been reported, for instance, that with benoxaprofen approximately 500,000 patients were exposed to the drug in the first 2 years after marketing in the United Kingdom. During that period the Committee on Safety of Medicines (CSM) received some 3500 reports of adverse reactions ("yellow card" reports), which included 61 deaths [23,24]. Against the background of this yellow card experience it is interesting to note that 5000 patients were followed postmarketing in a study utilizing record-linked methodology, but no instances of hepatic dysfunction were observed.

This experience emphasizes several important points with respect to postmarketing safety surveillance. It illustrates the extent to which the damage due to drug may be augmented by a failure to detect the initial occurrences of the toxicity. In addition, it very graphically makes the point that it is unwise to base a PMS strategy entirely on one approach.

Postmarketing evaluation is not confined exclusively to safety issues but extends to encompass all aspects of a drug's activity. Such aspects may be summarized as follows:

1. Efficacy
   a. Confirmation of the use and indications in the approved labeling
   b. Discovery of new information relating to efficacy
2. Safety
   a. Confirmation of the safety profile in the approved labeling
   b. Discovery of new information relating to safety

Potential new indications for a new drug may have been noted, or anticipated, during the preapproval phase. Postmarketing studies will then be required to fully document this use as a basis for amending the existing product labeling to provide guidance with respect to its use in the new indication. Alternatively, there may have been no suspicion of the new indication during the preapproval stage and such information may have been developed entirely as a result of postmarketing experience. It is not uncommon for such efficacy discoveries to originate entirely from empirical observations made during the normal course of treatment and not from formal studies designed to test a pharmacological hypothesis. These empirical observations are then subjected to the rigors of formal proof in a controlled study. For example, lidocaine was originally marketed as a local anesthetic and only subsequently found to have extensive use as an antiarrhythmic for ventricular arrhythmias. Similarly, the antihypertensive potential of propranolol arose from empirical observations made subsequent to the initial marketing and while the drug was being used for the approved indication in the ordinary treatment setting. These experiences emphasize that postmarketing surveillance can and often does lead to the reporting of events that may have efficacy as opposed to safety implications. In other situations a reaction that was initially regarded solely as adverse may prove ultimately to be the basis of a new indication. Diazepam, for instance, ultimately proved to be extremely useful in the treatment of a condition (e.g., status epilepticus) for which it was originally contraindicated in the labeling based on safety concerns.

With respect to safety, postmarketing surveillance serves at the very minimum to confirm the safety profile that emerged from the clinical research studies. It provides confirmation, in both a qualitative and a quantitative sense, that the safety profile reflected by the labeling is accurate and appropriate to the drug as used in the real-life treatment situation. This may not necessarily follow and, quite apart from the possibility of new adverse events emerging, the incidence or severity of known events may ultimately prove to be different from the experience derived from the clinical research program. The safety profile derived from a carefully selected patient population studied in the controlled environment of a research program may not extrapolate to the population at large who will receive the drug after marketing in an uncontrolled treatment setting. The drug may be used in different doses and for greater periods of time than are reflected in the preapproval program and there is the possibility of unanticipated drug interactions and other effects of concomitant therapies. There is also the possible contribution of other, coexisting pathology and the possibility of differences in response in different patient subpopulations. These subpopulations may not have been represented in the clinical research program or, if represented, the numbers may have been too few relative to the frequency of the reaction to have permitted any meaningful conclusions with respect to safety.

Subsequent to marketing the safety profile of the drug may actually be responsible for its disproportionate use in a specific patient population that itself is at risk for a particular effect. This in turn creates the spurious impression of a safety hazard that was not observed in the research program. For instance, upon marketing a nonsteroidal anti-inflammatory drug (NSAID) that has been found to be well tolerated by the gastrointestinal tract is likely to receive preferential use in patients at high risk of gastrointestinal problems. Such high-risk patients are commonly excluded from a clinical research program prior to approval or, alternatively, the use of such patients is carefully controlled. As a result the first substantial exposure of this susceptible patient population to the drug will occur postmarketing leading to questioning of the accuracy of the clinical research safety profile. In point of fact the profile was correct for the population in which it was studied but this has lead indirectly to its use in a spectrum of patients not represented in the research program.

These observations extend beyond the scope of the specific example cited since, as a general rule, high-risk patients are commonly excluded from clinical research programs prior to approval. These facts emphasize the importance of efficient postmarketing surveillance to provide the earliest possible warning of any impact the use of a drug in a different patient population may have on its safety profile as represented in the labeling.

Pregnant patients will also have been excluded unless the intended use of the drug is specifically associated with pregnancy. Nevertheless, in the average treatment situation it has been estimated that 93% of pregnant patients receive as many as four to five drugs during pregnancy [25].

Finally, there is the very difficult question of drug toxicity that manifests not in the actual patient receiving the drug but in the next generation. This aspect of potential drug toxicity is not normally explored in the clinical research program since in most instances the study protocols will have called for the exclusion of pregnant women unless they constitute the target population. The labeling at approval will describe the findings in preclinical animal reproductive studies and carry appropriate warnings with respect to balancing the potential benefit to the pregnant woman against the potential risk to the unborn fetus. The relevance of data derived from animal reproductive studies to the human situation is most often hypothetical and conjectural. In most instances definitive data relative to humans will only arise as a result of postmarketing experience obtained retrospectively in an uncontrolled setting.

The difficulties inherent in detecting second-generation drug toxicities are potentially compounded by two additional factors. These are the extent to which the drug effects mimic other non–drug-induced effects and whether or not the effects are apparent immediately after birth or require a considerable latent period to emerge. Certainly the existence of the drug effect at birth is calculated to favor early detection but this is not necessarily true. The thalidomide anomaly was detected very rapidly due to the severity and uniqueness of the effect. It is much less certain how long it would have taken to determine that the drug was responsible if the toxicity had manifested as a small but significant increase in the normal background incidence of spina bifida occulta or cleft palate. It would not seem unreasonable to conclude that it might well have escaped detection completely.

A somewhat comparable problem is presented by drug toxicities that require a long latent period before they ultimately manifest in the next generation. The remoteness in time of the drug-induced effect relative to drug exposure in the mother presents an almost insuperable problem for a safety monitoring system to overcome. But, once again, if the effect is unique and distinctive, e.g., diethylstilbestrol (DES) induced clear cell vaginal adenocarcinoma in young women, then its detection will be greatly facilitated notwithstanding the long latent period. The unusual nature and rarity of the particular type of event may be anticipated to prompt a review of the maternal history of drug exposure during pregnancy. But once again, if the DES effect had manifested in the second generation as a small increase in the normal incidence of carcinoma of the cervix in the appropriate age group, then the effect would most probably have gone undetected.

This is clearly a very important aspect of postmarketing safety surveillance. Nevertheless, in spite of its importance, it does not appear to have achieved the prominence accorded to conventional postmarketing safety surveillance. One might speculate that this is because of the magnitude of the problems to be confronted. An ad hoc approach can probably be relied on to detect future thalidomides or DESs but not the more subtle drug effects in the second generation. However, some countries, such as the United Kingdom, have recognized the limitations of conventional safety reporting systems in this context. The United Kingdom responded to the thalidomide disaster by establishing a Registry for Congenital Anomalies anticipating that the recording of such anomalies when correlated with the history of antenatal drug exposure would help to detect such problems. But even if one makes due allowance for the possible problems of detection already mentioned, this approach only deals with one aspect of the problem, specifically congenital anomalies. As the DES experience so graphically illustrates, the drug-induced effect in the next generation may not necessarily manifest at birth as a congenital abnormality.

Furthermore the problem must be viewed as having an international as opposed to a purely national dimension and there are cogent reasons why this is so. For example, national differences in the mode of use of a particular drug may have a profound impact on the extent and manner in which a drug toxicity manifests in a particular country. Consequently a purely national focus that ignores the broad international perspective can miss important information and generate erroneous conclusions. For instance, DES-induced vaginal carcinoma appeared to be predominantly a problem in the United States, almost certainly due to the much wider use in first-trimester pregnancy that the drug received in this country. In other countries in which such use was not as widespread the likelihood of the toxic effect being detected would be considerably diminished.

In some circumstances, quite aside from such differences in national use patterns, the total experience within one country may not be sufficient to permit safety conclusions. The patient exposure on a national basis may be so low that international pooling of data is essential if meaningful and valid safety conclusions are to be drawn. For instance, conception by in vitro fertilization is becoming increasingly accepted and cryopreservation of the 4- to 8-cell "embryo" for future implantation is an integral part of this technique. It is believed that cryopreservation does not lead to intracellular ice formation and consequently there is no risk of damage to the "embryo" as a result of this storage technique. While this is the prevailing view, it has not been established with any degree of certainty that damage will not occur. On the basis of present knowledge one is not able to exclude the possibility of subtle damage that becomes manifest after a latent period in one or more ways not currently predictable. This is another example of the potential inadequacies and unreliability of experimental safety evaluation and the consequent need for continuing safety surveillance. However, given the relative infrequency of the procedure on a national basis a safety surveillance approach would have limited merit if confined to one country. The numbers would be too small to permit conclusions for all except the most overt and unique effects. An effective PMS approach for a situation such as this should mandate an international registry of all children conceived by this technique so as to permit their subsequent development and medical histories to be followed.

The challenge presented in designing any effective PMS program is twofold. The first is to develop methodologies that seek to effectively utilize the large numbers of patients in the general population exposed to drug but at the same time attempt some compensation for the inevitable loss of the controlled study environment. The second is to incorporate the available methodologies into an effective overall strategy.

V. METHODOLOGY

Efficient postmarketing safety surveillance must address three sequential objectives. These are:

1. Recognition of the adverse reaction
2. Causality attribution
3. Quantification of risk

The first objective requires the provision of an early warning system to promptly identify adverse reactions or events that may potentially represent an unsuspected drug-induced toxicity. The second calls for a causality judgment in which the adverse event or reaction is causally related to drug. And finally, having attributed the adverse reaction to drug attempts must be made to obtain a precise estimate of the incidence and magnitude of the safety risk. A PMS system is not meeting its primary overall objective if it does not seek to determine the incidence and potential severity of the reaction in order to ensure that the magnitude of the risk is adequately reflected in the labeling. The primary purpose of postmarketing surveillance is to ensure that at all times the labeling provides the most up to date and accurate information for the benefit of the patient and the prescribing physician.

A variety of PMS techniques have been developed to address these objectives but no one system can address each of these objectives in the most efficient manner possible. The most efficient early warning system is one that gathers data from all patients exposed to the drug in question. However, the very fact that the system seeks to encompass all patients exposed to drug is counterproductive to the other objectives, which are most appropriately pursued in a controlled study environment.

It is not unexpected therefore to find that the generic term "postmarketing safety surveillance" encompasses a broad spectrum of different methodological approaches (Fig. 1). Each method has its own particular strengths and weaknesses and in a general sense they may be regarded as being listed in descending order with respect to the precision of the conclusions they are able to generate. An inevitable tension will always exist between the desire to include the large numbers of patients appropriate to low-incidence events and the desire to retain a controlled study environment to ensure data reliability.

At one extreme are the phase IV postmarketing studies. These experimental approaches comprise well-controlled studies or open uncontrolled studies. Here the emphasis is on the retention of the study environment at the expense of patient numbers. At the other extreme is the relatively unstructured methodology of a voluntary reporting system for spontaneous events/adverse drug reactions (VRSE), which seeks to make maximum use of all patients exposed to the drug worldwide. However, it achieves the benefit of maximum patient numbers at the expense of a controlled study environment. Data quality may suffer and the system is potentially susceptible to generating spurious impressions. Epidemiological-type studies utilizing observational methodology, e.g., cohort and case control studies, occupy a middle ground and represent an attempt to

STRUCTURED METHODOLOGY

Experimental.
      i. Phase IV Postmarketing Controlled Studies.

Observational.
      i. Cohort Studies.
      ii.Case Control Studies.

RECORD-LINKED METHODOLOGY

      i. Prescription Linked Monitoring.
      ii. Hospital Pharmacy Monitoring.

UNSTRUCTURED METHODOLOGY

      i. Voluntary Reporting of Spontaneous ADR's.

Figure 1   Postmarketing surveillance methodology.

resolve this tension between the need for a controlled study environment to ensure data reliability and the need to include the larger numbers of patients appropriate for the study of infrequently occurring events. Although not as burdensome as large phase IV controlled studies, their implementation does nevertheless impose appreciable economic and logistical demands.

A VRSE has immediate appeal not only because of its simplicity but because potentially it derives its data from the total patient population exposed to drug. Therefore in statistical terms it provides the highest probability of detecting very low-incidence toxicities. In a well-organized system its reach transcends national boundaries and encompasses all patients exposed to the drug. The international component can be very important. This is not only because of the augmentation of patient numbers that a global approach provides but also because national differences in safety profile may be discernible and related to national differences in the mode of drug use or other factors. However, the benefits that the broad scope of this approach confers are not available without a price. The data, and therefore the conclusions derived from the data, are impacted to a varying and often unknown extent by deficiencies relating to the number and quality of the adverse reaction reports received (numerator problems) and similar deficiencies with respect to the subjects exposed (denominator problems). There are also other factors that may operate and that therefore require that certain caveats attach to any conclusions drawn from such data. These factors will be discussed more fully later. Nevertheless, these problems notwithstanding, such systems do serve as a very useful and important function. They provide the early warning system that is mandatory to detect the possible existence of significant safety problems, the nature or extent and magnitude of which may have been previously unknown or unsuspected.

A. Experimental vs. Observational Methodology

The comparative merits of these two types of approach will be discussed in greater detail later in connection with the different types of studies. However, a few preliminary comments with respect to these two categories of study are in order by way of introduction. The key difference between these two methodologies lies in the primary purpose for which the drug is administered and the consequences that naturally flow from this. The generic term "experimental" refers to studies in which the drug is given for the primary purpose of acquiring new knowledge. Nonexperimental or "observational" studies, on the other hand, are distinguished by the fact that the drug is given with the sole intent of treating the patient. Any new research knowledge is acquired secondarily to this primary purpose and this may impact on the completeness and quality of the data collected.

In the experimental study patient selection, drug administration, the nature and frequency of the observations, and the setting in which these observations are made are strictly proscribed by the study protocol. However, in the observational study patient selection and drug administration are much more flexible and observations are made in the uncontrolled treatment setting. The extent of these observations is governed entirely by what is considered essential to the treatment of the individual patient, not what is required to serve the overall needs of a research objective. Experimental study design is therefore more conducive to the generation of accurate data addressing specific questions with respect to the drug. However, questions may be raised regarding the validity of extrapolating from such an artificial experimental setting to the population at large. Nonexperimental or observational studies, on the other hand, represent an effort to collect meaningful data from large numbers of patients who are being exposed to drug in the real-life treatment setting. While such studies have the practical advantage of being the only setting relevant to the actual use of the drug they suffer from potential deficiencies with respect to the availability and quality of important data.

Another important difference between experimental and nonexperimental methodology is the ability to control bias. Drug studies should be capable of generating accurate and reliable data from which valid conclusions may be derived, but this process may be compromised by the introduction of bias. Bias is usually considered to be related to the conduct of the study per se but Sackett has pointed out that it may be introduced prior to the initiation of the study or following its completion. In a review of the biases that may be introduced into a clinical study he concluded that this could occur at any stage from the conception of the study to the final publication of the results [26]. In his view biases could be introduced at any of the following points:

1. In the literature research prior to the study
2. In the specification and selection of the study sample
3. In the conduct of the study
4. In the measurement of relevant parameters and outcome variables
5. In the analysis of the data
6. In the interpretation of the analysis
7. In the publication of the results

He also pointed out that there is a very real danger of perpetuating bias. Bias introduced into the publication of study results may subsequently influence the literature research conducted prior to the design and conduct of the next study addressing this same point.

Since bias may be a factor in the selection of the study groups, in the conduct of the study, in the measurement of the data points, and in the analysis of the data, and study design must seek to minimize these biases. In experimental methodology this is accomplished by the use of the controlled clinical trial in which the protocol regulates the conduct of the study, specifies selection criteria, employs a control group(s), randomly assigns patients to treatment groups, requires double-blind observation, and specifies in advance the analytical techniques to be employed in data analysis. The controlled randomized study, which is the basis of the experimental method, exhibits the greatest propensity for minimizing bias, whereas observational methodology (cohort studies, case control studies) or uncontrolled experimental studies probably have the greatest likelihood of introducing bias.

Another important consideration is whether or not the study is prospective or retrospective. Experimental methodology is based on prospective, randomized, controlled studies. Such a design, however, mandates that precise information be available with regard to the nature and magnitude of the effect to be studied. While this is invariably the case in establishing efficacy, it is very commonly not the case when evaluating safety. On the other hand, observational methodology may be either prospective or retrospective. As a general rule observational studies are less precise than experimental and those that are retrospective are subject to a great deal of bias.

While these abstract theoretical observations may be correct they must be tempered by more pragmatic considerations. If one seeks to take advantage of the maximum patient numbers available then this fact alone, aside from any other factors, determines the methodology based solely on considerations of feasibility and practicality. This is particularly true in the postmarketing situation when safety evaluation is the issue.

B. Experimental Methodology

Postmarketing (phase IV) controlled studies have their maximum utility in addressing those additional efficacy issues that need to be explored during the postmarketing period. To a large extent the limitations that apply to the evaluation of safety issues in controlled studies during the research program apply equally to phase IV studies. Phase IV postmarketing safety studies present exactly the same problems as controlled studies in the preapproval stage and their usefulness is constrained by the same factors. First, there must be a safety hypothesis to test, and they are clearly of little use when the nature and magnitude of the safety risk is still unknown. Second, the constraint on sample sizes is a very real limitation with respect to the sensitivity of the study to differentiate between treatment groups with respect to low-incidence events.

In certain situations the constraint on patient numbers may not be operative to the same extent as during the preapproval research phase. For instance, a large multicenter study of many thousands of patients may be initiated primarily for efficacy purposes. Studies exploring the effects of a hypolipemic drug on morbidity and mortality or the prophylactic use of β-blocker therapy following an initial myocardial infarction would be relevant examples. In such cases the use of patient numbers far in excess of those customarily included in preapproval studies would provide greater power with respect to the less common toxicities. While this would apply particularly to the probability of rare infrequent toxicity manifesting in the drug group, it should be emphasized that the numbers may still not be large enough to differentiate treatment groups if confusing background noise is present in the control group.

While large phase IV postmarketing studies directed toward safety issues may incorporate a controlled design, they are much more commonly established as large uncontrolled studies involving approximately 10,000–20,000 patients. Typical studies would be those conducted immediately postmarketing with cimetidine [27], captopril [28], cyclobenzaprine [29], and prazosin [30]. Such studies are usually conducted with the objective of confirming the qualitative aspects of the drug's existing side effect profile or to confirm the frequency of an already identified adverse reaction. Of the four studies cited, not one revealed any new adverse reactions that had not been observed in the preapproval research program. The prazosin study was specifically designed to address the side effect of syncope and served to confirm the incidence (1%) that had previously been observed in the preapproval clinical research program.

It is important to note, however, that although these study sizes were large (7000–22,000) they could not be relied on to detect hitherto unreported side effects. In point of fact other additional new adverse events were subsequently identified for two of these drugs through spontaneous reports to the VRSE database. For this reason it is generally concluded that such phase IV studies are not adequate for the detection of safety events that have an incidence of less than 1 in 10,000. Since these sample sizes are of the same order of magnitude as those commonly employed for the other forms of structured PMS methodology, e.g., case control and cohort studies, these same strictures will also apply. These findings further serve to underscore the fact that, for really low-incidence toxicities, such as those occurring with a frequency of 1 in 100,000 or less, the VRSE system may be the only viable approach to their detection in spite of the potential problems inevitably associated with the collection of data from an uncontrolled setting.

C.   Nonexperimental or Observational Studies

Observational studies provide a practical approach to the study of large patient populations in the normal treatment setting. A setting that may properly be regarded as the only one relevant to the use and safety of the drug in question. Although the observational approach has certain obvious advantages over the experimental, most especially with regard to patient numbers, there are some disadvantages to this approach that the study methodology must seek to circumvent.

Developments in the field of observational studies have been mainly in the direction of increasing the precision of the safety hypotheses generated. This not only facilitates the improved design of subsequent confirmatory controlled studies, but it provides for greater confidence in the conclusions of the observational study in those situations in which the logistics of patient numbers involved make a subsequent controlled study impractical.

In addition to these design issues there are also attitudinal issues that need to be considered. In sharp contrast to design issues, which tend to be specific to the different types of observational study, attitudinal issues are generic to all types of observational studies. They also have their impact in the unstructured setting of VRSE systems. Attitudinal issues have their genesis in the fact that medical practice is outcome-oriented whereas clinical research is data-oriented. In an experimental study the focus is primarily on data acquisition. It is on the measurement of the different parameters of drug effect, both beneficial and adverse, as required by the protocol rather than on the needs of the individual patient for treatment purposes. The relationship is more oriented toward investigator and patient-volunteer and the pursuit of research knowledge than physician and patient and the optimum treatment outcome for the individual patient.

By contrast, in the observational study the relationship begins and remains exclusively one of physician–patient in the ordinary treatment setting. The focus is on the treatment needs of the individual patient, no more and no less. It is not on the individual patient as a study subject and the collection of data according to protocol. Certain important sequelae flow from this subtle but important distinction. It can significantly impact on the quality and completeness of the data available and also on physician feedback relative to potential safety events. For instance, in a controlled study full evaluation is always mandatory in an attempt to determine causality of an adverse reaction. In a treatment setting with its primary focus on the treatment needs of the patient there will be instances when this could justifiably be regarded as irrelevant to treatment needs and an undue burden on the patient. In such instances data are likely to be less than complete.

D. Cohort Studies

In a cohort study a group or groups of patients are identified and then followed forward, prospectively in time, and observed for the occurrence of certain events. The primary focus for the purposes of selection and information gathering is on the patient. A cohort of patients is identified on the basis of certain predetermined selection criteria that are not related, at least not directly, to the issue under investigation. For instance, when the matter under investigation is an adverse drug reaction profile a cohort of patients might be identified that comprises all patients falling within certain defined categories without reference to the type and pattern of their drug exposure. Subsequent to the identification of the cohort their drug exposure and adverse experience history is recorded. It is inherent in the methodology of the cohort study that it incorporates its own control group but it is nevertheless essential to confirm the comparability and homogeneity of the two groups. As a general rule both cohort studies and case control studies (vide infra) depend on the existence of a hypothesis to be tested. However, while case control studies may on occasion be used for hypothesis generation, cohort studies are not appropriate as "fishing expeditions" for the detection of unknown and as yet undescribed reactions. They are appropriate for hypothesis confirmation as opposed to hypothesis generation.

Most often a cohort study is prospective in nature and will identify the group to be studied (cohort) according to certain preset criteria before the events to be monitored develop. It may, for instance, call for the selection of all female patients over 65 years of age with rheumatoid arthritis attending certain clinics. The scope of the information sought may be as broad as a complete drug history and all adverse events experienced, or, alternatively, it may be more focused and concentrate only on the use of one or two NSAIDs and the occurrence of peptic ulcer.

However, cohort studies are nevertheless sometimes conducted retrospectively. In such studies the adverse event to be monitored will already have occurred and patient recall becomes an extremely important factor with the potential to bias the results.

1. Potential Sources of Error

There are several potential sources of error in the interpretation of cohort studies. As already noted, problems associated with deficiencies in patient recall are predominantly a feature of the retrospective form of cohort study. This problem is largely alleviated if a prospective design is followed in which monitoring and the elicitation of information is on a current and contemporaneous basis. Within the cohort of patients studied there will be one group of patients who develop the reaction under study and another who are unaffected and may be regarded as the control group. A careful check should be made for comparability and lack of heterogeneity between the groups since this may impact on the reliance that can be placed on the conclusions drawn from the study.

A final consideration is that the cohort as a whole should be fully representative of the population at large and the one to which the results are to be extrapolated. Patient selection is also an issue in experimental methodology where it is addressed by random allocation of patients to treatment. Nevertheless there must always remain a question with regard to the extent to which the results in the drug group of an experimental study may be extrapolated to the general population.

E. Case Control Studies

The case control study employs a group of "case" patients and a group of "control" patients. For each case patient studied a matched control must be located. These matched pairs of patients should be comparable with respect to all relevant factors, except for the condition under study which is present only in the case patient and not in the control patient. A retrospective examination of the two groups is then conducted to determine whether any significant differences exist between the two groups. It is important that the controls be selected from the same population as the cases and defined in such a way that, had they manifested the condition under study, they would have qualified as case patients too. The population from which the patients are drawn may vary. It may comprise all patients admitted to a given hospital or hospitals, all patients treated at a particular clinic or clinics, or all patients from a given geographic locality. Similarly, the comprehensiveness of the case group may vary. It may represent all patients with that particular reaction or disease or it may be simply a subset of that population.

The key requirement for the selection of the control patients is that they should be as representative as possible of the population from which the cases are drawn. But they should exclude any patients who manifest the type of reaction being investigated. The control group should not include patients with conditions that are an absolute contraindication for therapy with the drug under study since drug exposure in the control group would not then be truly representative of drug exposure in the case group. The variables of age and sex are basic variables that should be matched with respect to the two groups.

The purpose of matching is to avoid a situation in which some factor associated with both drug exposure and the adverse reaction under investigation could operate to confound the results and show an apparent but spurious association between the drug and the reaction. For example, it is well documented that elderly patients fare significantly worse than younger patients with respect to the complications of peptic ulcer. Accordingly, a case control study of osteoarthritic patients in which the groups were not well matched for age might generate the erroneous conclusion that the complications of peptic ulcer were aggravated by NSAID therapy whereas the real reason was the disparity in age distribution of the two groups. This same type of problem can also be associated with the interpretation of results from a VRSE system. The major difference is that while the problem can be directly addressed in the case control study by matching the case and control groups, there is no means of addressing the problem in the VRSE system. Clearly it may not be possible to address all factors that might have an impact by matching. Those that have not been addressed must be dealt with in the analysis of the study.

A case control study to test for the association of a drug and a particular adverse reaction may proceed in one of two ways. Patients using the drug in question may be compared with controls who are not using the drug, for the emergence of the adverse reaction. Or, alternatively, a group of patients manifesting the reaction may be compared in terms of drug intake history with a group who do not manifest the reaction. Appropriate selection requires that, in the event that no association between the reaction and the drug exists, the controls should be as likely to use the drug as the patients, or the controls should be as likely to manifest the reaction as the patients.

The distinguishing feature of the case control study is its retrospective nature, which means that the logic flow of the cause-and-effect reasoning is the reverse of that obtained in the (prospective) cohort study. In studies relating to drug safety the cohort study identifies a cohort exposed to the putative cause of the reaction (the drug in question) and then follows it prospectively for the emergence of the adverse reaction. By contrast, the case control study identifies a group with the adverse reaction to be studied and retrospectively evaluates their drug exposure history. Memory recall is of paramount importance in eliciting items of information vital to the success of the study. This is inherent in the retrospective nature of the study design and can play an important role in introducing an element of bias. It is a factor that is largely outside the capabilities of the investigator to influence or the study design to control. It is therefore something that cannot be completely discounted when considering the results of the study.

Notwithstanding these caveats, case control methodology has proven to be an invaluable and practical approach to generating and testing hypotheses with respect to the adverse reactions to drugs. For instance, case control studies have been utilized to document the risk of thromboembolism associated with oral contraceptives and the incidence of bone marrow suppression as a result of amidopyrine therapy [31]. This particular type of retrospective analysis may also be able to provide vital information regarding the reasons why the case patients developed a specific adverse reaction to a particular drug. The retrospective case control study has a greater utility in generating safety hypotheses than testing them and for this reason is particularly useful for rare but important and serious adverse events. However, it should not be overlooked that prospective data are less biased than retrospective data since they do not place a primary reliance on memory recall and therefore do not incorporate any bias from this standpoint.

Nevertheless case control studies may be conducted prospectively and the various studies that were carried out to define the relationship between oral contraceptive therapy and certain pathological events provide excellent examples of the two contrasting types of case control study. A number of British studies that sought to define an association between such therapy and thrombotic events utilized a retrospective approach in which all defined events over a specified period in the past were identified and studied [32]. By contrast the American Collaborative Study used prospective methodology in which the cases and controls were identified and investigated as the study proceeded [33]. The latter approach has certain advantages over the former. With the retrospective approach the historical nature of the information means that one is constrained by the adequacy of the data records as they exist and by the clinical and laboratory investigations that were actually carried out at the time.

These past inadequacies in data generation do not necessarily reflect any deficiencies in patient management. They are more appropriately viewed as a failure to do those things that are not strictly relevant to proper patient care but would be necessary if the primary objective was to serve a research purpose. Patient evaluation and testing that is more than adequate for optimum patient treatment may well stop short of that minimum of data required if the primary purpose of patient treatment is a research objective. Conversely, the patient evaluation and testing required to serve a meaningful research purpose may be far more than is required for optimum patient care. Data deficiencies of this nature will have a lasting impact on the value of any subsequent retrospective study. The prospective approach by contrast allows one to actively pursue complete and comprehensive information at the time and to ensure that whatever investigations and procedures are required and relevant are in fact carried out. There is an opportunity to control and influence the generation of appropriate relevant data that is totally absent in the retrospective study. The results of the study are not inevitably constrained by the limitations in the data as they exist.

The great attraction of case control studies is that they can be carried out in a very expeditious fashion and with a minimum of financial expenditure. Indeed, if extensive personal interviewing is not a consistent requirement, but only on an ad hoc basis, then computer technology can be utilized to scan records, select cases according to predetermined criteria, and derive the relevant data. It is not surprising to find, therefore, that retrospective case control research has become extremely popular as an epidemiological tool and it has achieved widespread scientific acceptance within the medical community.

However, this enthusiasm should be tempered with the knowledge that this methodology can at times produce contradictory results. The classic and well-known examples are the erroneous conclusions that were originally derived from case control studies concerning the prophylactic effect of circumcision on carcinoma of the cervix and the association of reserpine therapy with carcinoma of the breast. In the latter instance, three case control studies initially purported to have demonstrated a causal relationship between reserpine and carcinoma of the breast [35–36]. But subsequently this conclusion was contradicted by an additional eight case control studies, all of which were consistently negative [37–44]. A detailed but by no means comprehensive review of the literature that was carried out revealed 17 scientific issues where the results of an initial case control study were subsequently contradicted by further case control studies or cohort studies [45]. This raises the question of whether there should be an unqualified acceptance of the conclusions of any single case control study as definitive in the absence of confirmatory cohort studies or further case control studies.

1. Limitations of Case Control Studies

A considerable staff effort is required in the interviewing process in such studies. Furthermore, if the study is of retrospective design, the study quality is inevitably limited by whatever deficiencies may exist in patient records, investigations, or other sources of information.

Case control studies are subject to bias from a number of sources, which in a controlled study may be minimized by the traditional methodological approaches to such studies. Reference has already been made to the potential for the introduction of bias due to a failure of recall. A patient's powers of recollection with respect to prior drug experience may be deficient and in some instances extremely selective. Such recall defects will impact adversely on the ability of the study to detect associations that may in fact be present. Another important source of bias in case control studies relates to the selection process. Within the framework of the controlled study this potential source of bias is minimized by the random assignment of patients to treatment groups in accordance with a randomization code. In the case control study this source of bias may be minimized if it is feasible to study a total patient population, as, for example, all patients in particular geographic location, e.g., in England and Wales in a study of oral contraceptives [46]. However, when the study involves a subset of a population, as is more commonly the case, then problems of selection bias will assume greater weight.

For example, the selection of all patients from one clinic or one hospital has the potential to introduce significant problems that may be related to certain determining factors associated with and specific to those locations. A preferred approach to circumvent this type of problem would be to draw the study population from a number of hospitals or clinics. But, depending on the nature of the determining factor leading to a spurious association, even this approach may not be sufficient to avoid the impact of selection bias. It is well established that elderly patients who develop peptic ulcer do less well with respect to the complications of the disease than younger patients. This is so to the extent that they can be expected to be hospitalized more frequently. Therefore a study that utilizes hospital admissions to determine the association of NSAID therapy with peptic ulcer disease may be biased with regard to any conclusions relating to apparent incidence.

Another factor to be considered in selection is that there should be no causal link between the adverse reaction studied and the drug prescribed, since this may bias results in either direction. If, for instance, an NSAID is widely promoted as being relatively free from gastrointestinal (GI) side effects then it is more likely than not that patients with a prior history of GI disease will figure prominently in the patient population exposed to the drug. This can result in an apparent incidence of GI side effects that is not representative of the population as a whole. Similarly in the study of a drug, e.g., an oral contraceptive, with the putative adverse effect of precipitating myocardial infarction a past history of recurrent infarction and/or ischemic heart disease constitutes a reason for excluding patients from the study. Otherwise a possible association of the drug with myocardial infarction might be concealed.

2. Analysis of Results

The results of case control studies may be expressed as the relative risk of the adverse reaction in question for users of the drug as compared with controls. When the study is designed to generate possible safety hypotheses rather than confirm a hypothesis the classical situation of multiple testing must be confronted. It then becomes necessary to avoid the possibility of chance alone finding a significant association from among the many associations tested. Therefore fairly strict criteria for the interpretation of results should be established for such studies. If the objective is to test for significance of the hypothesis at customarily accepted levels ($p \leq .05$) this will provide reasonable confidence of the result.

As already indicated, it is not possible to address all potential confounding factors when matching the control and case patients. These other factors, which are not addressed in the selection process, remain as potential sources of bias. They may, however, be explored post hoc in the analysis of the data for any contribution they may make with regard to the association being tested.

F. Voluntary Reporting of Spontaneous Events

The VRSE approach to monitoring drug safety is often referred to as "postmarketing surveillance" (PMS), but in many ways this is not the most appropriate choice of terminology. The term *postmarketing surveillance* is probably more correctly used in a generic as opposed to a specific sense to encompass all of the various techniques available to monitor drug safety in the postmarketing environment and of which this particular approach is but one. VRSE is a more descriptive term in that it more accurately conveys the true focus of the reporting efforts of the system. VRSE represents one extreme of the variety of methods available for postmarketing surveillance.

It may be viewed as an attempt to collect the clinical observations made during the ordinary course of medical treatment and incorporate those relevant to safety into an efficient system of postmarketing safety surveillance. Historically, experience teaches that routine observations of this type made in the unstructured treatment setting have certainly been responsible for the discovery of some significant therapy-related safety problems. In this context one might cite the microcephaly associated with irradiation [47], carcinoma of the thyroid following irradiation of the thymus in childhood [48], cataracts with rubella [49], clear cell vaginal carcinoma with DES [50], and phocomelia due to thalidomide [51]. It would seem to follow that a more organized approach to the collection of this type of data can only be anticipated to provide a more effective postmarketing safety surveillance system. However, the benefits accruing from careful clinical observation for potential safety issues cannot be fully realized unless the information is collected from all potential sources and brought together at one point for review.

An international approach to VRSE is mandatory and confers an advantage that goes beyond the question of numbers of patients exposed. It provides an opportunity to monitor safety issues that may be largely a function of distinctive national patterns of drug usage. For instance, clear cell adenocarcinoma of the vagina is thought to occur with a frequency of $1/1000$ in the daughters of mothers who received DES during the early stages of pregnancy. The occurrence of this pathology unrelated to drug is quite rare and occurs in a completely different age group. In the United States the drug enjoyed fairly widespread use in early pregnancy and the first recognition of this form of DES toxicity was undoubtedly facilitated by the fact that several million pregnant women were exposed to the drug in this country. However, it did not receive the same level of enthusiastic use in early pregnancy in Europe, and in Denmark and Finland it was not used at all in pregnancy. If the more conservative attitudes and use patterns had also been prevalent in this country the result would probably have been a great delay in the recognition of this toxicity. There would appear to be little doubt that national differences in the pattern of drug usage can influence its toxicity profile. Safety surveillance must therefore be organized on an international as opposed to a national basis in order to anticipate such an eventuality.

However, the fact that the observations are collected from a routine treatment setting are both a strength and a weakness. Whilst this is responsible for the significant advantages of VRSE it is also responsible for some of its limitations.

1. The Advantages

VRSE systems possess two significant advantages that justify their routine use in spite of the problems associated with interpreting the data generated. The first advantage relates to the number of patients exposed to drug. Unlike studies using structured methodology, there is no practical limit on the number of patients encompassed by a VRSE system. It is the only system with the potential to collect data from the total population exposed to the drug worldwide. This advantage is so overwhelming that this approach should be employed as a standard routine for all drugs and no effort should be spared to improve on its operation.

The exact number of patients exposed is simply a function of the degree of market use that the drug achieves. If the drug gains fairly rapid acceptance by the medical community, then these numbers may reach figures in excess of 1 million in a comparatively short space of time. Such exponential increases in patient accrual place a great emphasis on the efficient performance of the VRSE system, particularly in the period immediately after approval. During that time hitherto unsuspected rare toxicity may manifest very rapidly. With rapid patient accrual the consequences of missing a safety problem may have a much more serious impact than if the population database was accumulating slowly.

The greatly augmented patient numbers available in an VRSE system provide the necessary power to detect very low-incidence toxicities. In fact this system is the only viable approach to detecting very infrequent events, such as the agranulocytosis associated with phenylbutazone therapy with an incidence as low as 1/50,000 to 1/100,000. In general the other PMS approaches such as record-linked and observational methodology have limited application for events occurring with a frequency of less than 1 in 10,000.

The second advantage relates to the fact that drug safety is being monitored in the only relevant population. This is the population that receives the drug in the routine course of treatment as opposed to a carefully selected subset in an experimental study environment. This is a matter of some importance since the clinical research database is often not representative of the spectrum of patients who will receive the drug after marketing. The safety conclusions are therefore not necessarily extrapolatable to the general population.

The population at risk comprises many different patient subsets that are differentiated by various characteristics. These include, among others, ethnic differences, extremes of age, pregnancy, patients in a weakened and debilitated state, patients with various coexisting diseases, and patients receiving different concomitant therapies. Some of these subsets may have been included in the clinical research program but in numbers too small to permit meaningful conclusions for more uncommon safety events. Other subsets may not have been represented at all in the clinical program. The postmarketing period provides the first opportunity to obtain data from reasonable sample sizes of these various patient subsets.

Pragmatically a clinical research program can only explore those variables or patient subsets that will be most commonly encountered in practice or where there is some theoretical reason to anticipate an interaction or difference in safety profile. For unanticipated safety issues, whether related to coexisting pathology, concomitant therapy, or other factors, the information must come from the postmarketing situation. Similarly, the clinical research program may not have revealed safety issues that are a function of total drug exposure. Preapproval programs for chronic use drugs typically include therapy durations of 1–2 years in a subset of patients, commonly of the order of several hundred. However, such patient numbers may not be adequate if the safety event related to duration of therapy is of low incidence. It was noted previously that the likelihood of detecting an infrequent adverse reaction of the order of 0.1% is high (95% probability) if at least 3000 patients are studied. If a toxicity of this same frequency (0.1%) is specific to a subset of the target population represented only to the extent of a few dozen or a few hundred patients in the research program, then the power of detection is considerably curtailed.

By utilizing these large numbers of patients VRSE is capable of generating important safety data, especially on rare events. However, the extent to which this theoretical advantage is a reality depends on the impact of a variety of factors including the patient, the various health care professionals involved, and a multiplicity of other possible variables. These variables are necessarily an integral part of any treatment setting. They may operate to delay recognition of a potential problem or to distort estimates of its true magnitude and seriousness. Therefore the very feature that makes the data so representative may also impact adversely on the ability to obtain complete and accurate data with respect to the numerator and denominator, thereby affecting the validity of the conclusions.

2. The Limitations

There are a number of imperfections in any VRSE system that are limiting with respect to the conclusions that may be derived from it. Some of these, such as the actual reporting of adverse reactions by the treating physician (numerator problems) and information relating to the composition of the patient population exposed to drug (denominator problems) cannot be effectively addressed and controlled. Others, such as the precision of estimates with respect to the numbers of patients exposed, can be partially addressed. And finally there are those factors, e.g., data collection and follow-up of cases, that are entirely within the capacity of those in charge of the system to control. The corollary of these observations is an even greater emphasis on the need to address those potential sources of imperfection that can be directly controlled.

3. Factors Relating to the Numerator

The factors affecting the numerator arise from two sources. There are those that relate to the organization and functioning of the system itself. This involves the efficient collection of the reactions that are reported, and the processing, analysis, interpretation, and reporting of the data. These factors are entirely within the ability of those administering the system to influence. And, as emphasized earlier, it behooves one to maximize the efficiency of this aspect of the system since it is the one that can be directly controlled.

But what happens prior to the point of actual receipt of the reports by the various company locations is something completely outside the control of those administering the system. This is essentially a function of the conscientiousness with which physicians and other health care professionals cooperate in the reporting of adverse reactions to the system. The maximum that a well-organized VRSE system can achieve is to deal very efficiently with those reports it does receive. It can do nothing about those that are, for any of a number of reasons, not submitted.

There is no question but that significant underreporting does exist, and as such, it does compromise the utility of the VRSE system as an early warning system. Some estimates have placed this as low as 1–10%, but any such estimates must remain conjectural and not susceptible to formal proof since this is inherent in the very definition of a spontaneous report [52]. A more formal survey of over 1000 physicians revealed results that do not differ significantly from these estimates. Only 37% of physicians reported having detected an adverse reaction in a given year; the remaining 67% claiming not to have done so. Of those who saw a reaction only one in five reported it [53]. The main reasons offered for not reporting were "the reporting forms were unavailable," "the reaction was not serious," and "it had already been reported for that particular drug." Physicians not infrequently saw it as unnecessary to report "one more" of an already documented effect. This reasoning of course reveals a profound ignorance of the true purpose of spontaneous reporting. The degree to which a physician is sensitized to a situation by the publicity concerning reactions [54], the scientific literature, the advertising material, or the activities of sales representatives can also impact on reporting. Reporter bias can also be a factor, occasioned by the fact that patients who cite particular problems are the ones physicians remember.

However, the evidence in recent years indicates a growing sensitivity by the practicing physician to the reporting issue in that reporting compliance has shown some improvement [55]. One report cited the common factors predisposing the physician to report an adverse reaction as severity of the reaction, a certain relationship to drug, and the mechanism of the drug reaction. Reactions with an idiosyncratic or an allergic mechanism were more likely to be reported than those with a pharmacological basis [56].

And finally the physician may be uneasy about having caused harm to the patient by use of the drug. This concern by the physician that the patient not be aware that the treatment was responsible has been cited as a factor influencing nonreporting. In this context some suggest that a fear of litigation can lead to underreporting in the more litigious medicolegal environments.

Perhaps the most subtle and pervasive of all the factors affecting physician reporting to VRSE systems is what may be described generically as the attitudinal factor. In the normal treatment setting, the attitudinal bias of the physician is oriented primarily in the direction of treatment outcome. The physician's focus is on the management of the patient to ensure a favorable outcome to treatment with a minimum of untoward effects. The physician's conduct is governed primarily by what is essential for proper patient care and not what is required to properly evaluate a suspected adverse reaction. This additional information may have no relevance to the immediate necessities of patient care.

If a suspected adverse event supervenes during therapy the primary concern of the practicing physician is whether or not it will resolve following discontinuation of the drug. If this in fact occurs his next concern is an alternative therapy. These concerns take precedence over further evaluation of the reaction or reporting it. Commonly the question of causality will only be pursued further if it has a direct relationship to the treatment of the individual patient. This will occur if the reaction does not subside promptly, its etiology is in doubt, or the information is relevant to the issue of alternative therapy. In the treatment context causality attribution is only occasionally relevant to proper patient care and the reporting of spontaneous events is never relevant. These attitudinal factors will clearly have an inevitable impact both on the completeness of the data collected with respect to an adverse reaction and on the consistency of reporting such reactions.

This attitudinal bias, which militates against compliance with reporting obligations, receives further reinforcement from other sources. Not only is it often irrelevant to treatment needs, but it always constitutes an additional and unwelcome burden on the practicing physician. It is one that the physician is not compelled to observe and, from a purely materialistic point of view, he or she is not reimbursed for the collection of such data.

In the clinical research setting, however, there is a motivation for full reporting. The primary concern of the physician-investigator is the collection of data to further the research objectives of the study. In addition to the intellectual motivation the physician is reimbursed for his or her efforts and furthermore study monitoring will provide protection against deficiencies in study conduct, data collection, and reporting.

It should be noted that problems may arise not only from a failure to report but also from misplaced priorities with respect to reporting such as the physician's desire to publish. Benoxaprofen-induced cholestatic jaundice, for instance, was first reported in the United Kingdom in a medical journal and not by a yellow card report to the Committee on Safety of Medicines. Similarly the first recognition of Stevens–Johnson syndrome associated with isoxicam was significantly delayed because the first account was submitted for publication rather than reported in the VRSE system. The problem was compounded by the fact that the publication was held up. The importance of these various elements is underscored by the fact that underreporting is a very real and universal phenomenon.

Studies have shown a clear temporal pattern with respect to voluntary reporting systems. This would appear to have its origins in attitudinal characteristics also. Data have been generated that indicate a fairly distinctive pattern independent of the drug involved. The number of reports to VRSE systems tends to reach its peak by the second year after marketing. Thereafter reporting tends to fall off to year 5 with as much as a fivefold drop-off during that period for specific adverse reactions. This phenomenon has been well documented for cimetidine [57]. This has great relevance for the comparisons of VRSE data between different drugs since it calls into question comparisons that are not made for the same time point after marketing. The prescription event monitoring (PEM) system in the United Kingdom is very careful to take this factor into account when selecting the appropriate control agent.

It is of interest to note that there are also some very clear national differences in physician compliance with respect to spontaneous event reporting and it would appear that these differences are real rather than artifactual (Table 3). The United States is tenth in a list of 16 countries with well-established drug regulatory systems. The two countries at the top of the list (Denmark and New Zealand) have a reporting rate that is approximately 2½ times the level in the United States. The United Kingdom and Australia, which are fourth and fifth, respectively, have a reporting rate that is approximately 1½ times higher. Of the six countries below the United States only five have levels of reporting compliance that are significantly less, France and Germany with 50% and Italy and Japan with approximately 5% of the U.S. rate. What is particularly interesting, in view

Table 3 Frequency of Adverse Event Reporting in 16 Countries

Country	Population of country (mill)	Year system instituted	Maximum reports annually	Maximum rate ADR reports per 10 of population	Rx items per Caput per annum (year)
Denmark	5.12	1968	2087	407.6	6.5(1980)
New Zealand	3.03	1965	1160	383.2	8.5(1983)
Sweden	8.32	1965	2785	334.7	4.7(1980)
United Kingdom	56.00	1964	14701	262.5	6.5(1982)
Australia	14.93	1964	3715	248.8	7.7(1981)
Norway	4.10	1970	909	221.7	—
Canada	23.00	1965	4891	212.6	—
Ireland	3.44	1967	702	204.1	—
Finland	4.81	1966	726	150.9	5.1(1980)
United States	226.54	1961	33314	147.0	16.6(1979)
Netherlands	14.29	1963	1912	133.8	—
France	54.09	1976	4198	77.6	10.0(1982)
Germany	61.66	1962	4516	73.3	11.2(1982)
Belgium	9.85	1976	655	66.5	—
Japan	117.88	1967	822	6.9	—
Italy	56.24	1980	359	6.3	11.3(1982)

Source: Adapted from Ref. 60.

of the sociocultural similarities between the two countries, is that the Canadian performance is almost 1½ higher than the U.S.

The United States therefore has the most intensely regulated system of drug research and approval of any country, yet paradoxically it has relatively poor compliance in spontaneous reporting. It would appear that the heavy emphasis nationally on the regulation of drugs has contributed little toward inculcating good habits with respect to reporting compliance in the postmarketing period. By contrast, countries with a less intensely regulated process show a far higher level of postmarketing compliance.

It is interesting to speculate on the possible reasons for this pattern. It does not appear to be simply a function of the higher level of prescription drug use within a country. If this were the explanation one would expect those countries toward the top of the list with a higher level of compliance to have the highest prescribing rates. This is not so. In fact, of the countries for which information is available the United States has the highest prescribing rate but one of the lower reporting rates. The countries with far superior reporting compliance have an average prescribing rate that is two to four times less than that of the United States. The conclusion would appear to be that although drug use is lower it appears to be monitored more effectively by physicians.

The data provided in Table 3 do, however, suggest a possible explanation for the phenomenon. It may not be coincidental that the United States is distinguished from these other countries by its political philosophy with respect to the provision of health care. In the United States primary reliance is placed on the private sector for the provision of health care whereas those countries placed higher on the list (Table 3) adhere to a political philosophy that favors very significant, if not total, government involvement. It is not altogether too fanciful to conclude that physicians working within a health care system in which there is major government participation would be more compliant with respect to reporting than those who function in a system in which they regard themselves as autonomous participants in a completely free and independent private sector. The latter are more likely to equate the demands of a reporting system with the nuances of control, government or otherwise, of their prescribing habits and professional freedom. The former, however, are more likely to accept and comply since reporting requirements are an integral part of their professional activities within a public sector health care system. Their whole concept of health care is that of a system that has a significant component of documentation and reporting. Evidence of this is seen in the PEM system in the United Kingdom, which owes its success not only to the centralization of records that characterizes a national health care system (vide infra), but also to the compliance of the busy physicians in completing the questionnaire.

There may be an additional contributing factor. The United States is unique with regard to the litigious environment in which the provision of medical care and the prescription of drugs are conducted. Indeed at times it might appear that scientific decisions relative to drugs and the standards of medical care are made primarily in the courtroom. There has been ample precedent to indicate that even the scientific decisions of a statutory body such as the FDA are not immune in this respect. Courts have preempted the scientific authority of the FDA by holding that the information contained in an agency-approved package insert is inadequate on a scientific basis. In such cases they have held the physician liable for a failure to obtain fully informed consent, even when such consent was based on the approved package insert. Recent statements by the agency with respect to the fluoxetine issue would appear to indicate that the FDA itself is prepared to accept this concept of resolving a scientific debate in the courts. Since the publication of the original article by Teicher et al. there has been a literal explosion of personal injury litigation with respect to this drug's alleged behavioral effects and they have been advanced as a criminal defense. Extensive expert data review and analysis has provided no scientific basis for the contention that the drug precipitates suicidal tendencies or violent criminal behavior. A senior FDA official speaking on behalf of the agency rejected such an association stating that the use of such an argument by an attorney does not constitute scientific evidence. However, this balanced statement is almost immediately negated by the additional and rather surprising comment that "an actual court finding of a causal relationship between Prozac and violent behavior would be relevant." The FDA official went on to add that no such court decision has ever been issued [58]. The logical conclusion would appear to be that in spite of an expert panel having rejected the association the agency would be prepared to give credence to a jury decision on this scientific issue. Against this background it would not be surprising if the nature of the medicolegal climate and a fear of litigation were not contributing in some subtle manner to the poor performance of physicians in the United States as compared with other countries.

4.   Factors Relating to the Denominator

A reliable estimate of the incidence of an adverse reaction requires reasonably accurate information with respect to the number of patients experiencing the adverse event (numerator) and the patients exposed to the drug (denominator). The Achilles heel of voluntary reporting systems lies in the imprecision and softness of the data relating to these elements when compared to the hard data available from experimental studies. It is for this reason that VRSE data that purport to quantify a safety risk should be viewed with some caution. It should be regarded as a tentative conclusion, a safety hypothesis that must then be tested using some other form of PMS methodology.

The deficiencies relative to the denominator may be both quantitative and qualitative. Since the number of patients exposed to the drug cannot be measured directly, some indirect measure of patient exposure must be utilized. The usual approach to the denominator issue is to utilize unit sales volume of the drug or number of prescriptions as an index of patient exposure. There are clearly limitations to these approaches. Sales volume is a function of both the number of patients exposed and the pattern of drug use or duration of therapy. If the side effect is associated with a short-term-use drug, e.g., antibiotic, in which single prescriptions tend to be given and not repeated, then the sales volume or prescription volume will provide a reasonable approximation of the patients exposed. If, however, the drug is used on a chronic basis or receives both chronic and acute use, then some distortion will be introduced. The time pattern of the adverse event associated with a chronic use drug also plays a part. If the occurrence of the adverse event is a function of total drug exposure per se rather than time on drug, the sales volume will provide a reasonable approximation of patient exposure for purposes of calculating incidence. However, with some adverse reactions the reaction tends to be associated with the initial doses. A typical example is provided by syncope occurring in association with antihypertensive therapy with α_1-antagonist drugs. Here the side effect is characteristically associated with the initial administration of the drug. The use of sales volume data for purposes of denominator estimates in this situation will have the effect of spuriously lowering the apparent incidence of the reaction. The most appropriate measure would be an estimate of new prescriptions.

Various approaches have been developed based on some system of record linkage to provide greater assurance with regard to the accuracy of the denominator (see below). But this advantage is not purchased without a price. There is a practical limit on the numbers of patients who can feasibly be included in such studies. Study size is limited by both the number of patients included in the computerized database and the number of studies to be conducted. If a national database is utilized, as in prescription event monitoring in the United Kingdom, the limitation is not the number of patients in the database but rather the maximum number of patients it is practical and feasible to study, from the point of view of physician cooperation, in order to obtain reasonably reliable data. As a result, although these methods possess the advantage of providing an accurate denominator and reliable data feedback, the constraint on patient numbers does have some impact on the ability to detect low-incidence events. It will be recalled that benoxaprofen was the subject of a record linkage study in the United Kingdom prior to approval but without any evidence of hepatotoxicity becoming apparent. In fact it only became apparent later subsequent to marketing through the mechanism of the government-sponsored VRSE system (yellow card system).

Even when these more precise methods of identifying the number of patients exposed to drug are employed there are other factors that may operate to affect the validity of the denominator obtained. A denominator is required as a measure of the total population actually exposed to drug and from which the subset experiencing the adverse reaction is drawn. In the uncontrolled treatment setting of a record-linked study it cannot be assumed that a patient identified as a drug recipient is actually compliant with therapy and represents a valid measure of drug exposure. In this respect the record-linked study does not differ from other uncontrolled studies. Unlike the controlled clinical trial setting there are no measures adopted to ensure an optimum level of patient compliance. In this respect regimen bias is a very real phenomenon in the treatment setting. It can operate to adversely affect the validity of denominator estimates used as a surrogate measure of drug exposure. It has been estimated that while there is an 80% compliance with once-daily treatment regimens there is only a 60% compliance with a qid regimen. Other factors that influence compliance include chronic use therapy as opposed to acute use and whether or not the condition being treated is symptomatic or asymptomatic.

In VRSE sales volume or prescription volume, in spite of the deficiencies, remains the only viable approach to denominator estimates. Although precise estimates of incidence based on such data must be approached with caution, they do nevertheless provide a basis for alerting to possible changes in incidence. The sales volume/prescription volume approach is generally accepted as representing an acceptable approximation particularly if the same approach is employed consistently and uniformly over time and is used as a basis for detecting any change in incidence over comparable time periods.

If the quantitative aspects of the denominator pose problems for VRSE, the qualitative aspects are even more problematic. A number of factors may be operative here. If the adverse effects of a drug are more prominent in a particular patient subset, then clearly apparent incidence will be impacted by the extent to which that subset is represented in the total population at risk.

Peptic ulcer disease and its complications tend to be more serious in elderly patients and accordingly the extent to which this patient subset is included in the population exposed will impact the impressions gained with respect to the magnitude and severity of the ulceration problem with an NSAID. It is also not unreasonable to assume that the advantages of once-daily administration for a chronic use drug will lead to its preferential use in the elderly population as a matter of patient convenience. This may lead to the preferential use of a once-daily NSAID in elderly patients and this dosage regimen preselection may give a misleading impression of the severity of the GI problem. In other circumstances the safety profile itself may lead to patient preselection. Osmosin was introduced with the claimed advantage of fewer GI side effects. This led to its preferential use in patients with GI problems and resulted in a spuriously high incidence of GI effects and their apparent persistence after drug withdrawal.

Knowledge of the exact composition of the patient population exposed to a drug is clearly important and may be critical to obtaining an accurate interpretation of the data. Unfortunately, it is beyond the capabilities of any VRSE system to provide such data. The best that can be achieved is for the system to provide the basis for tentative hypotheses to be subjected to testing by one of the other PMS methodologies.

In summary, a variety of confounding factors and other biases may cause VRSE systems to yield spurious conclusions. No VRSE system, no matter how efficiently it is organized, is able to completely eliminate all factors that are likely to confound the interpretation of the data. It would be unrealistic to expect otherwise since the data are being provided on a voluntary basis by the physician during the course of his or her primary interest: patient care. However, it is not invariably or necessarily the case that the signals from a VRSE system are spurious and misleading.

The proper use of VRSE data mandates that an open mind be kept at all times with respect to both the validity of the conclusions and the need to utilize other PMS methodology to test their validity. Whenever such data are considered one should be alert to the possible contribution of one or more of the possible variables or biases and their capacity to influence the conclusions.

It is for this reason that the major contribution of VRSE systems is safety hypothesis generation. Their main purpose is to alert to the possible existence of a safety problem. In general they do not provide a suitable vehicle for hypothesis testing and primary reliance should not be placed on them for this purpose. While this may be possible in some situations, such systems are more appropriately viewed as early warning systems in the first instance. Most commonly there will be a need to employ more structured methodology for subsequent hypothesis testing and verification.

VI. ADVERSE REACTIONS VS. EVENTS

This question of adverse reactions vs. events has relevance to VRSE systems as well as to the particular form of record-linked methodology termed prescription event monitoring. It therefore provides a convenient link between the preceding discussion of VRSE systems and the next section on record-linked methodology.

The preference for the term *events* over *adverse reactions* has more than semantic significance and directly addresses one of the most important issues with respect to safety monitoring. In many situations the causal relationship of a particular adverse reaction to drug may be clear since it has already been established. In other circumstances it may be suspected based on the clinical presentation. This is typically the case when there is a temporal relationship to drug and the reaction in question is so rare or so distinctive that a causal relationship seems certain.

Very often, however, an adverse reaction is not suspected. This is particularly likely to occur when the same clinical picture may be present in the general population for reasons unrelated to drug. When this happens serious problems of detection and causality attribution arise and there can be considerable delay before it finally becomes apparent that the particular clinical syndrome may also be caused by drug. This situation is most likely to occur when definitive diagnostic tests are not available for differentiation. In such circumstances the only indication of a drug-induced etiology may be a temporal relationship to drug administration and an apparent increase in the incidence of the reaction in patients receiving the drug. This type of situation is very likely to go undetected in a safety monitoring system, such as VRSE, which is based on the spontaneous reporting of known or suspected adverse reactions. Furthermore, if there is the possibility that some patients may manifest a more serious or fatal form of the reaction, this may occur in some patients long before the drug is finally impli-cated as the cause but long after the milder manifestations of the reaction have first begun to appear. In effect, this difficulty in identifying an event as a drug-induced reaction can seriously compromise the effectiveness of VRSE as an early warning system.

This is more than a purely theoretical consideration and the experience with practolol in the United Kingdom provides an excellent illustration of the se-quence of events that may occur and their practical relevance. The ocular toxicity of this drug was not recognized until the drug was established on the market and in widespread clinical use. The first indication of a potential problem occurred when a number of patients with ocular syndrome were reported from an ophthal-mology clinic. However, although the severe form of ocular syndrome was a relatively infrequent occurrence, a milder manifestation of practolol-induced ocular toxicity was subsequently found to occur.

A formal study was conducted to test the hypothesis that a much larger proportion of patients receiving practolol manifested a less severe manifestation of the drug-induced eye disorder. This study, which comprised less than 100 patients, revealed that the milder form of the eye disorder was present in 20% of the patients exposed to drug. But of even greater importance, an identical syndrome completely unrelated to drug was found to be present in at least 6% of the control group.

Certainly the occurrence of the more serious forms of ocular toxicity with blindness could have been anticipated and their impact minimized if the much more frequent and milder manifestation of toxicity had been detected in a prompt and timely manner by the VRSE system in place (yellow card reporting system of the Committee on Safety of Medicines). It would seem reasonable to conclude that this resemblance between the manifestations of drug toxicity and a sponta-neously occurring condition had a significant impact in delaying final recognition of practolol's role in inducing ocular toxicity.

It may also be significant that the practolol ocular syndrome was first recog-nized by ophthalmologists working in a specialist clinic that was a focal point for the referral of patients in the area with ocular problems. This suggests the

Table 4 Frequency of Eye Complaints and Rashes with Practolol
(71 Patients)

Complaint	Number of patients	
	Before treatment	During treatment
Eye complaint	4 (6%)	14 (20%)
Skin rash	8 (11%)	16 (23%)
Eye complaint and rash	1 (1%)	7 (10%)
Mean duration of therapy (MO)	19.1	19.1

Source: Adapted from: Skegg DCG, Doll R. Frequency of eye complaints and rashes among patients receiving practolol and propranolol. *Lancet* 1977;2: 475.

possibility that the confusion caused by the resemblance to a spontaneously occurring syndrome was compounded by the fact that, to a great extent, the treating physicians were not experts in ophthalmic diseases and therefore were less likely to make the subtle distinction. The consensus view is that earlier detection of the milder manifestations of toxicity could have prevented the severer forms of the condition and the associated visual loss.

The practolol experience clearly exposed a potential weakness of the United Kingdom's yellow card reporting system since there was considerable delay in recognizing the ocular event as an adverse reaction causally related to drug. But this is not specific to the yellow card system. It is a weakness that is generic to all VRSE systems. These systems are designed to collect spontaneous reports of reactions that are known or suspected to be causally related to drug. The bias of the whole system is in the direction of reporting only those events for which there is a reason to suspect a causal relationship to drug. An adverse occurrence only becomes an ''adverse reaction'' when causality is established or suspected; prior to this it is an ''event.''

Apart from an expectation that some events may be submitted as spontaneous reports on the basis of a vague and ill-defined impression of possible drug involvement there is little that can be done by way of modification of the VRSE system to address this problem. It is not a practical or feasible solution to the ''practolol type of problem'' to attempt the routine collection of ''event'' data into a VRSE system. With current reporting requirements VRSE systems are hard pressed to achieve a reasonable level of compliance in reporting known or suspected adverse reactions. It would be completely unrealistic to expect that all events be reported even though there is presently no suspicion of any relationship to drug.

In recognizing that VRSE systems could not be modified to correct this obvious weakness, the United Kingdom took a completely different approach. The system of prescription event monitoring was developed. In this system advantage is taken of the centralization of records in the health service and, accepting smaller patient numbers than are available to VRSE systems, events are monitored from actual patient records. It is intended as a complement to the yellow card system, not a substitute for it.

VII. RECORD-LINKED METHODOLOGY

The record-linked techniques represent an attempt to bring some elements of the reliability of formal structured pharmacoepidemiological studies to a VRSE system. As with VRSE they utilize the larger numbers of patients available for safety monitoring in the normal treatment setting. But they seek to do this in a manner that addresses one of the main deficiencies of VRSE, a lack of precise information with respect to the denominator, i.e., the number of patients actually exposed to drug. It is the methodology used to provide a more accurate estimate of the numbers of patients exposed that constitutes the salient characteristic of this type of study.

The introduction of centralized databases of patient health care records, and in particular the advances in data storage and retrieval consequent to computerization, have combined to create an environment that facilitates this approach. Understandably, this type of approach is ideally suited and well adapted to the highly centralized and structured environment of government-sponsored health care systems, which potentially have the ability to encompass the entire patient population exposed. In view of this it is not surprising to find that record-linked methodology was pioneered by Professor Inman in the United Kingdom. This approach is also followed in Saskatchewan, a province that has adopted a government-sponsored health care system.

But the approach has not been limited to government-sponsored health care systems. It has also been adopted in this country where the provision of health care is predominantly a function of the private sector (Fig. 2). Since there does exist within the system a number of organizations that may be regarded as constituting separate discrete microcosms of a state system. Over the last two decades various types of health care organizations, medical payment schemes, and reimbursement schemes have been established. This in turn has necessitated the development of extensive computerized systems for data storage in order to support their activities. As a result of this the records available to Medicaid, health maintenance organizations, hospital pharmacies, and insurance plans (Blue Cross) have become available for drug safety studies and are able to provide fairly accurate information relative to denominators. The power of the computer has been harnessed to provide reliable information from these databases on the number of patients exposed and the safety events that occur. Like VRSE there is the statistical power of large numbers of patients exposed to drug in the normal treatment setting. But unlike VRSE there is reasonable

Governmental.

        Prescription Event Monitoring (UK)
        Saskatchewan Provincial Plan (Canada)

Private.

        Puget Sound Health Maintenance Organization (H.M.O.)
        Los Angeles, Kaiser Permanent Plan
        Portland, Kaiser Permanent Plan

Figure 2   Record-linked systems.

precision with respect to the patients actually exposed (denominator) and a greater assurance of the completeness of safety event information (numerator).

Computer assisted record linkage techniques can be utilized in a variety of ways. They can be used as a safety monitoring system per se for the generation of safety hypotheses. One example of this would be its use to provide a further refinement of the yellow card reporting system of the CSM in the UK. This is the Prescription Event Monitoring (PEM) system developed by Professor Inman in the UK. Alternatively they may be used as a means of facilitating the conduct of case control and cohort studies which may serve the objectives of both safety hypothesis generation and safety hypothesis testing.

A. Prescription Event Monitoring

Prescription event monitoring (PEM) evolved as a response to certain deficiencies in the United Kingdom's national system of voluntary reporting of adverse reactions (yellow card system). These were highlighted in dramatic fashion by the practolol experience (vide supra). It should be emphasized that these were not deficiencies of the U.K. system per se but deficiencies that are inherent in any system of voluntary reporting.

There are a number of problems associated with voluntary reporting systems that have the potential to impact on the reliability of the data and the conclusions drawn. These are well recognized and include cooperation in reporting reactions consistently and reliably, the completeness of the data received, and reasonable accuracy of information regarding the qualitative and quantitative aspects of the patient population from which the reports are received.

The practolol experience, however, served to draw attention to another potentially serious deficiency of a voluntary reporting system. Even when a reasonable level of cooperation in reporting has been achieved reactions are never reported unless and until the reporting physician or health professional suspects that the reaction is in fact caused by the drug. As the practolol experience demonstrated, this can cause serious delay in detecting the adverse event when the clinical manifestations of the drug reaction closely resemble other clinical syndromes that may arise from a non–drug-induced etiology.

Practolol was approved in the United Kingdom and had been on the market for 4 years with an accumulated experience of 250,000 patient-years before the ocular syndrome was recognized as an adverse reaction due to the drug. Approximately 619 reports were eventually collected postmarketing of which 20 cases represented near blindness [59]. Earlier detection could have averted these more serious manifestations of ocular toxicity. But this did not occur because the "dry eye" syndrome due to practolol superficially resembled that occurring spontaneously in many elderly people. The drug did not reach the market in the United States but this was not because of knowledge, or even a suspicion, of the ocular toxicity. In point of fact this delay was attributable to what eventually proved to be a misplaced concern on the part of the FDA regarding a carcinogenicity risk generic to all β blockers—a view that was not shared by European agencies.

Clearly, when an drug-induced event mimics a non–drug-induced condition recognition of the true etiology may take some time. While it is equally clear that the reporting of events associated with drug as opposed to recognized or suspected adverse reactions would lead to an earlier detection of such toxicities, this is almost impossible to achieve in any voluntary reporting system. The reporting burden on the health professional would be extreme and in an environment in which even the reporting of known or suspected adverse reactions is characterized by relatively poor compliance. In the final analysis events are not going to be considered for reporting to a VRSE system unless there is at least a suspicion that they may be drug-induced. That being the case the routine use of PEM may be regarded as a perfect complement to routine use of VRSE. But it is not a replacement for VRSE since the patient numbers involved in PEM are necessarily much smaller than those available to VRSE and the power to detect rare events correspondingly reduced. PEM is not appropriate for events with an incidence lower than 0.1%. VRSE theoretically provides unlimited power to detect rare adverse reactions but only those that are known or suspected to be adverse drug reactions are likely to be reported. PEM, on the other hand, has reduced power with respect to the rarer reactions but does possess the advantage that adverse reactions are accessible when they are only events and their causal relationship to drug is unknown and completely unsuspected.

1. Drug Surveillance Research Unit

This unit is a nongovernmental group established by Professor Inman at Southampton University in the United Kingdom. Prescription event monitoring (PEM) was developed by this unit as a form of postmarketing surveillance that sought to address the defect in conventional spontaneous reporting systems exposed by the practolol experience.

PEM draws on the resources of the U.K. National Health Service (NHS) to identify the patient databases to be used for safety monitoring. Most prescriptions in the United Kingdom are written under the NHS and the collection of these prescriptions is centralized within the Prescription Pricing Authority. Copies of these prescriptions are made available to the Drug Surveillance Unit on a confidential basis. In this way a cohort of patients is identified who are receiving the drug to be studied, most commonly one that just recently received a product license approval. Another group of patients is selected to receive a control drug, one that is chemically or pharmacologically similar to the study drug and that has already been marketed for the same indication. Great care is taken in the selection of the control group so as to ensure that the control drug selected is more or less contemporaneous with the study drug. For instance, comparisons of the study drug with a control drug that has been marketed for the past 15 years are avoided. The reason for this is that studies have shown that the reporting of adverse reactions for a drug are maximal in the early years after approval and thereafter show a steady decline. This phenomenon is generic to all drugs and is completely independent of the safety profile. As a consequence of this a comparison of the newly approved drug with one that had been on the market for many years would be a biased comparison.

The numbers of patients involved in PEM studies represents a compromise. Since the basic characteristic of this approach is to collect data on all events occurring in association with the drug rather than identified or suspected adverse reactions, there is a limit on the number of patients it is practical to include. On the other hand, the number of patients included is critically related to the sensitivity of the method to detect low-incidence events. It is these types of event that are of key interest since they are the ones most likely to elude detection during the preapproval clinical program.

Arbitrarily the PEM system is based on the ability to detect events with an incidence of 0.1% or higher. A database of 3000 patients provides a 95% probability of seeing at least one event if the underlying incidence is at least 0.1%. In point of fact PEM records data on the first 10,000 patients to receive the newly approved drug, as well as a comparable group receiving the control drug. The selection of the larger figure is to allow for the inevitable attrition that will occur due to lack of patient or physician cooperation or any one of a number of other factors.

Once the drug groups have been selected a fixed period of drug administration of up to 1 year is allowed to elapse. At the expiration of this period a questionnaire is sent to each patient's physician requesting certain information from the patient's records. The key information collected is that relating to events occurring during the treatment period. Information is sought on all events. These include identified or suspected adverse reactions but also new diagnoses, unexpected change in previous condition, and any injury or symptoms that were not present before treatment was started.

PEM has proved to be a highly successful methodology for safety surveillance, but its utility is largely a measure of the high level of cooperation shown by the practicing physicians. The existence of a government-sponsored health care system is clearly fundamental to a system such as PEM, but one must also ask the question of whether or not working in such a system is determinative of the cooperation shown by the treating physicians. This would appear to be a not unreasonable assumption since the level of physician cooperation with the U.K. yellow card reporting system is significantly higher (twofold) than that seen with the FDA spontaneous reporting (1639) system in this country [60].

Professor Inman has suggested that had practolol been subjected to PEM with propanolol as the control drug, the skin/ocular syndrome could have been detected with as few as 100,000 patients exposed to drug. This would have been apparent as an excess number of referrals to dermatology or ophthalmology clinics for skin and eye complaints without any causality attribution having been made by the treating physicians [61].

B. COMPASS (Computerized On-Line Medicaid Pharmaceutical Analysis and Surveillance System)

In the United States the Medicaid Program is a 50-state network of federally funded medical services for the poor and indigent. The Medicaid database provides a central repository of billing information on Medicaid patients provided by the various health care providers, physicians, pharmacies, hospitals, nursing homes, and laboratories. In addition to information relative to the specific drugs prescribed, the database also contains information on diagnoses and other items of data relevant to postmarketing safety surveillance studies.

Under a contract with the FDA, Health Information Designs developed the linkage system known as COMPASS to access the Medicaid data of patients. The relevant elements of data for postmarketing surveillance purposes are extracted from the state's Medicaid information system and forwarded to the offices of Health Information Designs in Washington, D.C.

Initially the project was established in Michigan and Minnesota but has now been extended to involve some 5.25 million patients in 10 states. It is a longitudinal database of medical histories extending back as far as 1980. It was established primarily for the purpose of providing a patient-specific drug-medical event-linked database suitable for postmarketing surveillance. As with the PEM system the emphasis is on treatment emergent events and not specifically on adverse reactions, "events" in which the reporting decision is based on a known or possible causal relationship to drug. Like that system, it is also intended to provide information on unanticipated beneficial effects as well as adverse events. Some preliminary work must always be undertaken prior to a study in order to create clusters of relevant clinical manifestations that will be interpreted as indicating the particular adverse event under study. Once this is done it is possible to search for a causal relationship between the adverse event and exposure to the study drug.

One important limitation to this approach stems primarily from the fact that the database employed is compiled exclusively for medical billing purposes. It is in no respect a clinical database, in which recourse can be had to actual medical records to provide further information or to validate or amend the computer database. In this respect it differs very significantly from a computerized database of the type of information contained in case report forms. The only guarantee as to the reliability of the medical data contained in the COMPASS database is the efficiency of the relevant state auditing program designed to detect false information supplied to support Medicaid billing requests. This absence of access to actual medical records can lead to serious deficiencies in the availability of information concerning past history, concomitant disease, smoking, alcohol, drugs, parity, etc. This constitutes a very significant difference from the PEM system, which provides greater assurance of being able to collect the relevant information. In the PEM system questionnaires are sent directly to the treating physician specifically requesting the relevant items of information. In marked contrast to the COMPASS type of system the information collected in the PEM system is primarily and exclusively for the purposes of safety surveillance and not for administrative billing purposes.

In addition, the theoretical advantage of a longitudinal database may be somewhat confounded by the fact that loss of the patient to follow-up may be a problem, in large part due to the fact that this is a Medicaid population. The database as a whole is very distinctive with respect to both economic and social variables and cannot be said to accurately reflect the U.S. population as a whole. This again is a very important difference from the PEM system. The system of government-sponsored health care provided by the National Health Service in the United Kingdom is one that favors stability of patient populations with their treating physicians. Consequently data loss as a consequence of patient mobility does not constitute the same problem.

The system's strongest feature is undoubtedly the reliability of the denominator information. Its limitations relate to the reliability of adverse reaction identification and the reliability of the numerator. The system certainly has the potential to provide useful information with respect to relative risk and the true incidence of events. However, for the reasons stated it would seem to have its main application in an adjunctive role. In this context studies employing the COMPASS database have produced results that are confirmatory of the results obtained in more formal pharmacoepidemiological studies, e.g., NASAID drugs and GI bleeding, and zomepirac and anaphylactic reactions.

C. Health Prepayment Schemes

The various forms of group health cooperative schemes or health maintenance organizations (HMOs) that have arisen in this country in an effort to contain the cost of health care provide another valuable source of data with which to conduct epidemiological studies of drug safety. Essentially the payments made by patients who are members of these organizations provide comprehensive medical coverage that includes physicians services, medication, and hospitalization. The computerized databases developed by these organizations differ from the COMPASS databases in two very important respects. First, since these organizations are in reality small private health care schemes the studies conducted are representative of quite a different patient population, in economic and social variables, than studies based on the COMPASS database. And equally important the data collected and computerized are more likely to be complete and accurate since they are being retained primarily for their medical accuracy and comprehensiveness as opposed to merely supporting medical billing requests. The other very important distinction from a COMPASS or Medicaid-based database is that, like a clinical trial database, actual medical records are available to validate and where necessary amend the information in the computer database. The data that can be generated from such databases are more comparable to those derived from the PEM system although the latter are likely to be more representative of the population as a whole.

D. Summarization

Experimental methodology in the form of controlled clinical trials provides accurate data regarding the nature and number of adverse events and the number of patients exposed. Such trials are therefore able to generate the most reliable conclusions with respect to safety issues. While they will be essential for some questions they have a limited role in the evaluation of certain safety issues. The limitations are most apparent in the area of greatest need, the study of infrequently occurring events.

Observational methodology, both case control and cohort studies, replicate the actual real-life treatment milieu. There is not the artificiality of the experimental setting. These types of study have their greatest application in testing safety hypotheses particularly when large patient numbers are required. Although they are not as powerful as the experimental study for identifying cause and effect, they serve a valuable purpose in providing confirmation of an early warning from a voluntary reporting system.

Although the generation of safety hypotheses is not their primary use they may be adapted to this purpose. Their strength is that they provide precise information, both quantitative and qualitative, regarding the denominator. However, a number of biases may influence the conclusions that are drawn and in the retrospective case control study memory recall is an important variable that can impact adversely on the value of the data collected.

Record-linked methodology certainly provides acceptable accuracy with respect to numerator, denominator, and data derived from actual records and is not subject to the potential distortion of imperfect memory recall. The purpose for which the data were collected does, however, impact on its utility for safety surveillance purposes. Accordingly, with some approaches e.g., COMPASS, the value of data may be limited by the fact that it was gathered for administrative as opposed to clinical purposes. Prescription event monitoring does overcome this problem in a way that allows for the collection of highly relevant data.

Finally, while patient numbers are not limiting with the observational methods to the same extent that they are with the experimental methods, they are nevertheless still limiting. A practical limit on the numbers of patients involved in such studies is somewhere in the region of 10,000. Even these numbers are not adequate for really low-incidence toxicities such as the marrow aplasia association with phenylbutazone. In the final analysis and notwithstanding its imperfections, a voluntary reporting system potentially covering all patients exposed to drug is the only method applicable to such events.

VIII. A STRATEGY FOR SAFETY SURVEILLANCE

Postmarketing safety surveillance (PMS) is a standard routine to be applied to all drugs following market approval. It is intended to compensate for the potential limitations with respect to safety evaluation that may be inherent in any preapproval research program regardless of its quality.

However, if the preapproval clinical research program has recognized limitations with respect to safety evaluation the same can certainly be said of the various methods employed for the conduct of postmarketing safety surveillance. Each PMS method has its own strengths and weaknesses and none is perfect.

In one sense the large number of patients exposed to drug postmarketing provides the optimum conditions for the detection of those toxicities that may hitherto have escaped detection. This larger patient exposure postmarketing may also serve to further refine estimates of the frequency or severity of those adverse events that were identified prior to drug approval.

However, the ability of each of the various PMS methods to achieve these objectives is a function of the extent to which the different methodologies are able to reconcile two conflicting principles. Unquestionably, the most reliable conclusions are those to be derived from a controlled study environment. But the greater the degree of control imposed in order to ensure this reliability, the greater the impact on the number of patients that it is practical and feasible for inclusion in the study. Conversely, the greater the number of patients involved, the less the degree of control that can reasonably be assured.

For these reasons an effective approach to PMS must be multifaceted in order to achieve its overall objective. It must combine several PMS methods into one overall strategy rather than rely on one particular method. If selected appropriately the different methods will complement each other and tend to cancel out their respective weaknesses while at the same time capitalizing on their respective strengths.

An effective PMS strategy is one that incorporates two or more PMS methodologies into a two-step sequential approach:

1. Generation of safety hypotheses:
   a. VRSE system
2. Testing and verification of safety hypotheses:
   a. Experimental methods; clinical research or phase IV trials
   b. Observational methods; cohort and case control studies
   c. Record-linked methodology

This strategy is implemented by employing a VRSE system to provide a timely warning of possible safety issues. The existence of the safety hazard thus identified is then verified, and the magnitude of the effect determined, utilizing one or more of the structured PMS methodologies.

The first step is the fundamental basis on which the whole strategy rests. It is based on a well-organized VRSE system that potentially covers all patients exposed to the drug worldwide. The primary function of the VRSE system is to act as an early warning system and alert to the existence of potential new safety hazards as rapidly as possible. These may be hitherto unsuspected toxicities or an apparent change in the incidence or severity of a known adverse reaction compared with the current description of this adverse reaction in the drug labeling.

Not uncommonly discussion of VRSE systems tends to focus almost exclusively on drug safety events from medical practice experience subsequent to marketing. However, in reality drug safety signals provided by a VRSE system arise from data that may derive from a composite of several possible sources. The actual blend of experience represented in the database at any time will depend on the exact stage of development that the drug has reached at that same point in time.

A VRSE database for a drug is first established when the drug enters its initial clinical research trials. During the research phase the events entered into the system are those that the sponsor requires to be reported promptly since they satisfy the criteria set forth in the federal regulations for expedited reporting to the FDA [62].

As the drug is sequentially approved in various world markets spontaneous safety reports will begin to flow into the VRSE database as a result of the use of the drug in medical practice. All such spontaneous reports from postmarketing use of the drug are entered into the system and the reportability of such reports to the FDA is determined in accordance with the criteria in the regulations [63]. Although safety event data in the postmarketing period are predominantly derived from medical practice experience with a component arising from phase IV trials, some data may continue to be derived from research trials. This arises because the VRSE database is a worldwide database and a drug never reaches the stage of market approval simultaneously in the various markets around the world. Also, of course, market status does not preclude the possibility of further research trials.

It is not the source of the safety data entering the VRSE system that changes over time but the relative contribution that each of these different sources makes to the total database. For this reason the term *postmarketing surveillance* is inappropriate since it conveys the impression that the data are derived exclusively from treatment use of the drug. The term *safety surveillance* is preferable since it conveys a better sense of the continuity of the process and the diversity of the sources from which the data are collected. VRSE is in reality a continuum of safety reporting that spans a drug's useful life as a therapeutic entity from the initial human studies to its use as a well-established market product.

The VRSE system may be able to contribute to the verification and quantification of a safety problem but this is not an essential requirement. As long as it warns of possible safety issues in a timely manner it will have served its primary purpose. In most instances, because of the deficiencies inevitably associated with VRSE databases, it will be necessary to turn to one or more of the other PMS methodologies for verification and an assessment of the magnitude of the risk.

This second strategic objective of verification is met by employing one or more of the structured approaches based on experimental, observational, or record-linked methodology. They are used to further explore the safety signals picked up by the VRSE system.

The precise detail of the approach taken will differ depending on whether the drug is still in the preapproval stage or has reached the postmarketing phase. However, the general format of the approach to verification is the same in both instances. It comprises the following sequential steps:

1. Reexamination of the current VRSE database
2. Reexamination of the current clinical trial database
3. Consideration of further studies

The first response of the group responsible for drug safety will be a reexamination of the VRSE database itself. This action is followed irrespective of whether the drug is still the subject of a research program or is now on the market. The objective is to seek any information contained in the total database that may assist in placing the new report in a proper perspective. This review of the existing VRSE database, in the light of the reported reaction, may well prompt a reassessment of the significance of earlier similar reports. At the time these earlier reports may not have been considered to have a relationship to drug or merit "expedited" reporting.

Following this, and before any consideration is given to the initiation of additional experimental or observational studies, attention is turned to the existing worldwide clinical trial database. This constitutes an invaluable resource of experimental data that are already available. The information, derived largely from controlled clinical trials, can be anticipated to be of uniformly good quality compared with that originating as spontaneous postmarketing reports. These latter reports may, and very frequently do, lack important information. The clinical trial data, on the other hand, are obtained from a data-oriented exercise with a monitoring function to minimize the possibility of missing data.

At any point in time the clinical trial database should contain reasonably current data from all company-sponsored trials worldwide, both research and postmarketing. And of particular relevance it contains safety data that are more extensive than can ever be duplicated in a voluntary reporting system.

For instance, if a report is received in the VRSE database relating to a suspected drug-induced agranulocytosis the database will be searched to determine whether any other similar events have been reported. If so the question of a possible increase in frequency will be explored. The clinical trial database will next be reviewed for similar types of reaction or any additional evidence that might tend to support a drug-induced etiology. In this particular example it may prove instructive to determine whether or not some patients have developed a fall in white blood cell (WBC) or granulocyte count, although not to levels that would have alerted the physician to discontinue drug and report the incident (e.g., to levels of $3000/mm^3$). If so, is this experience different from that seen in the control groups in the database. Alternatively, there may be subtle evidence of a downward trend in the WBC or granulocyte count for drug relative to control groups which, while demonstrable statistically, was not of such a magnitude as to be clinically evident to the treating physician.

Another situation might involve one or two incidents of unexplained and severe hepatic dysfunction that are reported to the VRSE database. The circumstances may be such that a non–drug-related etiology is a strong possibility. Once again, if subsequent examination of the clinical trial database reveals any suggestion, albeit subclinical and statistical, that transaminase levels are behaving differently in the drug group vs. the controls, then the possibility of a drug-induced etiology becomes more likely. The review of the two databases in parallel clearly has the potential to be much more informative on the issue of causality than the use of the VRSE database alone.

Following this initial review of the two databases any further action undertaken will depend on the status of the drug, whether it is still in the research phase or marketed. If the drug is still in the research phase consideration will be given to any additional experimental studies it may be feasible to conduct at this point. But, depending on the numbers of patients who might be required for any further exploration of the safety issue, there may be a practical limitation on what it is feasible to do prior to approval.

In these circumstances a commitment to larger phase IV studies postapproval may be the most appropriate course of action. During the prazosin research program, for instance, there were scattered reports of syncope with the initial doses of drug, which appeared to be influenced by initial blood levels as they related to the magnitude of the initial dose, dosage form, and drug bioavailability. Data developed during the research program placed the incidence at not greater than 1%. A phase IV study undertaken postmarketing in approximately 10,000 patients confirmed that the incidence established in the research program was correct as it applied to the starting dose of the marketed formulation [64].

If the drug is already on the market when the safety issue arises the scope and size of any further studies that may be implemented expands considerably. There is now an opportunity to employ one or more of the other PMS methodologies with much larger numbers of patients than are feasible during the research program. These may include large-scale phase IV studies of various types, observational studies, or one of the various forms of record-linked methodology. The constraints relative to study size are not absolute, however, and while they do not operate to the same extent as during the research program, they are nevertheless a factor to be considered.

As the practolol experience so graphically demonstrates, confusion of an adverse reaction with a similar spontaneously occurring event can significantly delay the recognition of a potential safety hazard. But all of the available PMS methodologies, with the exception of PEM, are directed toward the detection of adverse reactions per se rather than the identification of events that may subsequently prove to be adverse reactions.

Accordingly, an excellent case can be made for actively trying to identify such situations prospectively rather than retrospectively, by allowing them to insidiously make their presence known, often with serious consequences for some patients due to this delay. Ideally, an effective PMS strategy is to arrange for the routine conduct of a PEM study shortly after marketing. This will serve two purposes. First, it will provide confirmation of the safety profile developed during the research phase. Second, it will actively search for potential toxicity, which at this point may be manifesting as events rather than adverse reactions.

In summary, the VRSE database provides a timely warning of new and serious adverse reactions or a change in the severity or incidence of known serious reactions. This alerting function is needed just as much during the course of the research program as during the postmarketing phase. Supplemented by such other studies as are appropriate, it is essential to provide the most current and up-to-date safety information to the following vitally interested parties:

1. The patients at risk who are receiving the drug in the research trials or as treatment postmarketing.
2. The physicians using the drug in the research trials or treating patients postmarketing. This is accomplished by suitable amendment of the investigator's brochure and informed consent statement during the research phase, or the product labeling and other informational material in the postmarketing phase.
3. FDA and other appropriate regulatory authorities.
4. The sponsor company, in order to keep the company current with respect to the safety profile and to enable it to meet its obligations under items 1–3.

IX. ORGANIZATION OF A SAFETY SURVEILLANCE SYSTEM

The strategy outlined above suggests a format for the organization of a safety surveillance system. The VRSE database and the clinical trial database must be monitored in parallel, in a continuing and ongoing fashion, in order to achieve efficient safety monitoring. Furthermore the responsibility for monitoring the VRSE database cannot logically be separated from responsibility for the total safety profile of the drug as reflected in the clinical trial database.

The group responsible for the VRSE database must have full access to both databases and use them concurrently in performing their safety monitoring function. This calls for the establishment of a safety evaluation group (SEG) specifically charged with the overall responsibility for drug safety rather than a very specific and limited responsibility for the VRSE database alone. The SEG works in a close interactive fashion with other relevant groups, e.g., clinical project teams. But whereas the project teams are involved in all aspects of the drug's activity, efficacy, and safety, the SEG is dedicated to drug safety and has a pivotal role in all matters related to this issue. For reasons to be explained later, the SEG is probably best located as a section of the Regulatory Affairs Department. It reports to the head of that department rather than being part of clinical operations.

The organization of a safety surveillance system is most conveniently addressed under the following headings:

1. Responsibility for VRSE system
2. The database
3. Custodial function
4. Communications

A. Responsibility for VRSE

The establishment of voluntary reporting systems should not be the sole responsibility of government regulatory agencies anymore than it should be the sole responsibility of the drug sponsors. There are very cogent reasons for arguing that the responsibility for collecting events for a VRSE system should be a collective endeavor of the various national regulatory agencies and the companies responsible for marketing the drugs. Such an approach would seem to ensure the most comprehensive reporting system.

Among the numerator problems that beset voluntary reporting systems *reporting preferences* are a very real phenomenon. Some health care professionals, for instance, will manifest a much greater tendency to report events to a government agency whereas others will tend to make their reports to the drug sponsor. There do appear to be national differences in these reporting preferences. In some countries, e.g., United Kingdom and New Zealand, the largest input to the national systems was found to be from practitioners whereas in others, e.g., United States, Germany, and Italy, the largest contribution to the national systems came from reports that had first been submitted to the pharmaceutical manufacturers themselves [65,66]. The data are consistent with a greater tendency to report direct to the national registry of adverse reactions in those countries with well-developed government-sponsored health care systems.

These facts, when taken together with the unavoidable imperfections of data collection by VRSE systems, support a duplication of effort by both government and industry. It can only contribute to a more comprehensive reporting of adverse reactions and minimize the number of reactions that go unreported.

Most of the countries with well-developed drug regulatory systems provide for some system of voluntary reporting of spontaneous events to the national agency. However, these national voluntary reporting systems do have the disadvantage of being just that, national. Each agency has direct access only to that microcosm of the total available database that derives from its own country. For a global perspective of drug safety the various national authorities must rely predominantly on information provided by the pharmaceutical companies. There is a real need for a central collecting point for adverse reactions reported to each of the different national authorities, one to which companies could turn in order to supplement the experience in their own global databases. Unfortunately, however, the concept of an efficiently functioning global safety database does not exist at the level of national government.

There are several ways in which such an international safety database could be derived and attempts have been made to implement one of these. This is one in which the World Health Organization plays a pivotal role in organizing a central database for worldwide safety data to which all countries would contribute. In 1978, a WHO Collaborating Centre for International Drug Monitoring was established in Uppsala, Sweden. It was organized as a foundation and funded by the Swedish government. Theoretically a total of 26 countries are participating in the WHO scheme, but it is probably fair to say that it has not developed and achieved its prime objective as an early warning system.

The reasons for this are varied and include, among other things, a small staff and a low level of funding. However, the major contributing factor relates to the delays involved in reporting. Unvalidated reports may be forwarded to WHO within weeks of their receipt by the national agency, but validated and evaluated reports may take up to 1½ years before they are received. Recognition of a significant safety problem in a particular country may lead to considerable delay in forwarding reports since they will not be forwarded until an extensive review at the national level has first occurred [67]. This may be traced to the inevitable priority accorded to purely national interests. It is probably not surprising to find that the reality of national attitudes on health matters is not conducive to the success of such a venture. For most governments matters concerning the public health of the nation are sensitive and highly charged political issues, to the extent that they frequently outweigh purely scientific considerations. Accordingly, governments are unlikely to willingly abrogate their autonomy on such sensitive issues.

In the absence of effective centralization of postmarketing safety reports to government systems the logical fall-back position is to ensure a free and full interchange of available safety information between the various national authorities. The Working Group on Adverse Reaction Reporting of the Council for International Organizations of Medical Science (CIOMS) has certainly made great strides in this direction by facilitating the interchange of such data. The approach taken has been the standardization of the collection and reporting of safety data by pharmaceutical companies to the various national authorities.

Against this background, it is clear that the primary responsibility for establishing a worldwide safety database must rest with the pharmaceutical companies themselves whether this is required by regulation or not. There is a logic to this that goes beyond the obligations owed to patients, the requirements of regulatory authorities, or the company's own desire to have available the most comprehensive and current assessment of product safety.

The breadth and scope of the organization that characterizes the activities of pharmaceutical companies confers significant advantages with respect to implementing an effective global safety surveillance system. They commonly operate on a worldwide basis with respect to both their clinical trial and marketing activities. As a consequence the large international infrastructure that is in place to support these activities may be utilized to support a global safety surveillance operation.

By contrast, national regulatory agencies are quite limited with respect to the manning available. This is usually limited largely to the agency headquarters staff and does not extend to field staff to assist in the collection of safety data. National agencies function more as passive recipients of data channeled to them whereas the field staff available to pharmaceutical companies allows them to adopt a more proactive role in the collection of safety data. Most importantly, they are in an excellent position to mandate reporting to one central database from all of their subsidiaries and affiliates in the various geographic locations. This represents a significant advantage over national agencies.

B. The Database

From the point of view of routine safety surveillance there are two databases to be considered. The VRSE database is a small subset of the total safety experience with the drug. It represents serious reactions reported promptly from clinical trials and spontaneous postmarketing reports. Furthermore, as far as spontaneous postmarketing reports are concerned, it represents only events that were reported. It is not possible to retrieve those that for some reason the physician did not report.

By contrast, the clinical trial database represents a much more extensive and detailed safety experience with the drug that may help to place events reported to the VRSE database into better perspective. Most importantly, reactions that should have been reported promptly at the time, but for some reason were not, may subsequently be retrieved from this database.

1. The VRSE Database

The VRSE database is characterized not by the origin of the reports it contains but by their nature. These reports may emanate from clinical trails or from the postmarketing treatment environment. Guidance with respect to those serious or alarming reactions from clinical trials that must be reported promptly is provided in the federal regulations. With respect to postmarketing experience a conservative approach is adopted. All events that are spontaneously reported by health care professionals or other sources are regarded as potentially reportable. All reports must be channeled into the VRSE system as expeditiously as possible and a categorization and reportability decision is then made.

This ensures that all events, regardless of source, which may merit prompt regulatory reporting are received into the system for evaluation, categorization, and a reporting decision by the SEG at the sponsor's headquarters location.

2. Events to Be Reported

With respect to clinical trials an appropriate standardized protocol section will outline for the physician-investigator those types of event that must be reported back promptly to the sponsor for evaluation, categorization, and possible regulatory reporting (see Appendix 1). This standard protocol section may be used for all clinical trials, both research trials and postmarketing phase IV trials, regardless of their geographic location. It specifically details the types of reaction that merit prompt reporting as defined in the federal regulations [68].

All serious or alarming reactions that meet the definition must be reported, whether or not the investigator designates the reaction an intercurrent illness or a side effect. A definitive causality determination by the investigator is not a requirement for reporting to the VRSE system. The regulations require only that the reaction is "both serious and unexpected" and "associated with the use of the drug" [69,70]. A reaction is defined as being "associated" if there is "a reasonable possibility that the experience may have been caused by the drug." This standard applies both to research trials [71] and to phase IV postmarketing trials [72]. The federal regulations do however allow different time frames for the reporting of serious events from research trials (10 days) and postmarketing trials (15 days). It is suggested that the 10-day rule should be the uniform standard to strive for in the operation of the VRSE system regardless of the type of trial. The adoption of the more restrictive time frame as a uniform requirement, as opposed to permitting the two standards to operate, serves to encourage a more efficient performance throughout the system.

In order to achieve an additional measure of flexibility and in the interests of more comprehensive safety monitoring this protocol section requests information on events that do not fall strictly within the definition set forth in the federal regulations. It is possible that events that are potentially important from the point of view of safety may not be reported promptly because in the investigator's view they do not fall strictly within the definition provided. To circumvent this possibility, however remote, the protocol section also requires the investigator to report events that he considers significant even though they do not appear to fall strictly within the criteria listed.

And finally, in some clinical programs there may be certain events that it would be advisable to follow very closely in the interests of patient safety. However, these events are such that they would not merit immediate reporting in their own right. They do not, for instance, result in drug discontinuaton or fall strictly within the regulatory definition for prompt reporting. Therefore the protocol section specifically requests that these events also be reported promptly by the investigator.

Such a situation could arise with a drug that has been shown to be responsible for several instances of hepatotoxicity. However, clinical evaluation has been allowed to proceed cautiously in order to further define the level of efficacy relative to the potential risk. In such circumstances the protocol section could require that all instances of transaminase levels ≥ 100 units be reported promptly in order that the hepatic profile of the drug be monitored more closely than would normally be the case. A somewhat similar situation could arise if there was a suspicion of myelotoxicity. In such circumstances the protocol section would specifically request the reporting of specified levels of leukopenia on a prompt basis.

With respect to postmarketing experience all spontaneously reported events from the use of the drug in medical practice are regarded as being potentially reportable on an urgent basis and must be entered into the VRSE as expeditiously as possible. This will occur regardless of whether they are serious or nonserious, expected or not expected, and irrespective of whether or not they are attributed to drug. Whether or not these events fall within the definition of events to be reported promptly to the FDA (or other regulatory authorities) is determined after the data are received, evaluated, and categorized by the SEG. The basis for this classification is set forth in the federal regulations [73].

The definitions contained in the federal regulations are fairly precise and comprehensive with regard to the type of safety information that must be reported promptly. In terms of medical science they define those types of safety events that any regulatory authority would wish a company to monitor closely. Those differences that might appear to exist with respect to the definitions of different regulatory authorities would seem to be semantic rather than scientific. The only real differences would appear to be procedural in nature and relate to the manner and timing of the reports of duly categorized events that are required by the different authorities.

The FDA criteria may therefore be used, in a centralized worldwide system, as a uniform standard for categorizing those types of events that are of concern to all regulatory authorities. However, the reporting requirements and the frequency of any reports, for reactions that have been duly categorized, is quite another issue. Here the requirements of local law or regulation will be determinative.

The approach suggested for postmarketing spontaneous events is to enter all reports received into the database and make a suitable notation with respect to categorization and the authorities to whom a report is made. A variant to this approach would be to enter into the database only those spontaneous postmarketing reports that are adjudged to fall within the definition of a reportable event. Superficially this approach has a certain amount of appeal with respect to reducing workload and may be further justified on the basis that a large volume of spontaneous postmarketing reports are completely irrelevant to any issue of drug safety. However, one can never preclude the possibility that information contained in the "nonreportable" events may ultimately prove relevant. Accordingly, the preferable approach is to enter all spontaneous reports and list at each reporting period total events received and the relative proportions falling into the reportable and nonreportable categories.

Since the VRSE database contains reports from both clinical trials and the postmarketing situation there will be duplication of reporting for the information deriving from the clinical trials. A serious reaction in a clinical trial patient will be recorded both in the VRSE and in the clinical trial database (CTDB). But the CTDB will contain the most comprehensive information on this particular patient. There will be information extending well beyond the period of the particular event reported. If the VRSE system is working efficiently the reaction will appear in this system before the CRF record is received from the trial center and the data entered into the CTDB. Such differences will of course tend to disappear as remote data entry (RDE) becomes more universal for clinical trial data.

Because of this duplication in the two databases there must be "electronic hooks" linking the VRSE record of a clinical trial patient with that same patient's full CRF record in the CTDB. One reason for this is to assist in data evaluation and the other is for quality assurance purposes. When the SEG is reviewing the VRSE record of a trial patient on the monitor screen for purposes of evaluation and categorization, they should be provided with the functionality of accessing in a window on the screen the full clinical trial record for that patient. This record may contain valuable additional information that is useful for purposes of categorization. With respect to quality assurance, the system should be set up to utilize these electronic hooks to monitor continuously for consistency between the two databases to ensure that a given clinical trial event is represented in both databases.

3. Data Entry

Reports must be channeled into one central database from all geographic locations worldwide. Given the primary function of a VRSE system prompt entry of data into the database must be emphasized. Operational procedures must not allow reports to be held up at peripheral locations pending the receipt of further data. No discretion whatsoever should be given to the peripheral reporting units to make such value judgments.

Consistent with this approach minimum requirements must be established for the basic units of data that must be available to justify the first entry of a reaction into the system. For instance, the occurrence of a reaction, its identification with a specific patient, and an "association" with the drug would represent the minimum data required to trigger a first entry into the system. The standard adverse reaction form, which is completed for the initial entry of data on a reaction into the system, will have provision for a suitable notation that additional information remains to be obtained.

This standard adverse reaction form will be used for the entry of all data into the system. Preferably this is done by remote data entry from the peripheral locations. The necessary uniformity of data entry will be further assured by the use of standard coding dictionaries for disease state, adverse reactions, concomitant medications, and other relevant units of information. SEG will be responsible for the upkeep and maintenance of these dictionaries and ensuring that all relevant parties have copies.

The SEG must promptly review all data entered into the system for completeness, accuracy, and coding errors. It is responsible for ensuring that the peripheral locations submit all relevant available data. The SEG may initiate requests for additional data, if available, and will monitor the system to ensure that the peripheral locations do submit all outstanding data. In addition to performing data entry, the peripheral locations will also have the necessary functionality for viewing the database and manipulating the data but will not be able to change or amend the data once entered. Correction of the database is the sole responsibility and prerogative of the SEG as the corporate custodians of the VRSE database and any changes must be made through it. The integrity of the database is one of its most important responsibilities.

Each day the SEG is provided with a printout of all new entries received into the database during the preceding 24 hours. This will comprise both new reactions and additional information on previously reported reactions. A weekly summary output will also be available that details the new events and new follow-up information received during the preceding week.

On a quarterly basis more detailed output will be required. This will provide cumulative totals of all events received and the totals considered to be expedited reports. The reactions will also be listed by type and by body system. Change with respect to previous quarters will provide the basis for determining whether there is a change in incidence.

4. Clinical Trial Database

One CTDB should be established for all company-sponsored trials conducted worldwide, both research trials and phase IV trials. A CTDB of this scope provides a resource of inestimable value to the SEG in its task of continually monitoring the safety of the company's drugs. It can easily be accessed for any contribution it may make to better understanding of safety signals received from the VRSE database.

For any specific drug the CTDB is established when the first clinical studies are initiated. It continues to accumulate data from the research studies as the process of drug evaluation proceeds. As the drug is approved in the different markets of the world phase IV trials will commence and the data derived from them will continue to be entered into this same database. Eventually, when the drug is approved in all markets the data entering the CTDB will be almost exclusively derived from phase IV trials.

At any given point in time, therefore, a cumulative CTDB exists that is reasonably current and up to date. It will contain the sum total of all trial experience with the drug worldwide from the initial clinical studies to those in progress at the current time.

There is a sound scientific rationale for including all clinical trials, both research and phase IV, in the same database. This rationale is simply that clinical research trials and phase IV trials are not separate and distinct entities. It is unfortunate, in a way, that the use of these particular descriptive terms has tended to encourage a contrary view. Logically one should not speak of "clinical research" trials and "phase IV postmarketing" trials but rather of "good" trials and "bad" trials. In both types of clinical trial patients are included for purposes other than their ordinary medical care. Therefore the same standard of study design, study conduct, and data quality should apply regardless of whether the trials are conducted prior to approval or subsequent to marketing. The exposure of patients in clinical trials carries with it an obligation that the trials be conducted with good purpose. This in turn mandates the observance of the necessary trial standards required to ensure valid scientific conclusions.

Certainly clinical research trials may utilize more sophisticated parameters and are more comprehensive and detailed with respect to the volume of data collected. But this does not militate against including the data from both types of trial in one common database provided that two essential preconditions are met. A certain standard of study design must be guaranteed and, while the same volume of data does not have to be collected in all trials, that which is collected must be recorded and entered into the database using a standard format. This concept is particularly important for safety surveillance purposes. The collection and recording of adverse reactions and laboratory data in a uniform and standard manner will permit the pooling of these data across the entire CTDB.

The required degree of uniformity with respect to study design may be achieved by careful control of protocol design for all company-sponsored trials. This may be implemented by assigning the conduct of all clinical trials, research and phase IV, to one clinical department in order to ensure this uniform standard. Alternatively, if research and phase IV trials are the responsibility of different departments the use of a protocol committee to monitor and control protocol standards will serve the same objective.

A uniform approach to data recording and collection may be achieved if the case report form (CRF) is standardized for all company-sponsored trials. This does not necessarily mean that all the data collected in a research trial must be collected in a phase IV trial but simply that whatever data are collected are obtained and recorded in a uniform manner.

The standardization of CRFs is best approached by establishing a library of CRF modules. This library would contain standard CRF modules for patient demographics, side effects, laboratory parameters of safety, various special safety parameters, and the various efficacy parameters. As new parameters are encountered with respect to safety or efficacy additional standard modules will be created and added to the library. It will be a requirement that the CRFs used in any study, whether research or phase IV, be compiled from the modules in this library.

It follows logically that a standard set of coding dictionaries, e.g., adverse reactions, concomitant therapy, disease state, etc., must be used by all locations that are responsible for data entry. If the side effect dictionary is based on the WHO dictionary then provision must be provided for translation into COSTART for those agencies, such as the FDA, which favor this system. Since these dictionaries are also of great importance to the VRSE database the SEG, as mentioned earlier, will have responsibility for their maintenance.

Relative to the timing of data entry, the conduct of clinical research trials will seek to ensure the most rapid entry of data into the database subsequent to its generation. This may be achieved by an appropriate level and intensity of monitoring or, as is increasingly the practice today, the use of remote data entry at the study sites. By comparison, less restrictive standards may be permitted for the phase IV trials. An acceptable approach would require that all phase IV trials be summarized and their data entered into the database within 3 months of the completion of the study. The conduct of any trial, research or phase IV, involves the voluntary participation of the patient in an experiment. This should mandate both a scientific interest and an ethical obligation to review the data and draw the necessary conclusions in the form of a study summary as soon as possible.

Finally, a study inventory should be compiled and maintained in connection with the CTDB. This additional feature will serve both an informational and a quality assurance function. For each drug a current computer-based inventory is maintained of all clinical studies sponsored by the company. This will list the key items of information relative to each study in the inventory. This will include such items of information as the location of the study, the study type (research or phase IV), the purpose of the study, the study design and size, age range, and sex of the patients, dosage form and doses employed, and the control agents. A notation will be entered when the study is complete and when the study summary is available.

Each study entry in the inventory should be crosslinked to computerized IND files for that study in the event that fuller information than is contained in the inventory is required. As an informational tool the study inventory has a number of applications. It will be of great assistance when it is necessary to pool data to address a specific issue since it will help to locate those studies that are suitable. It will also assist in the location of studies involving specific patient groups. The inventory will also serve a quality assurance function. It serves as a useful cross-check that all sponsored studies are represented by data in the database and it serves as a reminder that studies have not been summarized.

C. Custodial Function

Although the SEG functions as the custodian of the central VRSE database its area of responsibility should be much broader than this. It should have overall responsibility for drug safety in the broadest possible sense. This is because there is little to justify separating responsibility for safety as it relates to serious adverse events from a responsibility for the total safety profile of the drug. The VRSE database is but one part of the total safety database and the safety profile represented by the VRSE database but one aspect of the complete safety profile of the drug. The responsibilities of the SEG must therefore extend beyond the categorization and reporting of serious reactions to include responsibility for evaluating the total safety profile of the drug. In order to be able to adequately discharge its duties in this respect the group must have access to both the VRSE database and the worldwide CTDB (Fig. 3).

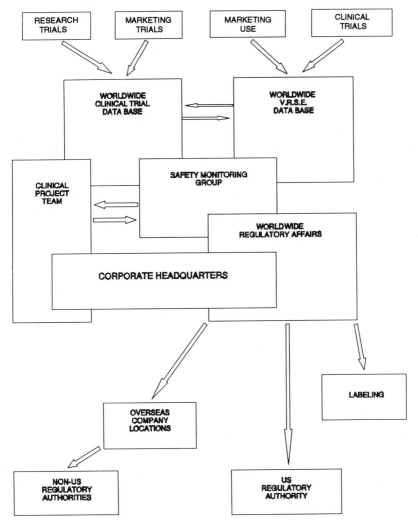

Figure 3 Organization of a safety surveillance system.

The SEG must be able to follow the developing safety profile of the drugs by monitoring these two databases in a continuing and ongoing fashion. A number of resources will be available to the SEG to assist in this function. The most extensive of these with respect to a scientific knowledge base regarding the drugs being monitored will be the respective clinical project teams. Accordingly, there must be a close interactive working relationship between SEG and these teams. In reaching safety decisions the two groups must work closely together to arrive at a consensus. However, the ultimate responsibility for the categorization of serious reactions and the decision on reportability rests with the SEG.

Within the context of this interactive working relationship between the two groups the function of the clinical project team is exclusively scientific. That of SEG, on the other hand, must be viewed as partly scientific and partly a regulatory or compliance function. For this reason the preferred location for the SEG is within the corporate Regulatory Affairs Department. The element of compliance associated with the SEG's responsibilities makes this a more appropriate arrangement than locating the group within clinical operations. As with the Regulatory Affairs Department, the objectivity and impartiality of the compliance function of the SEG could be regarded as being compromised if it is part of, and reports to, the clinical operations group.

1. Safety Evaluation

The SEG is responsible for reviewing all adverse reaction reports from clinical trials and spontaneous reports from postmarketing experience entered into the database. They are initially reviewed for quality of data, appropriateness of coding terms used, and any missing information. The SEG will interact directly with the reporting location with respect to missing items of information or any additional facts that they may consider relevant to a proper assessment.

The group is responsible for categorization of the event, causality, and the determination of whether or not the incident requires expedited (3-, 10- or 15-day) reporting to the FDA. These conclusions relative to categorization, causality, and reportability to the FDA are entered into the database as a permanent part of the record. Ideally these conclusions will be reviewed and approved by a safety committee which, in addition to the SEG, will have representation from the clinical project team, clinical operations management, and Regulatory Affairs.

This determination with respect to categorization and causality is binding on all reporting locations of the company. As already noted, the categorization of events is based on the federal regulations. The actual reportability of the event, however, will depend on local law, regulation, or requirement. To assist in this process and ensure a consistent approach corporate Regulatory Affairs is responsible for issuing a "Manual of Regulatory Reporting Requirements." This is done in cooperation with the country locations to ensure the currency and accuracy of the manual. It sets forth the regulatory reporting requirements of those countries in which the company operates and whenever they lack the desired level of specifity the manual will set forth the company's interpretation.

The SEG's decision on FDA reportability will, subject to approval by the safety committee, lead to the necessary report being submitted. Through Regulatory Affairs the SEG will provide copies of the material supplied to the FDA to the various country locations. Corporate Regulatory Affairs will recommend the action to be taken with respect to local reporting based on the manual. Such recommendation is not binding on the local affiliate, which should be given discretion to make the final decision with regard to local reportability. The local country organization may wish to use CIOMS forms for reporting locally, in which case they will be able to obtain output in this format from the system. The final action taken on a reaction at the local level will be entered into the database. There will therefore be a record in the database of all reports received, their categorization, and which reports were sent to the FDA and which to the various other national regulatory authorities.

It is important to remember that drug safety information may arise from sources other than spontaneous postmarketing reports or company-sponsored clinical studies. One possible source relates to publication in the literature. It was noted earlier that the first indication of the toxicity of isoxicam was an anecdotal report in a journal in the absence of any notification to the company or national authorities. In other instances adverse reaction reports may surface for the first time in the publication of a study that was not sponsored by the company. For these reasons the SEG is not adequately discharging its safety-monitoring responsibilities if it does not make arrangements to follow the world literature with respect to the company's drugs. This may be done by library search but a more efficient approach is to use one of the several commercial services available.

The Regulatory Affairs Department plays a key role in ensuring the consistency and uniformity of safety labeling worldwide. It also oversees regulatory interactions and the reporting on safety issues to the various regulatory authorities and is a major participant in labeling discussions within the company and with regulatory agencies. For these reasons it will be most convenient if both the SEG and the group responsible for labeling are located within the Regulatory Affairs Department.

2. Audit Function

There are at least two levels of audit activity involved with respect to safety surveillance. While these two functions are to some extent coextensive, they are not completely so. The audit function of the SEG is carried out on a continuing basis and relates to those parts of the overall operation that are responsible for channeling the safety information into the VRSE.

To a large extent the systems already in place to support the prompt and accurate reporting of safety events will provide the SEG with the mechanism for auditing the system. Many of the tasks required of the SEG as part of its normal duties will also serve an audit function. This is certainly true of the checking of data entered peripherally for accuracy and completeness, and the verification of coding. Certain items of information of a nonmedical nature are incorporated into the various reporting forms to facilitate this audit function. These include the items designed to monitor incomplete files and track the response to requests for missing or additional data. Periodic checks, at least quarterly, will be made to determine the time frames of the various steps in the reporting and data retrieval process to determine whether there are delays, and if so where they are occurring and what is the source. Appropriate corrective action will then be instituted.

However, there must be another level of audit activity that is completely independent of the SEG. This may be a corporate audit group that is part of the legal division of the company. This group will also repeat the audit of those activities leading to the receipt of information by the SEG, including on-site visits at the various country locations. But, in addition, it will audit the activities of the SEG in the final stages of the categorization and reporting of reactions.

D. Communications

The corporate Regulatory Affairs Department, with its two component sections the Safety Evaluation Group (SEG) and the Product Labeling Group, is the focal point for all internal and external communications and reporting functions with respect to drug safety (Fig. 4). These functions cover a spectrum of different needs and may be considered under three broad headings:

1. Housekeeping communications
2. Internal communications
3. External communications

1. Housekeeping Communications

The SEG produces such reports for both informational and audit or compliance purposes. Where these reports disseminate information to the various locations responsible for submitting data in the form of a weekly status report they also assist the SEG in monitoring the efficiency with which the system is working.

Weekly output is generated that lists all new events entered during the past week, their categorization, and their disposition with regard to FDA reporting. New follow-up information received during the previous week is listed and there is a listing of all follow-up information still outstanding. A monthly cumulative status report is also produced and distributed to these same locations.

2. Internal Communications

The quarterly reports produced by the SEG are primarily formal internal status reports regarding the different drugs. The quarterly cumulative status report

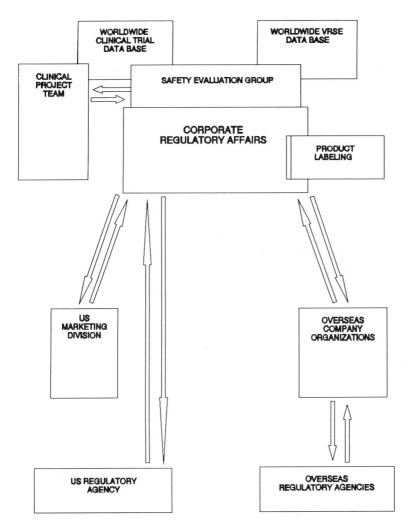

Figure 4 Regulatory communications.

provides a cumulative total of all reports entered into the VRSE database to date. This total is provided as ''all reports received'' and ''expedited reports.'' The latter figure is that proportion of the total considered to merit prompt (10- or 15-day) reporting. In addition the same totals, ''all reports'' and ''expedited reports,'' are shown for the last quarter and as the average for the last four quarters. The events are also broken down by body system and type of adverse reaction. The data are also examined for evidence of any change in incidence of any of the adverse reactions. A detailed listing is provided of the key items of information with respect to each of the expedited reports received over the last quarter. In addition to providing the cumulative data as patient totals, these totals are also be broken down into the four possible subgroups: U.S. spontaneous reports, international spontaneous reports, U.S. clinical trials, and international clinical trials.

When appropriate these quarterly internal reports will be used to provide the quarterly safety reports that are required to be filed to the NDA for the first 3 years subsequent to NDA approval.

In addition, the SEG will send an informational report on the functioning of the system to each location responsible for collecting data. This report will review the experience of the last quarter relative to data collection performance and compare this with previous quarters. It will explore performance with respect to three different time frames:

1. Time from occurrence of the reaction to receipt by the company
2. Time from first receipt by company to entry into database
3. Time from entry into database to FDA reporting

This information enables the performance of the system to be continuously monitored. It will highlight any problems that exist and help to focus corrective action at the appropriate point in the system.

The annual safety reports required by the FDA (see below) will be used as internal informational reports for the overseas locations.

3. Regulatory Communications

The SEG is responsible for categorizing the safety events reported to the VRSE system from all sources worldwide. Where appropriate a causality judgment is made along with a decision of whether or not the report meets the criteria for expedited reporting to the FDA. In performing this function the SEG works closely with the relevant clinical project team.

This central categorization of the report is binding on all country locations, and while corporate Regulatory Affairs will suggest whether the event is reportable in each country the final decision will rest with the local country organization. A computer-generated copy of the FDA report or a computer-generated CIOMS report will be used for regulatory reporting overseas. This approach ensures an internal consistency of all regulatory safety reporting.

As already noted the quarterly cumulative reports will serve both as regulatory reports (FDA) and as internal reports. They will also serve as the basis of any interim safety report that may be requested by a non-U.S. regulatory agency. In all instances safety reports requested by non-U.S. regulatory agencies will be based on the reports submitted to U.S. regulatory authorities to address a similar question.

An annual cumulative safety report will also be produced. This will serve the purpose of the annual safety report for the FDA but will also serve the purpose of an internal information report for overseas locations. It will follow the same format as the quarterly report, but in this instance it will also contain a current summarization of the complete safety profile, both side effects and laboratory parameters, in addition to dealing with the VRSE events.

When specific safety questions are posed by the regulatory agency, SEG working closely with the clinical project team will play a key role in drafting the response for review and approval by other headquarters staff. Such reports will be made available to country locations and will be used as the basis for responses to similar safety questions by overseas regulatory authorities. If it is an overseas regulatory authority that first raises a particular safety question, then the drafting of a response will again be the responsibility of the SEG working with the clinical project team. This will be forwarded to the local country headquarters for their input and submission. No submissions will be made without central approval. In this way there is assurance of a consistent position on safety issues by those most familiar with the particular drug and the worldwide safety database.

And finally, Regulatory Affairs in close conjunction with SEG and the Product Labeling Group will continually monitor the developing safety base against the current labeling (or the investigator's brochure if the drug is still in research). It will interact with clinical research management or the marketing divisions regarding the implications of any changes in safety profile and the labeling.

E. Conclusion

Safety surveillance is one continuing process that commences in the research phase and continues on during the postmarketing period. While one of the primary purposes of the research program is to establish the safety profile of the drug prior to approval, there can never be complete assurance that all potential safety hazards have been identified.

Safety surveillance during the postmarketing period is therefore no less important than during the research phase. However, the challenges inherent in collecting reliable data in the postmarketing period are greater. The study methodologies that are appropriate to address the safety problems encountered postmarketing are not capable of replicating the reliability obtainable with experimental studies.

In the postmarketing period a large number of potential variables may impact the data and the conclusions that are drawn. Many of these will be unknown and therefore cannot be effectively controlled. This places an even greater emphasis on the need to control the variables that are known. The magnitude of the task of effectively monitoring drug safety also demands the optimum use of available resources. A large degree of centralization is mandatory in order to reduce unnecessary reduplication of effort and to guarantee a uniform and consistent approach to the interpretation of the data.

Appendix 1

Protocol Section
for Serious Event Reporting

Immediate Reporting of Significant Adverse Experience

All deaths, serious adverse experiences, and study drug discontinuations whether
due to adverse experience or concomitant disease occurring during the study
period or the posttherapy period must be reported immediately. Such reports will
be made regardless of treatment group or suspected relationship to drug.

All reports will be made by telephone to the Clinical Monitor, Dr.
_____ at the following location, Tel. _____.

Such serious adverse experience includes but is not restricted to the following
events:

1. Fatal events
2. Life-threatening or potentially life-threatening events
3. Permanently disabling events
4. Events requiring inpatient hospitalization
5. Congenital anomaly, cancer, or the effects of drug overdose

It should be emphasized that, regardless of the above criteria, any additional
adverse experience which the investigator considers significant enough to merit
immediate reporting should be so treated.

Special Reporting Requirements

For this particular compound the all instances of the following type should be reported immediately even though they do not fall within the definitions given above, regardless of whether or not they result in drug discontinuation.

———————————

———————————

REFERENCES

1. Quoted in Penn, *Br J Clin. Pharmacol.* 1979;8:293, 300.
2. Pareti, *The History of Mankind: The Ancient World.* New York: Harper & Row; 1965.
3. Goldberg, *Br J Clin Pharmacol.* 1986;22:67S–70S.
4. Blake, *Safeguarding the Public: Historical Aspects of Medicinal Drug Control.* Baltimore: Johns Hopkins University Press; 1970:103–109.
5. McKendrick et al., *Br Med J.* 1980;2:957.
6. McKendrick et al., *Br Med J.* 1980;2:957.
7. Mann, *J Roy Soc Med.* 1986;79:353.
8. Medical Research Council, Special Report. Series of the Medical Research Council, no 66. London: Her Majesty's Stationery Office; 1922.
9. Worster-Drought, *Br. Med. J.* 1923;1:148. Short et al., *Ann Intern Med.* 1933;6:1449.
10. 34 Stat. 768. 1906. Universally referred to as the "Pure Food and Drug Act" although its full official title was "An Act for preventing the manufacture, sale or transportation of adulterated or mis-branded or poisonous or deleterious foods, drugs, medicines, and liquors, for regulating traffic therein, and for other purposes."
11. Food and Drug Act. 1875.
12. Goldberg, *Br J Clin Pharmacol.* 1986;22:67S,68S.
13. Kracke et al., *J Lab Clin Med.* 1934;19:799.
14. Referring to the incident, Commissioner George P. Larrick of FDA stated that a simple experiment on animals would have revealed the toxic properties of the "elixir." *Thalidomide and the Power of the Drug Companies*: 21.
15. Griffin, In: Wardell, ed. *Controlling the Use of Therapeutic Drugs: The United Kingdom.* Washington, DC: American Enterprise Institute; 1978:101.
16. *J Roy Coll Phys.* 1937;11:000.
17. Medicines Act 1968 (1968 c 67).
18. Federal Food, Drug and Cosmetic Act §505(d)(5), 21 USC §355.
19. Federal Food, Drug and Cosmetic Act, §505(d)(7), 21 USC §355.
20. *Thalidomide and the Power of the Drug Companies*, p. 27.
21. Strom BL, Miettinen OS, Melmon KL. *Clin Pharm Ther.* 1983;34:1.

22. Strom BL, Melmon KL. *JAMA*. 1978;242:2420–2423.
23. Shedden WIH. Side effects of benoxaprofen. *Br Med J*. 1982;284:1630.
24. Editorial comment. *Br Med J*. 1982;285:459.
25. Doering PL, Murphy FA. *JAMA*. 1978;239:843–846.
26. Sackett DL. *J Chron Dis*. 1979;32:51.
27. Gifford LM, Aeugle ME, Myerson RM, et al. Cimetidine postmarket outpatient surveillance program: interim report of phase I. *JAMA*. 1980;243:1532–1535.
28. Chalmers D, Dombey SL, Lawson DH. Post marketing surveillance report for captopril (for hypertension): a preliminary report. *Br J Clin. Pharmacol*. 1987;24:343–349.
29. Nibbelink DW, Strickland SC. Cyclobenzaprine (Flexeril) post marketing surveillance program: a preliminary report. *Curr Ther Res*. 1979;25:564–570.
30. Report on Experimental Techniques of Post Marketing Surveillance, attachments to a letter dated Oct. 14, 1976, from Pfizer Pharmaceuticals to Associate Director for New Drug Evaluation (FDA), available from Freedom of Information (HFI-35) Rockville, Maryland, FDA.
31. Vessey MP, Doll R. Investigation of relation between use of oral contraceptives and thromboembolic disease. *Br Med J*. 1968;2:199–205.
32. Inman WHW, Vesey MP. *Br Med J*. 1968;2:193. Vesey PM, Doll R. *Br Med J*. 1968;2:199.
33. Collaborative Group for the Study of Stroke in Young Women. *JAMA*. 1975:231:718.
34. Boston Collaborative Drug Surveillance Program. Reserpine and breast cancer. *Lancet*. 1974;2:669.
35. Heinomen OP, Shapiro S, Tuminen L. Reserpine use in relation to breast cancer. *Lancet*. 1974;2:675.
36. Armstrong B, Stevens N, Doll R. A retrospective study of the association between Rauwolfia derivatives and breast cancer in English women. *Lancet*. 1974;2:672.
37. Laska EM, Siegel C, Meisner M, et al. Matched pairs study of reserpine use and breast cancer. *Lancet*. 1975;2:296.
38. Mack TM, Henderson BE, Gerkins BR, et al. Reserpine and breast cancer in a retirement community. *N Engl J Med*. 1975;292:1366.
39. Lilienfeld AM, Chang I, Skegg D, et al. Rauwolfia derivatives and breast cancer. *Johns Hopkins Med J*. 1975;139:41.
40. Aromaa A, Hakama M, Hakulinen T, et al. Breast cancer and the use of Rauwolfia and other antihypertensive agents in hypertensive patients. A nationwide case control study in Finland. *Int J Cancer*. 1976;18:727.
41. Kewitz H, Jesdinsky HJ, Schroter PM, et al. Reserpine in breast cancer in women in Germany. *Eur J Clin Pharmacol* 1977;11:79.
42. Christopher LJ, Crooks J, Davidson JF, et al. Multicenter study of Rauwolfia derivatives and breast cancer. *Eur J Clin Pharmacol*. 1977;11:409.
43. O'Fallon WM, Labarthe DR, Kerland LT. Rauwolfia derivatives and breast cancer. *Lancet* 1975;2:292.
44. Armstrong B, White G, Skegg D, et al. Rauwolfia derivatives and breast cancer in hypertensive women. *Lancet*. 1976;2:8.
45. Horwitz RI, Feinstein AR. *Am J Med*. 1979;66:556.

46. Mann JI, Inman WHW. *Br Med J*. 1975;2:245.

47. Murphy DP. The outcome of 625 pregnancies in women subjected to pelvic radium or roentgen irradiation. *Am J Obstet Gynecol*. 1929;18:179.

48. DeGroot LJ, Paloyan E. Thyroid carcinoma and radiation: a Chicago endemic. *JAMA*. 1973;225:487–491.

49. Gregg N. Congenital cataract following German measles in the mothers. *Trans Ophthalmol Soc Aust*. 1941;3:35.

50. Herbst AL, Ulfelder H, Poskanzer DC. Adenocarcinoma of the vagina: association of maternal stilboestrol therapy with tumor appearance in young women. *N Engl J Med*. 1971;284:878.

51. McBride WG. Thalidomide and congenital abnormalities. *Lancet*. 1961;1:1358.

52. Wilson AB. *Pharmaceuz Industrie*. 1979;41:691–695.

53. Rogers AS, Ebenezer I, Smith CR et al., *Arch Intern Med*. 1988;148:1596–1600.

54. Wardell WM. *J Clin Pharmacol*. 1979;19:89–94.

55. Faich GA, Knapp DE, Dreis M, et al. *JAMA*. 1987;257:2068–2070.

56. Koch-Weser J. *N Engl J Med*. 1969;280:20–26.

57. Davis TG, Pickett DL, Sclosser JH. *JAMA*. 1980;243;1912–1914.

58. FDA Deputy Director Gerald Meyer in a July 26, 1991 letter to the Citizen's Commission on Human Rights (CCHR). Quoted in *F-D-C Reports*. 1991;53:31; T & G 7.

59. Editorial, *Br Med J*. 1977;1:861.

60. Griffin JP, Weber JCP. *Adv Drug React Ac Pois Rev*. 1986;1:23–55.

61. Inman WHW. *Br Med J*. 1981;282:1216–1217.

62. 21 CFR §312.32.

63. 21 CFR §314.80.

64. Report on Experimental Techniques of Post Marketing Surveillance, attachments to a letter dated Oct 14, 1976, from Pfizer Pharmaceuticals to Associate Director for New Drug Evaluation (FDA), available from Freedom of Information (HFI-35) Rockville, Maryland, FDA.

65. Griffin JP, Weber JCP. Voluntary systems of adverse reaction reporting. II. *Adv React Ac Pois Rev*. 1986;1:23–55.

66. Faich GA, Knapp D, Dreis M, Turner W. National adverse drug reaction surveillance: 1985. *JAMA*. 1987;257:2068–2070.

67. Strandberg K. *Experiences from the WHO Collaborating Centre for International Drug Monitoring*. 1985;19:385–390.

68. 21 CFR §312.32.

69. 21 CFR §312.32(c).

70. 21 CFR §314.80(a) & (c)(i).

71. 21 CFR §312.32(a).

72. *Fed Reg*. 1987;52:37935 Oct. 13.

73. CRF §314.80.

15

Postmarketing Surveillance: Applications and Limitations, with Special Reference to the Fluoroquinolones

Robert Janknegt

Maasland Hospital
Sittard, The Netherlands

Yechiel A. Hekster

University Hospital
Nijmegen, The Netherlands

I. INTRODUCTION

The fluoroquinolones are a group of antimicrobial agents, structurally related to nalidixic acid. They were introduced on the market in the late 1980s. The first drug to reach the market was norfloxacin, which could only be used in urinary tract infections. Modifications of the chemical structure yielded compounds with more favorable pharmacokinetics, which could also be used for the treatment of systemic infections. Nowadays several fluoroquinolones, such as ciprofloxacin, enoxacin, norfloxacin, ofloxacin, and pefloxacin, are marketed all over the world. They have a wide spectrum of antimicrobial activity, including almost all gram-negative aerobic bacteria, such as Enterobacteriaceae and *Pseudomonas aeruginosa*, and are active also against staphylococci and *Legionella pneumophila* [1]. A very important aspect of these drugs is that they are well absorbed after oral administration and can also be given by intravenous infusion.

The fluoroquinolones are usually well tolerated and the most frequent side effects include gastrointestinal reactions, skin disturbances, and central nervous system (CNS) side effects. A summary of the incidence of side effects observed in clinical trials is given in Table 1. These data cannot be compared directly due to methodological differences in study design (the methods of inquiry as to incidence of side effects is usually not described in detail), comedication, and patient population. The incidence of adverse events is relatively low in Japanese

Table 1   Adverse reactions (%) with Fluoroquinolones in Clinical Trials

System	Ciprofloxacin $n = 9473$ (200–2000 mg)	Norfloxacin $n = 1841$ (800 mg)	Ofloxacin $n = 13,717$ (300–600 mg)	Pefloxacin $n = 1181$ (800 mg)
GI	4.2	3.6	1.9	5.6
Metabolic	4.4			
CNS	1.4	4.4	0.7	0.9
Skin	1.1	0.5	0.4	2.2
Hematological	0.9	3.0		
Urogenital	0.8			
Senses	0.2			
Cardiovascular	0.2		0.1	
Joints and muscles	0.06			
Other	0.6			

Data from Refs. 2–4.

studies, higher in European studies, and highest in studies performed in the United States [5]. No clear-cut explanation for these differences has been found.

One of the major limitations of the use of fluoroquinolones is the fact that they are not allowed for use in children below 18 years of age. It has been shown in young beagle dogs that fluoroquinolones induce histopathological changes on articular cartilage [6].

Some fluoroquinolones, especially enoxacin, show important drug interactions. Enoxacin (and to a lesser extent also ciprofloxacin and pefloxacin) inhibit the metabolism of theophylline and caffeine, resulting in relatively high levels of these drugs with potential toxicity [5].

A drug interaction that has caused some concern is the observation of convulsions in patients receiving both enoxacin and the nonsteroidal anti-inflammatory drug (NSAID) fenbufen in Japan [7].

Soon after the introduction of fluoroquinolones on the market, several case reports of severe CNS reactions (hallucinations, depersonalization, psychosis, convulsions) and hypersensitivity reactions were published. Therefore the postmarketing surveillance (PMS) of fluoroquinolones has focused on three items:

1. With special emphasis on joint evaluation, how safe are fluoroquinolones in children?
2. Does the observed interaction between enoxacin and fenbufen also apply to other quinolones and other NSAIDs?
3. What is the incidence of (serious) adverse reactions with fluoroquinolones during the postmarketing phase, under real-life conditions?

These studies will be described below.

II.   SAFETY OF FLUOROQUINOLONES IN CHILDREN

In 1977 Ingham and coworkers [8] showed that nalidixic acid, oxolinic acid, and pipemidic acid induced changes in articular cartilage development in young beagle dogs. These effects have also been found for the new fluoroquinolones, such as ciprofloxacin, although higher dosages were needed to obtain these effects [9]. The fact that higher dosages were needed is relevant, as these drugs are used in much lower dosages than nalidixic acid in humans. The safety margin appears to be much higher for the fluoroquinolones than for nalidixic acid.

This potential toxicity limits the use of these drugs in children below 18 years of age. This is unfortunate because the fluoroquinolones are a very valuable group of agents for the treatment of young patients with cystic fibrosis (CF), due to their oral availability and their activity against *P. aeruginosa*.

Several investigators have studied the incidence of side effects of fluoroquinolones in children.

A.   Ciprofloxacin

Recently the data from a study on the tolerance of ciprofloxacin in children were published. Physicians who requested ciprofloxacin for use in children on a compassionate use basis received the drug as well as a case report form, and were requested to monitor the safety of the drug. Special emphasis was given to joint evaluation. The manufacturer used this catch-all system for investigation of side effects to gain insight on the incidence and severity of side effects in children [10]. A total of 634 children and adolescents aged 3 days up to 17 years were studied. The majority of patients were in the age group 10–17 years. Detailed records were kept on all relevant patient data and also dosage regimen, duration of treatment, comedication, and a detailed description of the adverse reactions and relation to therapy with ciprofloxacin. The methodology of inquiring into the adverse reactions during ciprofloxacin was not mentioned. The period between the introduction of ciprofloxacin and the observation of adverse events was recorded. The incidence of adverse reactions is shown in Table 2.

The incidence of adverse reactions is this study was relatively high in comparison with clinical studies in adult patients. It must be kept in mind that the mean daily dose was relatively high (25 mg/kg body weight per day, with a very wide range of 3.1–93.8 mg/kg/day) in the children compared to the usual adult daily dose of 1000–1500 mg. Most of the children who were included in this study were relatively ill. The mean intravenous dose was 7 mg/kg body weight per day (range 3.2–11.5 mg/kg). Eight of 634 patients (1.3%) complained of arthralgia. The intensity was mild in three cases, moderate in four cases, and not reported in the last case. The time that elapsed between start of ciprofloxacin and the development of arthralgia ranged from 1 to 23 days. All eight patients were female, while in the whole group of 634 patients 51.1% were female. No cases

Table 2 Adverse Reactions (ADR) Related to Ciprofloxacin in Children Under 18 Years

No. of patients treated	634
No. of patients with ADR	80 (12.6%)
No. of drug related ADR	122
GI	31 (4.9%)
Metabolic	15 (2.4%)
Skin	21 (3.3%)
Whole body	25 (2.5%)
Urogenital	8 (1.3%)
Cardiovascular	8 (1.3%)
Joints and muscles	8 (1.3%)
Nervous system	5 (0.8%)

of arthralgia were observed in boys. No explanation for this finding was given. All joint complaints were transient.

The relationship between the arthralgia and ciprofloxacin was highly probable in two cases, probable in two cases, and possible in the four others. Five of the eight patients were CF patients.

B. Norfloxacin

Yu et al. [11] studied the safety of norfloxacin in children. Norfloxacin (15–20 mg/kg/day) was given to 433 patients with diarrhea in China. Their ages ranged from 20 days to 12 years, one third of the patients being less than 1 year old. Special attention was given to the possible effects of the drug on cartilage. Head circumference, body weight, and height were documented and the length of the legs was measured. The joints of knees, hips, and wrists were examined by x ray. No obvious damage was observed to any of the joints studied, even after a 9-month to 4.5 year follow-up in 32 children.

C. Ofloxacin

Pertuiset and coworkers [12] studied the joint tolerance of ofloxacin and pefloxacin in children aged 2–20 years suffering from CF. None of the 37 children treated with ofloxacin showed any joint complication. No arthralgia was observed. It was an interesting observation that five patients, who had shown arthropathy after treatment with pefloxacin, tolerated ofloxacin without any joint problems.

D. Pefloxacin

A relatively high incidence of arthropathy was found in 63 children and adolescents suffering from cystic fibrosis, who were treated with pefloxacin (9–16 mg/kg/day). A total of nine cases of arthralgia were observed, mainly affecting the knees, elbows, and wrists. A very high incidence of this adverse reaction was found in the age group 15.5–20 years, in which 6/13 (46%) of the children suffered from arthralgia. Contrary to the cases observed with ciprofloxacin, both boys and girls suffered from arthralgia. Five of nine cases were found in boys [12].

E. Conclusions

The incidence of cartilage toxicity of fluoroquinolones in children appears to be low, with the possible exception of pefloxacin. More data are needed on the relative risks of various age groups, boys and girls, and whether there are significant differences between the fluoroquinolones with respect to cartilage toxicity.

Fluoroquinolones have to be used with caution in children, but the available data do not support a contraindication for the use of these drugs in children, again with a possible exception of pefloxacin.

It should be reminded that arthralgia is found in a relatively high frequency in children with CF, whether or not they are being treated with antimicrobial agents [13].

III. INTERACTION BETWEEN FLUOROQUINOLONES AND NSAIDs

The induction of convulsions by quinolone antibiotics is related to the inhibition of γ-aminobutyric acid (GABA) receptors. All quinolones inhibit GABA receptor binding in a dose-dependent manner. The concentration that inhibited 50% of the binding ranges between 1.4×10^{-5} M, about 4.5 mg/L, for norfloxacin and 1×10^{-3} M, about 300 mg/L, for ofloxacin. These concentrations are lowered over 1000-fold in the presence of biphenylacetate, a metabolite of the NSAID fenbufen. The effects of other NSAIDs, such as flurbiprofen and diclofenac, are far less pronounced [7]. In Japan a high incidence of convulsions was observed in patients receiving enoxacin in combination with fenbufen [14].

Although a serious interaction between other quinolones and other NSAIDs seems less likely than for the combination enoxacin-fenbufen, a potential interaction between ofloxacin and NSAIDs has been subject of PMS studies.

A. Ofloxacin

The incidence of psychotic reactions (such as agitation, confusion, depersonaliz-ation, depression, hallucinations, hostility, etc.) and convulsions in patients on ofloxacin therapy with our without NSAID comedication were studied from spontaneous reports in the Hoechst PMS study in Germany, from a request to report such symptoms in Switzerland, and from phase IV studies [15].

1. Spontaneous Reports

Since the launch of ofloxacin in Germany, Hoechst has received 1691 sponta-neous reports of adverse reactions to oral ofloxacin in this country. On the assumption that the mean dosage regimen of ofloxacin was 400 mg daily for 7 days, it is estimated that 6.4 million patients were treated with the drug in the study period.

There was one report of a suggested interaction with the NSAID tiaprofenic acid. The patient showed restlessness and transient anxiety and unreal feelings.

Of the 1691 patients experiencing side effects, 151 were given concomitant treatment with at least one NSAID. The other 1540 patients were not reported as receiving NSAIDs.

Of the 1540 patients without NSAID comedication, 337 (21.9%) showed at least one "psychotic" side effect. The frequency of these side effects in the 151 patients receiving NSAIDs was only marginally higher, 25%, with very similar results for the individual NSAIDs: acetylsalicylic acid 24% (12/51 cases), diclofenac 27% (6/22 cases), ibuprofen 25% (1/4 cases), indomethacin 17% (1/6 cases), and the analgesic drug paracetamol 27% (11/41 cases).

It is a well-known fact that elderly patients often suffer from CNS side effects, induced by various agents, such as the β-blocking drugs. These may also contribute to psychotic side effects observed with ofloxacin.

From the spontaneous reports, there is no evidence that a higher frequency of psychotic reactions or convulsions is observed with the combination of ofloxacin with NSAIDs.

2. Phase IV Studies

Three prospective, open, noncomparative studies with oral ofloxacin were taken into consideration. These studies comprised a total of 10,578 patients. Of these 705 (7.3%) had comedication with NSAIDs. The total incidence of side effects was 7.8% in the patients without NSAIDs and 8.5% in the patients with NSAIDs. The incidence of psychotic reactions was low in both groups: 0.46% in patients without NSAIDs and 0.3% in patients with NSAIDs [15].

Similar results were obtained from phase IV studies with ofloxacin in Japan. A total of 2522 patients received a combination of ofloxacin with a variety of NSAIDs (no details of specification, dosage, and duration were given). There was no event of convulsion in any of these patients [16].

The phase IV studies also do not evidence an important drug interaction between ofloxacin and NSAIDs.

B. Conclusions

There are only data available on a possible interaction between ofloxacin and NSAIDs. Results show no evidence of an increased incidence of CNS side effects when these drugs are used in combination. No published data are available on a potential interaction between other fluoroquinolones and NSAIDs.

IV. POSTMARKETING SURVEILLANCE STUDIES WITH FLUOROQUINOLONES

It has been generally agreed that postmarketing surveillance (PMS) must be noninterventional. PMS must be conducted under real-life conditions. Spontaneous reports continue to be central to the generation of signals. However, it is important that the quality and quantity of spontaneous reports be increased. Education, information, and monitoring are important variables to be considered.

The number of side effects and the frequency of reporting varies with the nature of side effects. Also the time period between penetration into the market and the assessment of a possible causal relationship between adverse events and drug use should be kept in mind. Severe and rare adverse reactions (ADRs) tend to be reported more frequently (in a relative sense) than mild gastrointestinal reactions.

Several pharmaceutical industries have undertaken PMS studies with fluoroquinolones during the first years of marketing. Generally the method of spontaneous reporting has been applied.

PMS is needed to detect adverse events with a low frequency. Usually only about 2000 patients participate in clinical trials during phases I–III. Company (phase IV) studies, such as postmarketing clinical trials, can include many more patients, but such ADRs are not detected.

Spontaneous reporting of side effects in real life may involve millions of patients. The methodology of the assessment and the evaluation of spontaneous reporting may be different for various companies. A relatively high rate of reporting of side effects has been observed for ofloxacin in Germany. This is at least partly due to the increased awareness of CNS side effects because of television programs in which the problem of CNS side effects of ofloxacin was discussed.

A. Ciprofloxacin

1. Phase IV Studies

A large-scale phase IV study, observance of applications (in German: *Anwendungsbeobachtung*), involving over 12,000 patients has been performed. Questionnaires were handed out to physicians working in hospitals or in private practice in Germany. These forms requested information on patient diagnosis, concomitant disease and medications, ciprofloxacin therapy, and laboratory tests. One fourth of the questionnaire was devoted to the acquisition of safety data [17]. The results of this study are shown in Table 3. The distribution of side effects is roughly similar to those observed in phase I–III clinical trials (see Table 1). Metabolic side effects, such as impaired liver function tests, serum creatinine, and blood urea nitrogen, were observed far less often during the phase IV study. This is not surprising, as these tests were performed in virtually all patients participating in the clinical trials and only in a few patients of the phase IV study.

2. Spontaneous Reporting

The transfer of all serious adverse drug events reported to the manufacturer to the central Institute of Drug Safety of Bayer Ltd. (Germany) is mandatory for all Bayer companies worldwide. In the period from 1987 until July 1989 an estimated 30 million patients were treated with ciprofloxacin all over the world.

The most frequent report of serious adverse drug events was anaphylaxis, which was observed in 43 patients (39 considered to be drug-related), followed by kidney failure in 26 (9 drug-related) and convulsions in 25 (13 drug-related). The serious Stevens–Johnson syndrome was observed in 4 patients (3 ciprofloxacin-related). No detailed data were given concerning the exact nature of these events and on the reporting of psychiatric side effects.

Table 3 Adverse Drug Reactions (%) During Phase IV Studies

System	Ciprofloxacin $n = 12,404$	Ofloxacin	
		$n = 28,887$ (Europe)	$n = 13,850$ (Japan)
GI	4.7	5.2	1.9
Metabolic	0.1		0.3
Body as a whole	2.3		0.1
Nervous system	1.4	2.9	0.4
Skin	0.8	1.0	0.3
Hematological	0.1		0.2
Cardiovascular	0.4	0.2	
Senses	0.1		
Urogenital	0.1		0.1
Other	0.2	0.3	

B.   Ofloxacin

1.   Phase IV Studies

The methodology of phase IV studies with ofloxacin performed in Germany is similar to that used for ciprofloxacin. The results of these studies and those performed in Japan are shown in Table 3. Because of the fact that the classification of side effects was not identical in these studies, the ofloxacin data cannot be compared directly to the ciprofloxacin data. All cases and events were included if the physician classified the causal relationship between definite and improbable.

As usual the incidence of ADRs was lower in the Japanese phase IV study. The majority of the Japanese patients (7965) received a daily dose of 600 mg, while 4679 patients received a dose of 300 mg. In the European study most patients received 400 mg daily.

Table 4   Adverse Drug Reactions During Ofloxacin, Spontaneous Reporting During 6.4 Million Courses in Germany

System	Reports number	ADR number	Most frequent ADR	
Nervous system	833	1829	Nervousness	130
			Hallucinations	121
Hypersensitivity	462	852	Rash	137
			Dyspnea	105
GI	293	455	Nausea	125
			Abdominal pain	73
Cardiovascular	171	234	Tachycardia	56
			Cardiovasc. disorder	20
Headache	119	119		
Joints and muscles	123	160	Arthralgia	40
			Myalgia	29
Blood cells	93	129	Thrombopenia	27
			Leukopenia	26
Liver	76	114	Test abnormal	58
			Liver damage	11
Skin	101	103	Sweating	30
			Skin disorder	19
Coagulation	77	105	Petechiae	20
			Purpura	9
Kidney	60	87	Creatinine increase	15
			Kidney failure	11

Source: From Ref. 18.

The incidence of neuropsychiatric side effects did not show any relationship to the daily dose of ofloxacin [16].

One patient showed moderate shock-like hypersensitivity symptoms, who had previously experienced a similar reaction to cefaclor. A relatively high incidence of total and hypersensitivity reactions was observed in patients with a past history of allergic reactions to food or drugs or with a history of allergic disease [16].

2. Spontaneous Reporting

An estimated 6.4 million patients have been treated with oral ofloxacin in Germany since its launch in June 1985 up to June 1990. A total of 1691 single reports were documented, involving 4659 events. The details of these reports are shown in Table 4.

The number of reports per quarter increased in the first 2 years, to reach a maximum of about 70 reports per million daily doses in the first quarter of 1987, and then gradually declined to 25 reports per million daily doses in the second quarter of 1990. The distribution of adverse events is completely different from those observed in clinical trials and in phase IV studies. Gastrointestinal reactions are reported less often than CNS reactions and hypersensitivity, due to the fact that gastrointestinal reactions are so common to most drugs that the rate of reporting for this "normal" side effect is relatively low.

In Japan the most frequently reported adverse reaction was hypersensitivity; in 17 patients shock or shock-like symptoms were observed. Neuropsychiatric side effects were infrequently reported in Japan, with only 31 spontaneous reports, including 3 cases of convulsions. No data on the use of ofloxacin (relating to number of patients treated with the drug) were given.

C. Pefloxacin

1. Spontaneous Reporting

A total of 192 adverse events was reported to Rhone-Poulenc France since its launch in 1985. The number of treatment courses on the assumption of a daily dose of 800 mg for 10 days was estimated to be approximately 350,000 [19]. The distribution of adverse events is again different from those reported with ciprofloxacin and ofloxacin. Skin reactions were observed in 50 patients and musculoskeletal reactions in 50 others. Of these, arthralgia was seen in 25 patients, 4 of whom were children under 16 years of age. Central nervous system reactions were found in 17 patients. Eleven cases of convulsions were reported, with most of the patients showing an epileptic history or preexisting brain lesions. None of these patients was reported to have received NSAIDs. Psychiatric side effects were observed in 16 patients; blood-clotting reactions in 33.

Table 5 Adverse Events of Fluoroquinolones in the First 120 Days After Introduction in the United States

Quinolone	No. of treatment courses	No. of adverse events		Adverse events per 100 treatment courses	
		Total	Severe	Total	Severe
Ciprofloxacin	196,000	25	11	13	6
Norfloxacin	104,000	21	4	20	4
Ofloxacin	267,000	67	8	25	3
Temafloxacin	174,000	188	48	108	20

Source: From Ref. 20.

D. Temafloxacin

The importance of postmarketing surveillance has been clearly demonstrated in the case of temafloxacin. About three months after its introduction in the United States many cases of severe adverse events, such as hypoglycemia, hemolytic anemia, anaphylactic reactions, and renal failure were reported to the FDA. At least three fatal cases of hemolytic uremic syndrome were described. The incidence of adverse events of fluoroquinolones in the first 120 days after its introduction in the United States is shown in Table 5. Because of this unfavorable side-effects profile, the drug was withdrawn from the market on June 5, 1992.

E. Conclusions

The most frequent adverse reactions following spontaneous reporting was allergy for all the quinolones studied. In Japan a distribution of spontaneously reported side effects was seen for ofloxacin similar to those for ciprofloxacin and pefloxacin. In Germany a high rate of reporting of CNS side effects was observed for ofloxacin, following attention for these adverse reactions in the mass media. Severe adverse drug reactions, such as shock or convulsions, which were rarely seen during clinical trials, have been observed during the postmarketing surveillance of these drugs. A different profile of adverse events (hemolytic uremic syndrome, renal failure, hypoglycemia, anaphylactic reaction) was observed for temafloxacin, leading to withdrawal of this fluoroquinolone.

REFERENCES

1. Verbist L. In vitro activity and mode of action of fluoroquinolones. *Pharm Weekbl Sci.* 1987;9:S2–S10.
2. Blomer R, Bruch K, Krauss H, Wacheck W. Safety of ofloxacin: adverse drug reactions during phase II studies in Europe and Japan. *Infection.* 1986;14 suppl 4:S332–S334.

3. Wang C, Sabbaj J, Corrado M, Hoagland V. World-wide clinical experience with norfloxacin: efficacy and safety. *Scand J Infect Dis.* 1986;48:81–89.
4. Schacht P, Arcieri G, Hullmann R. Safety of ciprofloxacin. An update based on clinical trial results. *Am J Med.* 1989;87 suppl 5A:98–102.
5. Janknegt R. Fluoroquinolones. Adverse reactions during clinical trials and post-marketing surveillance. *Pharm Weekbl Sci.* 1989;11:124–127.
6. Schluler G. Ciprofloxacin: toxicologic evaluation of additional safety data. *Am J Med.* 1989; 87 suppl 5A:37–39.
7. Janknegt R. Drug interactions with quinolones. *J Antimicrob Chemother.* 1990;26 suppl D:7–29.
8. Ingham R, Brentvall DW, Dale EA, McFadzean VA. Arthropathy induced by antibacterial fused N-alkyl-4-pyridone-3-carboxylic acids. *Toxicol Lit J.* 1977;1:21–26.
9. Stahlmann R, Merker HJ, Hinz N, et al. Ofloxacin in juvenile non-human primates and rats. Anthropathy and drug plasma concentrations. *Arch Toxicol.* 1990;64:193–204.
10. Chysky V, Kapila K, Hullmann R, et al. Safety of ciprofloxacin in children: worldwide clinical experience based on compassionate use, emphasis on joint evaluation. *Infection.* 1991;16:289–296.
11. Yu A, Li D, Han T et al. Studies on safety of norlfoxacin in children. Third Int Symp on New Quinolones, Vancouver, 1990, abstr 4A.
12. Pertuiset E, Lenoir G, Jehanne M, et al. Tolerance articulaire de la pefloxacine et de l'ofloxacine chez les enfents et adolescents atteints de mucoviscoidose. (Articular tolerance of pefloxacin and ofloxacin in children and adults suffering from cystic fibrosis.) *Rev Rhum Mal Ostesartic.* 1989;56:735–740.
13. Philips BM, David TV. Pathogenesis and management of arthropathy in cystic fibrosis. *J Roy Soc Med.* 1986;79 suppl 12:44–50.
14. Hori S, Shimada J, Saito A, et al. Comparison of the inhibitory effects of new quinolones on GABA receptor binding in the presence of antiinflammatory drugs. *Rev Infect Dis.* 1989;11 suppl 5:1397–1398.
15. Juengst G, Weidmann E, Breitstadt A, Huppertz E. Does ofloxacin interact with NSAIDs to cause psychiatric side effects. 17th Int Congr Chemother, Berlin, 1991, abstr 412.
16. Sawada M, Nakamura S, Yamada A, et al. Phase IV study and postmarketing surveillance of ofloxacin in Japan. *Chemotherapy.* 1991;37:134–142.
17. Reiter C, Pfeiffer M, Hullmann RN. Brief report: safety of ciprofloxacin based on phase IV studies (*Anwendungsbeobachtung*) in the Federal Republic of Germany. *Am J Med.* 1989;87 suppl 5A:103–106.
18. Juengst G, Russwurm R, Weidmann E, et al. Update on spontaneous reporting of adverse reactions to ofloxacin in Germany 1985–1990. Third Int Sympos on New Quinolones, Vancouver, 1990, abstr 21.
19. Simon J, Guyot A. Pefloxacin safety in man. *J. Antimicrob Chemother.* 1990;26 suppl B:215–218.
20. Wiedemann B. Zum Rückruf von Temafloxacin. (The withdrawal of temafloxacin.) *Chemother. J.* 1992;1:182–183.

Index

427

DATE DUE

SE 23 '87			

Demco, Inc. 38-293